Clinical Management
of Binocular Vision

Heterophoric, Accommodative, and Eye Movement Disorders

Second Edition

Clinical Management of Binocular Vision

Heterophoric, Accommodative, and Eye Movement Disorders

Second Edition

Mitchell Scheiman, O.D.

Professor
Director, Pediatric and Binocular Vision Programs
Pennsylvania College of Optometry
Philadelphia, Pennsylvania

Bruce Wick, O.D., Ph.D.

Associate Professor
College of Optometry
University of Houston
Houston, Texas

Illustrations by

Barbara Steinman, O.D., Ph.D.

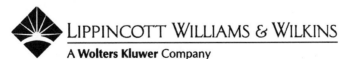

LIPPINCOTT WILLIAMS & WILKINS
A **Wolters Kluwer** Company

Philadelphia • Baltimore • New York • London
Buenos Aires • Hong Kong • Sydney • Tokyo

Acquisitions Editor: Jonathan Pine
Developmental Editor: Joanne Bersin
Production Editor: Thomas Boyce
Manufacturing Manager: Benjamin Rivera
Cover Designer: Christine Jenny
Compositor: TechBooks
Printer: Maple Press

© 2002 by LIPPINCOTT WILLIAMS & WILKINS
530 Walnut Street
Philadelphia, PA 19106 USA
LWW.com

First Edition 1993

Printed in the USA

Library of Congress Cataloging-in-Publication Data

0-7817-3275-1

Care has been taken to confirm the accuracy of the information presented and to describe generally accepted practices. However, the authors and publisher are not responsible for errors or omissions or for any consequences from application of the information in this book and make no warranty, expressed or implied, with respect to the currency, completeness, or accuracy of the contents of the publication. Application of this information in a particular situation remains the professional responsibility of the practitioner.

The authors and publisher have exerted every effort to ensure that drug selection and dosage set forth in this text are in accordance with current recommendations and practice at the time of publication. However, in view of ongoing research, changes in government regulations, and the constant flow of information relating to drug therapy and drug reactions, the reader is urged to check the package insert for each drug for any change in indications and dosage and for added warnings and precautions. This is particularly important when the recommended agent is a new or infrequently employed drug.

Some drugs and medical devices presented in this publication have Food and Drug Administration (FDA) clearance for limited use in restricted research settings. It is the responsibility of the health care provider to ascertain the FDA status of each drug or device planned for use in their clinical practice.

10 9 8 7 6 5 4 3 2 1

To Maxine,
for her love, patience,
and understanding.
—M.S.

Contents

V. Vision Therapy and Optometric Practice

Appendices

Preface

It has been eight years since this book was first published. We have received very positive feedback from colleagues and students. They have remarked that this book is easy to read and understand and that it provides valuable information about the diagnosis and treatment of binocular vision. We have also received some excellent constructive criticism and suggestions.

The two most important suggestions were to add several topics and to modify the organizational approach we used in the first edition to present vision therapy procedures. The topics most often mentioned for inclusion in a new edition are:

1. Binocular vision, accommodative and eye movement disorders related to computer use
2. Binocular vision, accommodative and eye movement disorders related to acquired brain injury
3. Binocular vision, accommodative and eye movement disorders related to reading

We have written three chapters that meet these requests. The format of these chapters is similar to the structure used in other chapters. For each topic we review the diagnosis and treatment of the most common non-strabismic binocular vision, accommodative and eye movement disorders associated with the given condition. We also provide a sequential treatment approach to allow clinicians to treat these conditions in an organized manner. Finally we use a series of cases to demonstrate some of the important concepts discussed in each chapter.

The most significant change we have made from the first edition is a reorganization of the chapters in which we present the various vision therapy procedures. Previously we had organized Part II of the book by the type of equipment being used. This classification included:

1. Anaglyphs and Polaroid filters
2. Lenses, prisms, and mirrors
3. Septums and apertures
4. Paper, pencil, and miscellaneous tasks
5. Stereoscopes
6. After-images, entoptic phenomena, and electrophysiological techniques

A number of faculty members from schools of optometry suggested that organizing the vision therapy techniques into vergence, accommodative and eye movement procedures would be more consistent with the way they organized their courses. In response to this suggestion we have re-organized Part II.

We also heard some criticism about the quality of the photography and illustration in the first edition and have made significant changes in this area. Almost all figures in the second edition have been re-designed by a professional illustrator, Barbara Steinman, OD, PhD. We believe that she has made a significant contribution to this new edition by improving the quality and value of the figures in this textbook.

Of course, over the course of eight years there have been new research studies and other new literature that are relevant to the topics covered in this text. We have carefully reviewed this new literature and have incorporated information from these studies when appropriate.

We hope that the new chapters, new organization, and new illustrations will make this second edition even more useful than the first edition for faculty designing courses, students studying these topics for the first time, and established practitioners looking for a practical, easy-to-use reference on accommodative, ocular motility, and nonstrabismic vision anomalies.

Preface to the First Edition

Our objective in writing this book was to provide students and clinicians with a comprehensive text covering accommodative, ocular motility, and nonstrabismic binocular vision disorders. The prevalence of these conditions in the clinical population is greater than any condition except refractive error. Given this high prevalence, we felt that a book devoted exclusively to these problems was warranted.

We have organized the book into five parts. The first three chapters (Part I) provide the foundation and general principles for diagnosis, case analysis, and management of accommodative, ocular motility, and binocular vision disorders. Chapter 1 covers diagnostic testing, but is not intended to stand alone. We have assumed a basic knowledge of testing administration. Our emphasis in this first chapter is on important issues and considerations for the various tests rather than how to administer the tests.

In Chapter 2 we describe a structured case analysis approach we call Integrative analysis. We believe that this approach builds on previous diagnostic systems such as analytical analysis, graphical analysis, and normative analysis. Our emphasis is on understanding the physiological basis for each test and relating or grouping tests that measure the same function(s). In this chapter we also present an updated, comprehensive classification of accommodative, ocular motility, and nonstrabismic binocular vision problems. In Chapter 3 we describe a structured, sequential management approach. One of our primary objectives is to emphasize the importance of considering all treatment options for every accommodative, ocular motor, and binocular vision anomaly that is encountered.

Part II of this book covers the topic of vision therapy in detail. Chapter 4 provides underlying theory and principles that apply to all vision therapy techniques. Our goal is to simplify the topic of vision therapy and to demonstrate that knowledge and clinical ability to use only a small number of procedures is sufficient to successfully treat all vision problems discussed in this book. Chapters 5 to 8 contain detailed descriptions of a variety of vision therapy procedures. With this background clinicians should be able to apply their knowledge to new procedures and techniques and continue to expand their skills.

Part III of the book, Chapters 9 to 15, is devoted to a detailed presentation of the diagnosis and management of each accommodative, ocular motility, and nonstrabismic binocular vision disorder described in our classification system. Each chapter follows the same format: overview of management, prognosis, background information, symptoms, signs, differential diagnosis, treatment, and case studies. If vision therapy is necessary for the condition being discussed, we provide a detailed vision therapy program. For each condition discussed we also provide case studies that serve to summarize and emphasize key concepts for that disorder. We have specifically attempted to write these chapters so that each stands alone. A student or practitioner seeking information about convergence insufficiency, for example, can turn to Chapter 9 and find all the information necessary for diagnosis and treatment of this condition. Although the use of this format has led to repetition at times, we purposely chose this style to create an easy-to-use reference and resource for students and clinicians.

Chapters 16 to 19 (Part IV) deal with subjects we consider "advanced management issues." Some of the topics discussed in these chapters fall into the category of new information that has not been totally integrated into routine clinical care, or lower prevalence problems not often encountered. Specific topics include interactions between accommodation and convergence, anisometropic amblyopia, nystagmus, and aniseikonia.

The final chapter, Chapter 20 (Part V), covers patient management and practice management issues related to the conditions covered in this text. Included in the chapter is a discussion on establishing vision therapy in a practice. Three Appendices at the end of the text include samples of forms, brochures, and letters used in a practice offering vision therapy, and Home Vision Therapy procedures.

We believe this book will be useful to students studying these topics for the first time and to established practitioners looking for a practical, easy-to-use reference on accommodative, ocular motility, and nonstrabismic vision anomalies.

Mitchell Scheiman, OD
Bruce Wick, OD, PhD

Acknowledgments

One of the authors (M.S.) acknowledges several individuals who have had a strong influence on my professional development:

Dr. Jerome Rosner, who was so instrumental in teaching me how to teach in the very early stages of my career and giving me the push I needed to get involved in didactic teaching;

Drs. Nathan Flax, Irwin Suchoff, Jack Richman, Martin Birnbaum, and Arnold Sherman, who inspired me to devote my professional career to the areas of vision therapy, pediatrics, and binocular vision;

Dr. Michael Gallaway, for his personal and professional support over the last 20 years, and for reviewing sections of this manuscript;

Dr. Andy Gurwood, for his work in developing many of the illustrations used in the first edition of this book;

Dr. Barbara Steinman, for her outstanding work in designing the illustrations for the second edition of this book;

My family, for their support, and for showing so much patience with me during my many months of writing.

PART I

Diagnosis and General Treatment Approach

1

Diagnostic Testing

After a thorough case history and determination of the refractive error, the first important step in the management of accommodative, ocular motor, and nonstrabismic binocular vision problems is the diagnostic testing routine. In this chapter, testing procedures for assessing accommodation, binocular vision, and ocular motor skills will be discussed. The emphasis will be on presentation of important issues, considerations, and expected values for the various tests. The setup and administration of these tests is summarized in the Appendix to this chapter and described in detail in other texts (1–5).

Determination of Refractive Error

All measures of alignment and accommodation require an accurate full-plus refraction with a binocular balance. It is useful to perform a binocular refraction technique that yields a maximum plus refraction. To perform such an examination often requires an initial objective determination of the refractive error. This can be accomplished with static retinoscopy, autorefraction, or even starting with the patient's previous refractive correction. To perform a modified binocular refraction, we recommend the following procedure:

- Use a 20/30 line (or an acuity line 2 lines above threshold).
- With the left eye occluded, add plus [0.25 diopters (D) at a time] to the objective findings, until the right eye is barely able to read the 20/30 threshold line. If too much plus is used, the next step will be difficult, so you may want to back off slightly (add −0.25 D, at most).
- Perform Jackson cross-cylinder (JCC) testing. Adding plus in the step above allows the patient to make more accurate JCC responses.
- Repeat for left eye, with right occluded.
- Add prism (3 Δ up before the right eye; 3 Δ down before the left) and +0.75 D to each eye.
- Perform a dissociated balance by adding plus to the clearer target, until both are reported to be equally blurred.
- Remove the dissociating prism and slowly add minus, until the patient can just read 20/20. DO NOT arbitrarily add some amount of minus!
- Place the Vectographic slide in the projector with analyzers in the phoropter. Place "I" target with letters on each side into patient's view and ask if both sides are equally clear. If not, add +0.25 D to the clearer side. This is a binocular balance—but not a true binocular refraction—where the JCC would be performed under these conditions as well; it is generally not necessary to perform a JCC here unless the patient has a significant astigmatism (>1.00 DC) and a torsional phoria is suspected.
- Perform associated phoria measures and stereopsis testing.
- Return to the standard slide and check visual acuity. If the patient cannot see 20/15, check whether −0.25 more OU improves the acuity. It is virtually never necessary to add more than −0.50 OU total. DO NOT arbitrarily add some amount of minus!

The maximum plus refraction technique breaks down when acuity is very unequal (e.g., amblyopia). In these instances, where often no refractive technique works well, use retinoscopy to determine balance after attempting to achieve maximum plus on the "good" eye (make the retinoscopic reflexes appear equal for the two eyes).

ASSESSMENT OF NONSTRABISMIC BINOCULAR VISION DISORDERS

General Considerations

The evaluation of binocular vision involves several distinct steps (Table 1.1). The first phase of testing is the measurement of the magnitude and direction of the phoria at distance and near, along with the AC/A ratio. Conventional procedures to accomplish this include tests such as cover testing, the von Graefe phoria test, and the modified Thorington test. Fixation disparity testing represents a more recent method of assessing binocular vision and provides additional information that should be considered in the evaluation of binocular vision status. The primary advantage of fixation disparity testing is that it is performed under binocular or associated conditions, in contrast to other tests that are performed under dissociated conditions.

The second step is the assessment of positive and negative fusional vergence using both direct and indirect measures. Direct measures refer to tests such as smooth and step vergence testing, whose primary objective is to assess fusional vergence. Indirect measures refer to tests such as the negative relative accommodation (NRA), positive relative accommodation (PRA), fused cross-cylinder, binocular accommodative facility (BAF), and monocular estimation method (MEM) retinoscopy that are generally thought of as tests of accommodative function. Since these procedures are performed under binocular conditions, however, they indirectly evaluate binocular function as well. The results of such testing, therefore, can be used to confirm or deny a particular clinical hypothesis of a binocular vision disorder. Chapter 2 describes the analysis of these indirect measures in detail.

The traditional evaluation of fusional vergence involves only measurement of smooth vergence ranges or vergence amplitude using a Risley prism in the phoropter. In recent years, additional ways of evaluating fusional vergence have been suggested. One method is step vergence testing, which is done outside the phoropter, using a prism bar (6,7). Another addition to the traditional approach to assessing fusional vergence is vergence facility testing (8–14). This test is also performed outside the phoropter, using a specially designed vergence facility prism (Fig. 1.1). The patient's ability to make large rapid changes in fusional vergence is assessed with this procedure over a specific period of time.

TABLE 1.1. *Important steps in the evaluation of binocular vision*

Measurement of the phorias AC/A and CA/C ratios	Cover test
	von Graefe phoria
	Modified Thorington
	Fixation disparity
Assessment of positive and negative fusional vergence	
Direct measures	Smooth vergence testing
	Step vergence testing
	Vergence facility testing
Indirect measures	Negative relative accommodation
	Positive relative accommodation
	Fused X-cylinder
	Binocular accommodative facility
	Monocular estimation method retinoscopy
Convergence amplitude	Near point of convergence
Sensory status	Worth four-dot
	Stereopsis testing

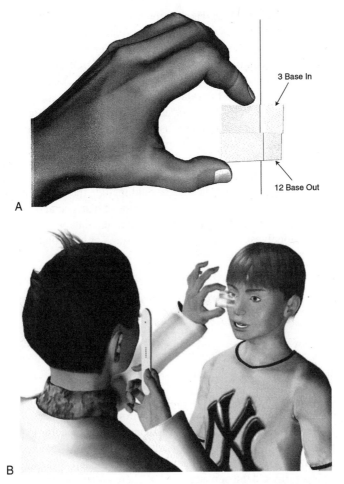

FIG. 1.1. A: Vergence facility prism (3 △ base-in/12 △ base-out). **B:** Vergence facility prism clinical procedure.

An important distinction among different methods of evaluating fusional vergence is the assessment of vergence amplitude versus vergence facility. Smooth and step vergence testing are designed to assess the patient's vergence amplitude, while vergence facility testing measures vergence dynamics. Grisham (11) found a relationship between vergence dynamics and symptoms in subjects he studied. His research indicated that vergence latency and vergence velocity are of diagnostic importance in a binocular evaluation. It is possible for a patient to have normal fusional vergence amplitudes and still have a problem in the area of facility or vergence dynamics. Using only the traditional smooth vergence evaluation approach would fail to detect such a problem. In a recent study, Gall et al. (12) found that the use of 3 △ base-in/12 △ base-out for vergence facility testing can be used to differentiate symptomatic from nonsymptomatic patients.

Another consideration in testing fusional vergence amplitude or facility is the issue of performance over time (8). The underlying question is whether the patient is able to compensate for a given amount of prism over an extended period of time. Traditionally, fusional vergence amplitude is measured just once. Recent research suggests that this may not be sufficient (11,12). Rather, these tests should be repeated several times, and testing that probes facility and ability to respond over time should be incorporated into the evaluation.

The third area that should be evaluated is convergence amplitude. Generally referred to as the near point of convergence, this test is particularly important in the diagnosis of one of the most common binocular vision disorders—convergence insufficiency. Important issues include the type of target(s) to be used and the issue of performance over time (15,16).

The last aspect of the binocular evaluation is sensory status. Assessment of suppression and stereopsis are the primary areas to evaluate. Information about sensory status can also be obtained from many of the other tests discussed above. On several of these tests, suppression can be monitored. A specific test that can be used to assess suppression is the Worth four-dot test. As a general rule, clinical measures of stereopsis are either not affected or only minimally affected in nonstrabismic binocular vision disorders. Slight suppression, however, is a common finding.

A complete assessment of binocular vision should include all four of the components described above. A suggested minimum database would include the near point of convergence, the cover test at distance and near, step vergence ranges at distance and near, and stereopsis testing. If a patient presents with symptoms and the minimum database does not yield conclusive information, additional testing using indirect measures of binocular function, along with facility testing and fixation disparity assessment, should be utilized.

Assessment of Size and Direction of the Phoria or Fixation Disparity

Cover Test (in the Absence of Strabismus)

1. Purpose The cover test is an objective method of evaluating the presence, direction, and the magnitude of the phoria.

2. Important issues

(a) Controlling accommodation The most important aspect of the cover test procedure or any other test of binocular alignment is control of accommodation. A recent study by Howarth and Heron (17) reaffirmed the significance of the accommodative system as a potential source variability in clinical heterophoria measurement. Underaccommodation will result in an overestimation of the degree of exophoria or an underestimation of the esophoria. Overaccommodation will yield the opposite results. There are two techniques that can be used to maximize control of accommodation during the cover test procedure. These refinements to the basic procedure tend to increase attention on the task. The examiner can use multiple fixation targets to maintain attention and accommodation on the task. This can easily be accomplished using Gulden fixation sticks that have 20/30 targets on both sides of the stick (Fig. 1.2). Periodically, the fixation stick is turned around to change targets. The patient is asked to identify the target during the cover test.

Another useful procedure is to move the target left to right very slightly (1 to 3 cm), between movements of the cover paddle. The examiner looks for a small pursuit movement in the uncovered eye. If a pursuit movement occurs when the target is moved left to right, it suggests that the patient is attending to the target. Attention on the target tends to encourage accommodation.

(b) The cover test is an objective test Because the cover test is an objective technique, it is one of the most valuable methods for assessing the motor characteristics of binocularity. It becomes particularly valuable when working with young children.

3. Expected values Although the expected finding for the cover test has not been specifically studied, we expect it to be similar to the values found during phoria testing. At distance, the expected value is 1 exophoria, with a standard deviation of ± 1 Δ. The mean expected value at near is 3 exophoria, with a standard deviation of ± 3 Δ (18).

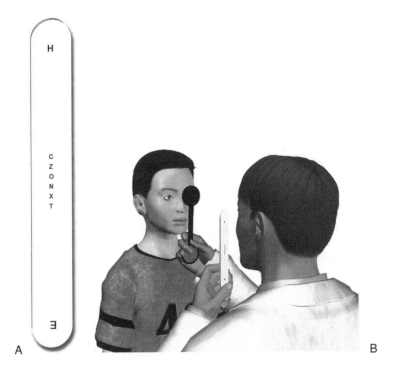

FIG. 1.2. A: Gulden fixation stick. **B:** Gulden fixation sticks with small targets used as a fixation target.

Phoria Measured Using the von Graefe Technique

1. Purpose The von Graefe phoria test is a subjective method of evaluating the presence, direction, and the magnitude of the phoria.

2. Important issues

(a) **Controlling accommodation** Controlling accommodation is also important when evaluating the phoria using the von Graefe procedure. It is vital to emphasize this in the instructional set to the patient. Often clinicians merely ask the patient to look at one image and report when the other is right above or below. To ensure more accurate accommodation, the clinician should state:

I want you to look at the lower image and it is very important to **keep it clear at all times.** While you keep it clear, tell me when the upper image moves directly above the lower image.

Although the instruction to keep the target clear is not always included in phoria testing, a lack of attention to this issue may lead to variability and poor reliability. Another issue that should be considered, particularly in young children, is whether the patient understands the task. Clinicians often use the following instructional set to try and explain the objective of the test.

Look at the bottom line and tell me when the top line moves directly above it, like buttons on a shirt.

Although this may be helpful in older children and adults, we have found that children who are 7 years old and younger do not perform well with this analogy. To promote an understanding in young children, we suggest an actual simple demonstration outside the phoropter using one's fingers. The young child is asked to look at the examiner's fingers, which are held one directly over the other. We use the following instructional set.

> Look at the finger on the bottom and tell me when my top finger is right over my bottom finger. (Demonstrate by misaligning your fingers and then bringing them back to alignment.) Now let's try it; tell me when to stop.

Using this method allows the examiner to determine whether the child has an understanding of what is expected.

Although the von Graefe procedure is commonly used in clinical practice, a recent study by Rainey et al. (19) indicated that this procedure is the least repeatable of the various tests used to measure the phoria.

3. Expected Values (Table 1.2). At distance, the expected value is 1 exophoria, with a standard deviation of ± 1 Δ. The mean expected value at near is 3 exophoria, with a standard deviation of ± 3 Δ (18) for children and young adults and 1 esophoria, with a standard deviation of ± 1 Δ at distance, and 8 exophoria with a standard deviation of ± 3 Δ at near for presbyopes.

Phoria Measured Using the Modified Thorington Technique

1. Purpose This technique is a subjective method of evaluating the presence, direction, and the magnitude of the phoria.

2. Important issues

(a) **Controlling accommodation** With the modified Thorington test, it is important for the clinician to emphasize that the patient keep the letters on the chart clear during the test procedure. In a recent study (19), the results of seven different procedures of assessing the phoria were compared to determine the repeatability of the clinical tests. The authors compared the estimated cover test, prism-neutralized objective cover test, prism-neutralized subjective cover test, von Graefe—continuous presentation, von Graefe—flash presentation, the Thorington method and the modified Thorington method. They found that the modified Thorington procedure was the most repeatable method, while the von Graefe methods had the poorest repeatability.

(b) **Testing outside the phoropter** An important advantage of this technique is that it can be used for patients that are difficult to test with a phoropter. For this reason, the modified Thorington technique has value with children under the age of 7 or 8. As indicated above, it has also been shown to be the most repeatable method of assessing the phoria.

3. Expected values (Table 1.2). At distance, the expected value is 1 exophoria with a standard deviation of ± 1 Δ. The mean expected value at near is 3 exophoria, with a standard deviation of ± 3 Δ (18).

Fixation Disparity Assessment

1. Purpose Fixation disparity testing is designed to evaluate binocular vision under associated conditions. This is in contrast to cover testing, the von Graefe phoria test, and the modified Thorington techniques, which are done under conditions in which either one eye is covered or the eyes are dissociated.

2. Important issues

(a) **Fixation disparity testing is performed under binocular conditions** The main deficiency of the typical phoria measurement is that the evaluation occurs under dissociated conditions. Wick (20) states that "the vergence error under binocular conditions is often not

TABLE 1.2. *Table of expecteds: binocular vision testing*

Test		Expected finding	Standard deviation
Cover test			
Distance		1 exophoria	±2Δ
Near		3 exophoria	±3Δ
Distance lateral phoria		1 exophoria	±2Δ
Near lateral phoria		3 exophoria	±3Δ
AC/A ratio		4:1	±2Δ
Smooth vergence testing			
Base-out (distance)	blur:	9	±4
	break:	19	±8
	recovery:	10	±4
Base-in (distance)	break:	7	±3
	recovery:	4	±2
Base-out (near)	blur:	17	±5
	break:	21	±6
	recovery:	11	±7
Base-in (near)	blur:	13	±4
	break:	21	±4
	recovery:	13	±5
Step vergence testing			
Children 7–12 yr old			
Base-out (near)	break:	23	±8
	recovery:	16	±6
Base-in (near)	break:	12	±5
	recovery:	7	±4
Adults			
Base-out (distance)	break:	11	±7
	recovery:	7	±2
Base-in (distance)	break:	7	±3
	recovery:	4	±2
Base-out (near)	break:	19	±9
	recovery:	14	±7
Base-in (near)	break:	13	±6
	recovery:	10	±5
Vergence facility testing			
(12 base-out/3 base-in)			
Near point of convergence	15.0 cpm		±3
Accommodative target	break:	5 cm	±2.5
	recovery:	7 cm	±3.0
Penlight/red-green glasses	break:	7 cm	±4.0
	recovery:	10 cm	±5.0

the same as it is under monocular conditions." As a result, there are situations in which a patient may be symptomatic, but the conventional phoria/vergence analysis does not produce a clear understanding of the cause of the patient's symptoms. Although some clinicians suggest the routine use of fixation disparity testing, we have found that in the majority of cases, phoria/vergence testing is sufficient to reach a tentative diagnosis and management plan. In those situations in which the diagnosis is unclear or a prism prescription is being considered, fixation disparity testing is a useful addition to the examination procedure.

   (b) Associated phoria versus forced vergence fixation disparity assessment Various instruments are available for the evaluation of fixation disparity. Older instruments such as the Mallett unit, the American Optical Vectographic slide, the Borish card, or the Bernell lantern (Chapter 14) are used to determine the associated phoria. The associated phoria is the amount of prism necessary to neutralize any perceived misalignment of the lines.

   Recent studies suggest, however, that the use of forced vergence fixation disparity testing is more likely to yield data that are useful for determining those patients who are likely to have symptoms (21,22). Based upon current information, forced vergence fixation disparity testing should be used when assessing a horizontal deviation. For a vertical deviation, associated phoria testing is sufficient.

(c) **Determination of prism correction** Fixation disparity is currently considered the method of choice for determining the amount of prism to prescribe for binocular disorders. Other methods tend to yield higher amounts of prism than fixation disparity analysis.

3. Expected values Refer to Chapter 14.

AC/A Ratio

1. Purpose To determine the change in accommodative convergence that occurs when the patient accommodates or relaxes accommodation by a given amount.

2. Important issues

(a) **Significance in diagnosis and treatment** Determination of the AC/A ratio is important in analysis of optometric data. The AC/A finding is a key characteristic in the final determination of the diagnosis. It is also one of the most important findings used to determine the appropriate management sequence for any given condition. For example, esophoria at near associated with a high AC/A ratio would generally respond well to plus lenses. If the same degree of esophoria is associated with a normal or low AC/A ratio, the recommended treatment approach would include prism correction and/or vision therapy.

(b) **Calculated versus gradient AC/A ratio** There are two methods for determining a patient's AC/A ratio. The first, referred to as the calculated AC/A ratio, is determined using the formula:

AC/A = IPD(cm) + NFD(m) (Hn − Hf)
IPD = interpupillary distance in centimeters
NFD = near fixation distance in meters
Hn = near phoria (eso is plus and exo is minus)
Hf = far phoria (eso is plus and exo is minus)

Example: IPD = 60 mm, the patient is 2 exophoric at distance and 10 exophoric at near (40 cm).

$$AC/A = 6 + 0.4(-10 + 2)$$
$$= 6 + 0.4(-8) = 6 + (-3.2)$$
$$= 2.8$$

When using this formula, one should remember to use the correct signs for esophoria and exophoria. A rule-of-thumb is that a high AC/A will result in more eso or less exo at near, and a low AC/A ratio will lead to less eso or more exo at near.

The second method, called the gradient AC/A, is determined by measuring the phoria a second time using −1.00 or −2.00 lenses. The change in the phoria, with the additional minus, is the AC/A ratio. For example, if the near phoria is 2 esophoria through the subjective finding and, with −1.00, it is 7 esophoria, the AC/A ratio is 5:1.

There may be significant differences between the two methods of determining the AC/A ratio. For instance, divergence excess and convergence excess patients both have high calculated AC/A ratios, but many of these patients have approximately normal gradient AC/A ratios (20). The same phenomenon may occur with convergence insufficiency. The calculated AC/A ratio will be low, but the gradient AC/A may be normal (20). The reason for these differences is the effect of proximal convergence and the lag of accommodation. The calculated AC/A ratio is usually larger than the gradient because of the effect of proximal vergence, which affects the near phoria measurement. Since the gradient ratio is measured by testing the near phoria twice at a fixed distance, proximal vergence is held constant and theoretically does not alter the final result. The lag of accommodation also accounts for differences between the calculated and gradient AC/A ratio measurements. Although the stimulus to accommodation is 2.50 D at near, the accommodative response is typically less than the stimulus. This difference between the stimulus and response of the accommodative system is called the lag of accommodation. The lag of accommodation is generally $+0.25$ to $+0.75$ D. Since the patient will tend to underaccommodate for any given stimulus, the gradient AC/A tends to be lower than the calculated AC/A ratio.

   (c) Controlling accommodation A source of measurement error in the AC/A evaluation is failure to control accommodation. The clinician should emphasize, in the instructional set, that clarity of the target is essential. It is easy to understand how variation in accommodative response from one measurement to another would adversely affect results. The gradient AC/A requires two measurements of the near phoria, first with only the subjective in place and then with -1.00 over the subjective. If a patient accurately accommodates for the first measurement, but underaccommodates for the second, the result will be an underestimation of the true AC/A ratio. It is, therefore, critical to ask the patient to maintain clarity and it is advisable to ask the patient to read the letters periodically.

   (d) Response versus stimulus AC/A ratio When evaluating the accommodative or binocular systems, we usually present the stimulus at 40 cm. This creates an accommodative demand of 2.50 D. This is referred to as the stimulus to accommodation. Although the stimulus to accommodation is 2.50 D, we know that the accommodative response will generally be about 10% less than the stimulus (23). The expected finding for MEM retinoscopy, for example, which assesses the accommodative response, is a lag of accommodation of about $+0.25$ to $+0.50$ D. It is important to be aware of the difference between the response and stimulus to accommodation, realizing that most patients will underaccommodate by about 10%. An instance where this becomes important is when comparing the calculated AC/A to the gradient AC/A ratios. The gradient AC/A ratio will tend to underestimate the AC/A ratio. For example, the phoria is measured as 10 exophoria at near and, when repeated with -1.00 lenses, the phoria is 6 exophoria. Based on this information, the gradient AC/A ratio would be 4:1. However, if we assume that the patient underaccommodates by 10%, the phoria has changed by 4 Δ while accommodation has changed by 0.75 D. This would be an AC/A ratio of about 4.45:1.

   3. Expected values The expected AC/A ratio is 4:1, with a standard deviation of ±2.

CA/C Ratio

   1. Purpose To determine the change in accommodation that occurs when the patient converges or relaxes convergence a given amount.

   2. Important issues

   (a) Significance in diagnosis and treatment The CA/C ratio is still not commonly assessed in the clinical situation. Determination of the CA/C ratio is important in analysis of optometric data. The CA/C finding is sometimes an important characteristic in the final determination of the diagnosis. It may also play a key role when one determines appropriate management. For example, divergence excess and other cases of high exophoria at distance may benefit from the use of added minus lenses. Analysis of the CA/C ratio helps in this determination.

   (b) Clinical determination of the CA/C ratio To measure the CA/C ratio clinically, we have to use either a blur-free target or pinholes to eliminate blur as a stimulus. There is still no widely accepted method for determining the CA/C ratio. One possible approach is to use a target called the Wesson "DOG" card ("DOG" or difference of gaussian) (24) along with dynamic retinoscopy. To use this technique, ask the patient to view this target at four different distances as you perform retinoscopy. You can determine the amount of accommodation with different vergence levels.

(c) **Stimulus versus response CA/C** Unlike the accommodative system in which there may be a significant difference between the stimulus and response, the vergence stimulus and vergence response are generally identical. There is, therefore, no need to differentiate between a stimulus and response CA/C ratio (25).

3. Expected values The expected CA/C value for young adults is 0.50 D per meter angle. In vision research, one meter angle equals 10% of the distance IPD (interpupillary distance) in millimeters; thus, for a patient with a distance 50 mm IPD, one meter angle is 5 Δ, for a patient with a 69 mm distance IPD, one meter angle is 6.9 Δ. For clinical purposes, it is satisfactory to consider one meter angle to be about 6 Δ. Because there is little difference between vergence stimulus and vergence response, there is very little difference between the stimulus and response CA/C ratio. The CA/C ratio is inversely related to age.

Direct Assessment of Positive and Negative Fusional Vergence

Smooth Vergence Testing

1. Purpose Smooth vergence testing is designed to assess the fusional vergence amplitude and recovery at both distance and near. This is considered a direct measure of fusional vergence.

2. Important issues

(a) **Amplitude versus facility** Smooth vergence testing is the most common method used for assessing the amplitude of the fusional vergence response for both positive and negative fusional vergence. The blur finding is a measure of the amount of fusional vergence free of accommodation. The break indicates the amount of fusional vergence and accommodative vergence. The recovery finding provides information about the patient's ability to regain single binocular vision after diplopia occurs. Although smooth vergence testing provides important information about the amplitude of fusional vergence, studies (11) have shown that it is possible to have normal fusional amplitudes and still have a problem referred to as fusion vergence dysfunction. Additional testing must be performed to assess fusional facility.

(b) **Smooth versus step vergence** Smooth and step vergence testing are both designed to evaluate fusional vergence amplitude. The primary value of step vergence testing is that it is administered outside the phoropter. This is an important advantage when examining young children. Before the age of 8 or 9, children tire quickly and may move around making testing with a phoropter difficult. Because it is impossible to see the child's eyes behind the phoropter, the clinician cannot be sure if the patient is responding appropriately. Recent studies (6,7) have demonstrated that expected findings are different for smooth versus step vergence.

3. Expected values Table 1.2 lists the expected values for the blur, break, and recovery for positive and negative fusional vergence using smooth vergence testing.

Step Vergence Testing

1. Purpose Step vergence is a method of evaluating fusional vergence amplitude outside the phoropter.

2. Important issues

(a) **Testing outside the phoropter** When a young child is evaluated who is either very active or not responding reliably, step vergence testing represents a useful alternative. The child's eyes can be seen because testing is done with a prism bar and the test becomes more objective. Instead of relying on the patient's responses, the examiner can observe when the child loses binocularity.

3. Expected values The expected values have been determined to be different for adults and children (6,7). Table 1.2 lists the break and recovery values for positive and negative fusional vergence testing for both children and adults.

Vergence Facility Testing

1. Purpose Vergence facility testing is designed to assess the dynamics of the fusional vergence system and the ability to respond over a period of time. This ability to make rapid repetitive vergence changes over an extended period of time can be referred to as a measure of stamina and is the characteristic that we assess clinically. Another characteristic that we indirectly evaluate using vergence facility testing is sustaining ability. This refers to the ability of the individual to maintain vergence at a particular level, rather than to rapidly alter the level, for a sustained period of time.

2. Important issues

(a) **Amplitude versus facility** Because it is possible to have normal fusional vergence amplitudes and vergence facility problems, both aspects should be evaluated with a symptomatic patient. We suggest using vergence facility testing when a patient presents with symptoms characteristic of a binocular disorder and other testing does not reveal any problems. Such a patient may have normal fusional vergence amplitudes but reduced facility.

(b) **Strength of prism to use/target to use** Until recently, there had been a lack of systematically gathered normative data and little consensus in the literature about the strength of prism that should be used for this test. Buzzelli (9) recommended the use of 16 base-out and 4 base-in. Another common recommendation (8) was 8 base-out and 8 base-in. Gall et al. (12) performed the first systematic study of vergence facility and found that the magnitude of choice is 3 Δ base-in/12 Δ base-out. This combination of prism yielded the highest significance for separating symptomatic from nonsymptomatic subjects. They also found that this combination of prisms produced repeatable results (R = 0.85) when used for near vergence facility testing.

In another study, Gall et al. (13) compared the use of three different vertically oriented targets for vergence facility testing. The targets tested were a vertical column of 20/30 letters, a back-illuminated anaglyphic target, and the Wirt circles oriented vertically. The study was designed to determine if it is important to use a target with a suppression control for vergence facility testing. They found that vergence facility is nearly independent of the target and a simple vertical row of 20/30 letters is an appropriate target.

3. Expected values Based on the work of Gall et al. (12), the expected findings for vergence facility, using values of 3 Δ base-in/12 Δ base-out, is 15 cpm at near (Table 1.2).

Indirect Assessment of Positive and Negative Fusional Vergence

Near Point of Convergence

1. Purpose The purpose of the near point of convergence is to assess the convergence amplitude. A remote near point of convergence was recently found to be the most frequently used criterion by optometrists for diagnosing convergence insufficiency (26).

2. Important issues

(a) **Target to be used** Different targets have been suggested for near point of convergence testing. Recommendations vary from an accommodative target, a light, and a light with a red glass before one eye, and a light with red-green glasses. Some suggest that a variety of targets should be used to determine if there are differences with various targets. We recommend repeating the near point of convergence twice—first using an accommodative target and then using a transilluminator or penlight with red-green glasses.

   (b) Does the repetition of the near point of convergence test yield additional useful clinical data? The near point of convergence test traditionally is performed by slowly moving a target towards the eyes until the patient reports diplopia or the examiner notices a break in fusion (3). This is recorded as the breakpoint. The target is then slowly moved away from the patient until fusion is reported or the examiner notices realignment of the eyes, signaling recovery of fusion.

   Several modifications to this traditional approach have been suggested in the literature to make the test more sensitive. Wick (27) and Mohindra and Molinari (28) recommend that the near point of convergence test should be repeated 4 to 5 times. Their suggestions are based on the claim of Davis (29) that asymptomatic patients manifest little change in the near point with repeated testing, while symptomatic patients have significantly less convergence with repeated testing. Thus, this recommendation is designed to improve the diagnostic sensitivity of the break of the near point of convergence test. Scheiman et al. (16) found a recession of the near point of convergence after repetition in both normals and convergence insufficiency patients. In the subjects with normal binocular vision, however, the amount of recession was small, less than 1 cm. In the convergence insufficiency group, the amount of recession was 1.5 cm after five repetitions and about 4 cm after ten repetitions (16). These findings suggest that repetition of the near point of convergence would have to be performed about 10 times to yield useful clinical information.

   (c) Does the use of the red glass or red-green glasses, along with the near point of convergence test, yield any additional useful clinical data? Another criterion utilized for assessment of convergence ability is the recovery point, or the point at which an individual regains fusion (after fusion has been lost) during the push-up convergence testing. Capobianco (30) reported that a recovery point greatly different from the break indicates greater convergence problems. She also suggested repeating the test with a red glass before one eye. She stated that greater recession with the red glass suggests a more significant convergence problem. Several authors (27,28,31,32) have suggested that this procedure be part of the standard assessment of convergence amplitude.

   Scheiman et al. (16) found a statistically significant difference between the break and recovery with an accommodative target and the results with a penlight and red-green glasses in patients with convergence insufficiency. For convergence insufficiency subjects, the mean break with an accommodative target was 9.3 cm and, with a penlight and red-green glasses, the mean break was 14.8 cm. The recovery finding with the accommodative target was 12.2 cm and with a penlight and red-green glasses it was 17.6 cm. For both the break and recovery, therefore, there was a difference of about 5.5 cm between the accommodative target and penlight and red-green glasses. Statistically significant differences were not found for an accommodative target compared to a penlight or a penlight compared to a penlight and red-green glasses.

   In the subjects with normal binocular vision, there were no significant differences for any of the conditions described above. The mean break was between 2.4 and 2.9 cm and the mean recovery was between 4.2 and 5 cm.

   (d) The value of assessing convergence ability using a jump convergence format Pickwell et al. (33) described another method of assessing convergence ability, which they termed "jump convergence." In this procedure, the subject first fixates a target at 6 cm and then changes fixation to a target at 15 cm. Pickwell et al. (33,34) reported that this jump convergence test appears to have more clinical significance and is a more sensitive way of determining the presence of convergence problems than the near point of convergence. In the original study (33), the authors compared the effectiveness of the standard near point test (pursuit convergence) and the jump convergence procedure in a group of 74 subjects with inadequate convergence. Fifty of the 74 showed normal pursuit convergence but reduced jump convergence. Only five subjects passing the jump convergence test failed the pursuit convergence procedure. The authors concluded that "this evidence clearly suggests that the jump convergence test is more likely to detect inadequacy of convergence than the measurement of the near point of convergence." In a second study, Pickwell et al. (34) found that in a sample of 110 subjects with inadequate convergence, poor jump convergence was more frequently associated with symptoms than was poor pursuit convergence. One problem with the jump convergence test is the lack of expected values for this test. In their recent study, Scheiman et al. (16) found a mean of 30 cpm (standard deviation = 10) for subjects with normal binocular vision and 23 cpm (standard deviation = 11) for subjects with convergence insufficiency (16).

3. Expected values Although this test is commonly used to diagnose convergence insufficiency, there had been no normative data for children or adults until recently. Hayes et al. (35) studied 297 schoolchildren and recommended a clinical cutoff value of 6 cm. Scheiman et al. (16) studied an adult population and suggested that when using an accommodative target, a 5 cm cutoff value should be used for the break and a 7 cm cutoff value should be used for the recovery. Using a penlight and red-green glasses, the cutoff value for the break is 7 cm and the recovery 10 cm.

Negative Relative Accommodation and Positive Relative Accommodation

1. Purpose NRA and PRA tests were designed to be used as part of the near point evaluation of accommodation and binocular vision. The primary objective of these tests is to determine if the patient requires an add for near work. In a pre-presbyopic patient, the two findings should be approximately balanced (NRA = +2.50, PRA = −2.50). A PRA value higher than the NRA suggests that a patient may benefit from an add (Chapter 10, High ACA). The test is also used with the presbyopic population in the same manner to determine if an add is necessary and to finalize the magnitude of the required add. The NRA can also be used to determine if a patient has been overminused during the subjective examination. The NRA is performed through the subjective prescription, which should eliminate all accommodation at distance. Since the test distance is 40 cm, the patient will accommodate approximately 2.5 D to see the target clearly. Therefore, the maximum amount of accommodation that can be relaxed is 2.50 D. Thus, an NRA finding greater than +2.50 suggests that the patient was overminused.

In this text, we will stress another use for the NRA/PRA tests. These tests can be used to indirectly analyze both accommodation and vergence. This is explained in detail in Chapter 2.

2. Important issues

(a) Instructional Set It is important to ask the patient to keep the target clear and single during these tests. Traditionally, the instructional set is:

"As I add lenses in front of your eyes, keep these letters clear for as long as you can. Tell me when the letters are blurry."

We believe it is important to also ask the patient to report diplopia, because these tests also indirectly probe the ability to maintain fusion using positive and negative fusional vergence.

(b) High NRA Finding A high NRA finding indicates that the patient has been overminused during the subjective.

(c) At what level should the PRA be discontinued? The maximum value that should be expected with the NRA is +2.50 for the reasons explained above. However, there is no consistent endpoint for the PRA. The endpoint for the PRA will vary, depending on the patient's amplitude of accommodation, AC/A ratio, and the negative fusional vergence. The examples below illustrate the variables that determine the endpoint for the PRA.

Test	Patient #1	Patient #2	Patient #3
Amplitude of accommodation	12 D	12 D	12 D
AC/A ratio	2:1	4:1	8:1
Base-in vergence (near)	12/20/12	10/20/10	8/12/8
Expected PRA finding	−6.00	−2.50	−1.00

In the first patient, we would expect the patient to be able to keep the target single and clear until about −6.00. As we add minus lenses binocularly, the patient must accommodate to maintain clarity. This is not a problem because the amplitude of accommodation is 12 D. At the same time, the patient must maintain single binocular vision. As the patient accommodates, the AC/A ratio causes convergence that must be counteracted using negative fusional vergence. For every 1 Δ of accommodation, the patient must use 2 Δ of negative fusional vergence. Since Patient #1 has 12 D of accommodation and 12 Δ of negative fusional vergence, he or she will be able to maintain clear single binocular vision until about −6.00 D. Using the same reasoning, the PRA endpoint will decrease as the AC/A increases, as demonstrated above for patients #2 and #3, who have higher AC/A ratios and lower negative fusional vergence ranges.

In contrast to the NRA where the maximum expected endpoint is always +2.50, the maximum endpoint for the PRA varies with multiple factors. Since the primary objective of the NRA/PRA tests is to determine if the two values are balanced, it makes sense to stop the PRA test after reaching a value of −2.50.

3. Expected values The expected values for NRA are +2.00, ±0.50; for PRA, the expected values are −2.37, ±1.00.

EVALUATION OF SENSORY STATUS

General Considerations

While sensory fusion anomalies can be very dramatic in cases of strabismus, in cases of nonstrabismic binocular vision disorders, sensory anomalies are much less severe. Most patients with nonstrabismic binocular anomalies have normal or only mildly reduced stereopsis. Suppression is common in heterophoria, but is less intense and the size of the suppression scotoma is smaller in size than in strabismus.

Although sensory status is not as significant an issue in heterophoria, the presence of suppression or loss of stereopsis is still important in determining the prognosis and sequence of treatment. In many cases, the presence of suppression can be determined by performing the binocular vision testing described above. During the near point of convergence, near lateral phoria, and fusional vergence testing, patients may be unable to appreciate diplopia in spite of misalignment of the visual axes, indicating suppression.

Evaluation of Suppression

Worth Four-dot Test

1. Purpose The Worth four-dot test is a subjective test designed to evaluate the presence and size of the suppression scotoma. It is considered one of the most accurate methods of evaluating suppression (36).

2. Important issues

(a) **Determining the size of the suppression scotoma** The size of the suppression scotoma can be determined by moving the Worth four-dot away from the patient. As the flashlight is moved away from the patient, the target subtends a smaller angle. For instance, at 13 in., the target subtends an angle of approximately 4.5 degrees. At 3 ft, the angle subtended is approximately 1.5 degrees. When performing the Worth four-dot, it is initially held at 13 in. and the patient, wearing red-green glasses, is asked to report the number of dots seen. If the patient reports four dots, the clinician should slowly move the flashlight from 13 in. to about 3 ft. If the patient reports four dots at 13 in., but two or three dots at 3 ft, a small suppression scotoma is present. If a three- or two dot-response is present, even at 13 in., the suppression scotoma is larger. The size of the suppression scotoma is important because there is a relationship between the size of the suppression scotoma and the level of stereopsis. As the suppression scotoma becomes larger, the stereopsis decreases (8).

(b) **Determining the intensity or depth of the suppression** It is important to evaluate the intensity of the suppression scotoma. It is possible to have a small suppression scotoma that is more intense and, therefore, more difficult to treat than a larger, less intense, suppression scotoma. To assess the depth of the suppression, the clinician can perform the Worth four-dot with normal room illumination and again with the room lights turned off. Normal illumination simulates the patient's normal visual conditions and is more likely to yield a suppression response. As the conditions are made artificial, the patient has more difficulty maintaining the suppression. The suppression is considered more intense, therefore, if it is present even with the room lights off.

3. Expected values The expected response with the Worth four-dot is four dots at both 13 in. and 3 ft.

Other Tests for Evaluating Suppression

Many other tests are available for testing suppression; these include both subjective and objective tests. Commonly used subjective tests include the AO (American Optical) Vectographic Chart, the near Mallett unit, Bagolini striated lenses, and cheiroscopic tracings. The 4 Base-out test is an objective method of assessing suppression. We suggest the use of the Worth four-dot because of its availability, low cost, ease of administration, and accuracy in detecting suppression. A complete discussion of instrumentation and specific clinical procedures is available in other texts (1,37).

Evaluation of Stereopsis

Randot Stereotest

1. Purpose The Randot Stereotest is a subjective test designed to evaluate the presence and degree of stereopsis using both global and contour (local) stereopsis targets.

2. Important issues

(a) **Global versus contour targets** Two types of targets are commonly used for the assessment of stereopsis. The first, called contour or local stereopsis, uses two similar targets that are laterally displaced. The Titmus stereofly, Wirt rings, and animals (Fig. 1.3) are examples of this type of target. A shortcoming of this type of stereopsis target is that patients with no stereopsis may be able to guess the "correct" answer using monocular cues. Cooper and Warshowsky (38) found that the correct response for the first four Wirt rings could be determined by looking for monocular displacement of one of the circles. Clinically this may

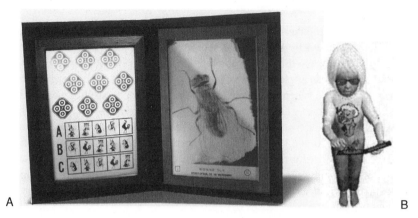

A   B

FIG. 1.3. A: Titmus stereofly. **B:** Child reaching for "fly" that appears to be floating in front of the page.

be significant when a clinician is examining a child who is trying to give the "right answer" to please the examiner. Of course, with a patient giving accurate responses and not trying to fool the examiner, this test works well.

The second type of stereopsis technique, called global targets, eliminates this problem. Global targets contain random dot stereopsis targets and have no monocular cues. As a result, the guessing that can occur with contour stereopsis is not a problem with global stereopsis.

Another important distinction between contour and global targets is their value in detecting the presence of a constant strabismus. Cooper and Feldman (39) investigated the use of stereopsis tests to detect strabismus and found that with random dot stereogram of 660 seconds of arc disparity, no constant strabismic could pass the test. Thus, even a gross random dot stereopsis target is effective at detecting the presence of a constant strabismus. With contour stereopsis targets, a constant strabismic can occasionally appreciate up to 70 seconds of arc stereopsis (36). Random dot targets can be used to rule out the presence of a constant strabismus, while contour stereopsis targets can be used to determine if peripheral stereopsis is present. Peripheral stereopsis is considered to be any value greater than 60 seconds of arc. Both types of stereopsis targets, therefore, have value and it is best to use both in the clinical evaluation of stereopsis. This can be accomplished using one test, such as the Randot Stereotest (Fig. 1.4A),

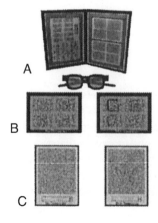

A

B

C

FIG. 1.4. Examples of random dot stereopsis. **A:** Randot Stereotest. **B:** The Synthetic Optics Circle, Square. **C:** The Synthetic Optics Butterfly target.

or by using two tests, such as the Synthetic Optics Circle, Square, and E targets (Fig. 1.4B) or Butterfly (Fig. 1.4C) and the Titmus stereotest or the Synthetic Optics Animals and Circles.

3. Expected values A patient with normal binocular function should be able to achieve 20 seconds of stereopsis with the contour stimuli and appreciate stereopsis with the gross random dot targets.

ASSESSMENT OF ACCOMMODATIVE DISORDERS

General Considerations

The traditional evaluation of accommodative function (Table 1.3) involves measurement of the amplitude of accommodation using either Donder's push-up method or the Optometric Extension Program (OEP) minus lens procedure. There are shortcomings to this limited approach, however. In recent years, many authors have reported the clinical significance of testing accommodative response and facility as well as amplitude (27,40–45). An important concept is that an individual may experience asthenopic symptoms and have an accommodative disorder even when the accommodative amplitude is normal (42,44). Several studies have investigated the relationship between accommodative facility and the presence of symptoms. Both Hennessey et al. (44) and Levine et al. (45) reported that symptomatic subjects perform significantly poorer than asymptomatic subjects on both monocular accommodative facility (MAF) and BAF testing.

Lui et al. (42) were able to objectively measure changes in latency and velocity of accommodative response before and after vision therapy. They found that accommodative dynamics changed significantly after vision therapy. The fact that accommodative facility results are related to symptoms, and that changes can be demonstrated after therapy, suggests that it is a valuable assessment technique. It should be part of the routine evaluation of accommodative function.

The third aspect of the evaluation, accommodative response, has also been studied (46–49). It has been demonstrated that the accommodative response is generally not equal to the stimulus. Since most optometric testing relies on stimulus measures and assumes equality between stimulus and response, a clinician might be misled when managing binocular or accommodative anomalies. It is, therefore, important to actually measure the accommodative response. MEM retinoscopy is a widely used procedure that can be utilized for this assessment. Rouse et al. (48,49) have demonstrated the validity of MEM retinoscopy and established normative data.

Wick and Hall (50) studied the relationship among the three areas of accommodation (amplitude, facility, and response) that are usually tested. They screened 200 children and, after eliminating those that had strabismus or significant uncorrected refractive error, found that only 4% had deficits in all three of the accommodative functions. Their results suggest that it is impossible to predict the results on one test based upon the results of another. Therefore, when accommodative dysfunction is suspected, all aspects of accommodation, amplitude, facility, and response must be considered.

A complete assessment of accommodation should include all three components described above. A suggested minimum database would include the amplitude of accommodation,

TABLE 1.3. *Important aspects of accommodative testing*

Accommodative amplitude	Push-up test
	Minus lens test
Accommodative facility	Accommodative facility
	Testing with ±2.00 lenses
Accommodative response	Monocular estimation method retinoscopy

TABLE 1.4. *Table of expecteds: accommodative testing*

Test	Expected finding	Standard deviation
Amplitude of accommodation		
Push-up test	18 − 1/3 age	±2 D
Minus lens test	2 D < push-up	
Monocular accommodative facility		
Children		
(±2.00 flippers, calling out numbers or letters on Accommodative Rock Cards)		
6 yr old	5.5 cpm	±2.5 cpm
7 yr old	6.5 cpm	±2.0 cpm
8–12 yr old	7.0 cpm	±2.5 cpm
Adults		
(±2.00 flipper lenses, saying now when clear)		
13–30 yr old	11.0 cpm	±5.0 cpm
30–40 yr old	not available	
Binocular accommodative facility		
Children		
(±2.00 flippers, calling out numbers or letters on Accommodative Rock Cards)		
6 yr old	3.0 cpm	±2.5 cpm
7 yr old	3.5 cpm	±2.5 cpm
8–12 yr old	5.0 cpm	±2.5 cpm
Adults (Use lens power based on amplitude scaled testing—refer to Table 1.5)		
	10.0 cpm	±5.0 cpm
Monocular estimation method retinoscopy	+0.50 D	±0.25 D
Fused X-cylinder	+0.50 D	±0.50 D
Negative relative accommodation	+2.00 D	±0.50 D
Positive relative accommodation	−2.37 D	±1.00 D

accommodative facility, and MEM retinoscopy. Table 1.4 lists the expected findings for all accommodative testing described below.

Assessment of Accommodative Amplitude

Push-up Amplitude

1. Purpose To subjectively measure the amplitude of accommodation under monocular conditions.

2. Important issues

(a) **Careful measurement of distance** It is critical to accurately measure the distance at which the patient reports a blur. Even small errors in measurement can lead to large differences in results. For example, an endpoint at 2 in. suggests a 20 Δ amplitude, while a blur at 2.5 in. suggests an amplitude of 16 Δ. To reduce this problem, the push-up amplitude can be measured through −4.00 D lenses. This modification moves the endpoint further away from the patient and allows more exact measurement of the endpoint.

(b) **Monitor patient response** With young children, it is important periodically to ask the child to read the letters to be sure that the print is not blurred. One modification in procedure that can be used is to begin the test with the chart very close to the child. Instead of asking when the print blurs, pull the chart away from the child until the patient can first read the letters. A recent paper compared the results of using the traditional push-up method of assessing the amplitude of accommodation to the pull-away method and found no significant difference in the measurement (51).

(c) **Relative distance magnification** A problem associated with the push-up method is that the letters no longer subtend the angle expected for a 20/30 letter because of relative

Procedure

1. Instructions to patient: "I will be changing the lenses in front of your eyes. Try to clear the print after each lens change. Tell me when you notice that the letters (examiner indicates appropriate print) are slightly blurred, still readable, but cannot be cleared by further effort."

2. Minus lenses are added in 0.25 D increments. When the patient reports "first sustained blur," the lens power is noted.

3. To obtain the amplitude in diopters, add 2.50 D for working distance to the amount of minus added.

Example

Minus added until first sustained blur	−6.00 D
Working distance (40 cm)	−2.50 D
Accommodative amplitude	−8.50 D

Important Points

1. Stress the importance of trying as hard as possible to clear the target.

ACCOMMODATIVE FACILITY TESTING

Equipment Needed:

Gulden fixation stick
+2.00/−2.00 flip lenses

Setup

1. If the patient wears glasses for close work, these should be used.
2. Hold Gulden fixation stick 40 cm from patient's face at eye level and place the +2.00 in front of the patient's eyes.
3. The test is initially performed binocularly.

Procedure (Child, Young Adult)

1. Ask the patient to try and get the letters clear and single as quickly as possible.
2. Instruct the subject to report (say "clear") as soon as the letters are clear.
3. When the letters are reported to be clear, quickly flip the flipper so the minus side is before the same eye, again instructing the subject to read the letters and report when the letters appear clear or if they disappear.
4. Continue alternating sides of the flipper lenses for 1 minute, calculating the cycles per minute achieved (1 cycle = plus and minus).
5. Repeat the procedure monocularly if the patient is unable to pass binocularly. The only difference in monocular testing is that the patient only has to report when the target is clear (diplopia is no longer an issue).
6. Record the cycles per minute. Record if one side (+ or−) of the flippers was more difficult, or if neither side was more difficult.

Procedure (30 Years and Older)

1. The differences in this age group are the working distance and the lens power to be used.

2. We suggest using the Amplitude Scaled Facility approach discussed earlier in this chapter (Table 1.5).

3. When using this method, select the lens power and working distance based on the amplitude of accommodation.

4. For example, if you are working with a 32-year-old patient with an amplitude of accommodation of 7.0 D, you would use ± 1.00 D lenses and the target would be placed 32.0 cm from the patient.

Examples

1. The patient can complete 18 flips in 1 minute. This equals 9 cpm.
2. If the patient cannot clear -2.00 at all, record as 0 cpm, fails minus.
3. If the patient cannot clear $+2.00$ at all, record as 0 cpm, fails plus.
4. If the patient reports diplopia, record as 0 cpm, diplopia with $+2.00$ or diplopia -2.00.

Important Points

1. Stress the importance of trying to keep the target both clear and single.

MONOCULAR ESTIMATION METHOD RETINOSCOPY

Equipment Needed:

Appropriate prescription (habitual or proposed near prescription)
Retinoscope
Age appropriate MEM graded cards (preschool to adult) affixed to retinoscope.
Loose lenses ($+0.50$, $+0.75$, $+1.00$, $+1.25$, etc.)

Setup

1. Patient is out of the phoropter, wearing his or her prescription.

2. The examiner sits opposite the patient, at eye level with the target, at either the patient's habitual reading distance (ask the patient) or Harmon distance.

3. Illumination must be sufficient so that the patient can easily see the words or pictures on the MEM card.

4. Select the appropriate MEM card corresponding to a grade or reading level closest to that of the patient. Card selected can be low demand (large print) or high demand (small print).

Procedure

1. Instructions: "With both eyes open, please read the words (or name the pictures) on the card out loud."

2. Make a sweep with the retinoscope and try to estimate the amount of "with" or "against" motion for each meridian. Repeat the sweeping motion as many times as needed. Repeat the measurements for the other eye.

3. To verify the estimation, a neutralizing trial lens is interposed *very briefly*, in front of one eye at a time, as the retinoscope light passes across the eye. If the motion is "with," interpose a plus lens. If the motion is "against," interpose a minus lens. When the true amount of lead or lag is measured in that meridian, a neutral response will be seen with the lens in place.

Important Points

1. Try to estimate the lens needed to neutralize the motion.
2. When using lenses, try to minimize the amount of time the lens is placed in front of the eye.

NSUCO OCULOMOTOR TEST—SACCADES

Equipment Needed:

Two Gulden fixation sticks (place a green circular sticker on one and a red circular sticker on the other)

Setup

1. Have the patient stand directly in front of the examiner.
2. No instructions are given to the patient to move or not to move his or her head.
3. Two modified Gulden fixation targets are used and held at Harmon's distance (distance from the patient's elbow to the middle knuckle) or no farther than 40 cm from the patient.
4. The examiner holds the targets so that each target is about 10 cm from the midline of the patient.

Procedure

1. Instructions to patient: "When I say 'red,' look at the red sticker and when I say 'green,' look at the green sticker. Remember, don't look until I tell you."
2. The examiner begins calling out red and green and repeats this so that the patient has to make ten saccades (five to the red target and five to the green target).
3. The examiner observes the saccadic eye movements and rates the performance in four categories including head movement, body movement, ability, and accuracy (Table 1.8).

Important Points

1. Do not make any statement in the instructions about head or body movement.
2. Have the patient stand during the procedure.
3. Keep the targets a maximum of 10 cm from the midline of the patient.

NSUCO OCULOMOTOR TEST—PURSUITS

Equipment Needed:

Gulden fixation sticks (place a red circular sticker on stick)

Setup

1. Have the patient stand directly in front of the examiner.
2. No instructions are given to the patient to move or not to move his or her head.
3. One modified Gulden fixation target is used and held at Harmon's distance (distance from the patient's elbow to the middle knuckle) or no farther than 40 cm from the patient.

Procedure

1. Instructions to patient: "Watch the red sticker as it goes around. Don't ever take your eyes off the ball."
2. The examiner moves the fixation target in a path no more than 20 cm in diameter, performed at the midline of the patient.
3. The examiner observes the pursuit eye movements and rates the performance in four categories including head movement, body movement, ability, and accuracy (Table 1.10).

Important Points

1. Do not make any statement in the instructions about head or body movement.
2. Have the patient stand during the procedure.
3. Move the target in a path no more than 20 cm in diameter, performed at the midline of the patient.

REFERENCES

1. Carlson NB, Kurtz D, Heath DA, et al. *Clinical procedures for ocular examination*, 2nd ed. New York: McGraw-Hill, 1996.
2. Eskridge JB, Amos JF, Bartlett JD. *Clinical procedures in optometry*. Philadelphia: JB Lippincott, 1991.
3. Benjamin WJ, Borish IM. *Borish's clinical refraction*. St. Louis: WB Saunders, 1998.
4. Rouse, Ryan. Clinical examination in children. In: Rosenbloom AA, Morgan MW, eds. *Pediatric optometry*. Philadelphia: JB Lippincott, 1990.
5. Rutstein RP, Daum KM. *Anomalies of binocular vision: diagnosis and management*. St. Louis: Mosby, 1997.
6. Wesson MD. Normalization of prism bar vergences. *Am J Optom Physiol Opt* 1982;59:628–633.
7. Scheiman M, Herzberg H, Frantz K, et al. A normative study of step vergence in elementary schoolchildren. *J Am Optom Assoc* 1989;60:276–280.
8. Griffin JR, Grisham JD. *Binocular anomalies: procedures for vision therapy*, 3rd ed. Boston: Butterworth-Heineman, 1995:49–50.
9. Buzzelli A. Vergence facility: developmental trends in a school age population. *Am J Optom Physiol Opt* 1986;63:351–355.
10. Scheiman M. Fusional facility. *Am J Optom Physiol Opt* 1986;63:76P.
11. Grisham D. The dynamics of fusional vergence eye movements in binocular dysfunction. *Am J Optom Physiol Opt* 1980;57:645–655.
12. Gall R, Wick B, Bedell H. Vergence facility: establishing clinical utility. *Optom Vis Sci* 1998;75:731–742.
13. Gall R, Wick B, Bedell H. Vergence facility and target type. *Optom Vis Sci* 1998;75:727–730.
14. Scheiman M, Wick B, Golebiewski A, et al. Vergence facility: establishment of clinical norms in a pediatric population. *Opt Vis Sci* 1996;[Suppl]:135.

15. Pickwell LD, Hampshire R. The significance of inadequate convergence. *Ophthal Physiol Opt* 1981;1:13–18.
16. Scheiman M, Gallaway M, Frantz KA, et al. Near point of convergence: test procedure, target selection and expected findings. *Optom Vis Sci* 2001 (in press).
17. Howarth PA, Heron G. Repeated measures of horizontal heterophoria. *Optom Vis Sci* 2000;77:616–619.
18. Morgan M. The clinical aspects of accommodation and convergence. *Am J Optom Arch Am Acad Optom* 1944;21:301–313.
19. Rainey BB, Schroeder TL, Goss DA, et al. Inter-examiner repeatability of heterophoria test. *Optom Vis Sci* 1998;75:719–726.
20. Wick B. Horizontal deviations in diagnosis and management in vision care. In: Amos J, ed. *Diagnosis and management in vision care*. Boston: Butterworth-Heineman, 1987:461–510.
21. Sheedy JE. Fixation disparity analysis of oculomotor imbalance. *Am J Optom Physiol Opt* 1980;57:632–639.
22. Sheedy JE, Saladin JJ. Phoria, vergence, and fixation disparity in oculomotor problems. *Am J Optom Physiol Opt* 1977;54:474–478.
23. Alpern M, Kincaid WM, Lubeck MJ. Vergence and accommodation. III. Proposed definitions of the AC/A ratios. *Am J Ophthalmol* 1959;48:141–148.
24. Wesson MD, Koenig R. A new clinical method for direct measurement of fixation disparity. *South J Optom* 1983;1:48–52.
25. Ciuffreda KJ. Components of clinical near vergence testing. *J Behav Optom* 1992;3:3–13.
26. Rouse MW, et al. How do you make the diagnosis of convergence insufficiency? Survey results. *J Optom Vis Dev* 1997;28:91–97.
27. Wick BC. Horizontal deviations. In: Amos J, ed. *Diagnosis and management in vision care*. Boston: Butterworth-Heineman, 1987:473.
28. Mohindra I, Molinari J. Convergence insufficiency: its diagnosis and management. Part I. *Optometric Monthly* 1980;71(3):38–43.
29. Davis CE. Orthoptic treatment in convergence insufficiency. *J Can Med Assoc* 1956;55:47–49.
30. Capobianco M. The subjective measurement of the near point of convergence and its significance in the diagnosis of convergence insufficiency. *Am Orthopt J* 1952;2:40–42.
31. Rosner J. *Pediatric optometry*. Boston: Butterworth-Heineman, 1982:258.
32. von Noorden GK, Brown DJ, Parks M. Associated convergence and accommodative insufficiency. *Doc Ophthalmol* 1973;34:393–403.
33. Pickwell LD, et al. Inadequate convergence. *Br J Physiol Opt* 1975;30:34–37.
34. Pickwell LD, Hampshire R. The significance of inadequate convergence. *Ophthal Physiol Opt* 1981;1:13–18.
35. Hayes GJ, Cohen BE, Rouse MW, et al. Normative values for the near point of convergence of elementary schoolchildren. *Optom Vis Sci* 1998;75:506–512.
36. Parks MM. *Ocular motility and strabismus*. New York: Harper & Row, 1975:73–84.
37. Wick B. Suppression. In: Eskridge JB, Amos JF, Bartlett JD, eds. *Clinical procedures in optometry*. Philadelphia: JB Lippincott, 1991:698–707.
38. Cooper J, Warshowsky J. Lateral displacement as a response cue in the Titmus Stereo test. *Am J Optom Physiol Opt* 1977;54:537–541.
39. Cooper J, Feldman J. Random dot stereogram performance by strabismic, amblyopic, and ocular pathology patients in an operant discrimination task. *Am J Optom Physiol Opt* 1978;55:599–609.
40. Scheiman M, Herzberg H, Frantz K, et al. Normative study of accommodative facility in elementary schoolchildren. *Am J Optom Physiol Opt* 1988;65:127–134.
41. Pierce JR, Greenspan SB. Accommodative rock procedures in VT—a clinical guide. *Optom Weekly* 1971;62(33):753–757; 62(34):776–780.
42. Lui JS, Lee M, Jang J, et al. Objective assessment of accommodative orthoptics: dynamic insufficiency. *J Am Acad Optom Physiol Opt* 1979;56:285–294.
43. Zellers JA, Alpert TL, Rouse MW. A review of the literature and a normative study of accommodative facility. *J Am Optom Assoc* 1984;55:31–37.
44. Hennessey D, Iouse RA, Rouse MW. Relation of symptoms to accommodative facility of school aged children. *Am J Optom Physiol Opt* 1984;61:177–183.
45. Levine S, Ciuffreda KJ, Selenow A, et al. Clinical assessment of accommodative facility in symptomatic and asymptomatic individuals. *Am Optom Assoc* 1985;56:286–290.
46. Haynes HM. Clinical observations with dynamic retinoscopy. *Optom Weekly* 1960;51:2243–2246, 2306–2309.
47. Bieber JC. Why near point retinoscopy with children? *Optom Weekly* 1974;65:54–57.
48. Rouse MW, London R, Allen DC. An evaluation of the monocular estimation method of dynamic retinoscopy. *Am J Optom Physiol Opt* 1982;59:234–239.
49. Rouse MW, Hutter RF, Shiftlett R. A normative study of the accommodative lag in elementary schoolchildren. *Am J Optom Physiol Opt* 1984;61:693–697.
50. Wick B, Hall P. Relation among accommodative facility, lag, and amplitude in elementary schoolchildren. *Am J Optom Physiol Opt* 1987;64:593–598.
51. Woehrle MB, Peters RJ, Frantz KA. Accommodative amplitude determination: can we substitute the pull away for the push-up method? *J Optom Vis Dev* 1997;28:246–249.
52. Hamasaki D, Onj J, Marg E. The amplitude of accommodation in presbyopia. *Am J Optom Arch Am Acad Optom* 1956;33:3–14.

53. Siderov J, DiGuglielmo L. Binocular accommodative facility in prepresbyopic adults and its relation to symptoms. *Optom Vis Sci* 1991;68:49–53.
54. Yothers TL, Wick B, Morse SE. Clinical testing of accommodative facility: development of an amplitude-scaled test. *J Am Optom Assoc* 2002.
55. Higgins JD. Oculomotor system. In: Barresi BJ, ed. *Ocular assessment.* Boston: Butterworth-Heineman, 1984:208.
56. Grisham D, Simons H. Perspectives on reading disabilities. In: Rosenbloom AA, Morgan MW, eds. *Pediatric optometry.* Philadelphia: JB Lippincott, 1990:518–559.
57. Maples WC, Ficklin TW. Interrater and test-retest reliability of pursuits and saccades. *J Am Optom Assoc* 1988;59:549–552.
58. Maples WC. *NSUCO oculomotor test.* Santa Ana, CA: Optometric Extension Program, 1995.
59. Richman JE, Walker AJ, Garzia RP. The impact of automatic digit naming ability on a clinical test of eye movement functioning. *J Am Optom Assoc* 1983;54:617–622.
60. Garzia RP, Richman JE, Nicholson SB, et al. A new visual-verbal saccade test: the developmental eye movement test (DEM). *J Am Optom Assoc* 1990;61:124–135.
61. Oride M, Marutani JK, Rouse MW, et al. Reliability study of the Pierce and King-Devick tests. *J Am Optom Assoc* 1986;63:419–424.
62. Rouse MW, Nestor EM, Parot CJ. A re-evaluation of the reliability of the developmental eye movement test. *Optom Vis Sci* 1991;61[Suppl]:90.
63. Colby D, Laukhanen HR, Yolton RL. Use of the Taylor Visagraph II system to evaluate eye movements made during reading. *J Am Optom Assoc* 1998;69:22–32.
64. Press LJ. *Computers and vision therapy programs.* Optometric Extension Program, Curriculum II, Series I, 1988;60:1–12.
65. Groffman S. Visual tracing. *J Am Optom Assoc* 1966;37:139–141.

2

Case Analysis and Classification

Several analytical approaches are presented in the optometric literature. All have their own unique characteristics, advantages, and disadvantages. Each of these systems also has short-comings that are significant enough to have prevented wide acceptance of any one approach by the profession. Rather, it is common for optometrists, during their early years of practice, to develop their own personal approach to case analysis that is often a combination of the various systems they had been taught during their education.

The four approaches that are most widely discussed in our literature are graphical analysis, the Optometric Extension Program (OEP) analytical analysis approach, Morgan's system of normative analysis, and fixation disparity analysis. In this chapter, we will briefly describe these four case analysis approaches. This discussion will lead directly into a detailed presentation of the case analysis approach that will be used throughout this text.

REVIEW OF CURRENTLY AVAILABLE ANALYTICAL APPROACHES

Graphical Analysis

Description

Graphical analysis is a method of plotting clinical accommodation and binocular findings to determine if a patient can be expected to have clear, single, and comfortable binocular vision (1). The test findings that are commonly plotted include the dissociated phoria, base-in to blur, break, and recovery; base-out to blur, break, and recovery; Negative Relative Accommodation (NRA), Positive Relative Accommodation (PRA), amplitude of accommodation, and near point of convergence (Fig. 2.1).

Advantages

The primary advantage of the graphical analysis system is that it allows one to visualize the relationship among several optometric findings and is, therefore, an excellent system to introduce the concepts of case analysis. The width of the zone of clear single binocular vision, the relationship between the phoria and fusional vergence, the AC/A ratio, and the relationship of the NRA and PRA findings to fusional vergence and/or accommodation are all clearly portrayed on the graph. For the student learning about accommodation and binocular vision for the first time, the ability to view a visual representation can be a very powerful learning tool. Over the years, graphical analysis has become a standard teaching approach in many optometric curricula.

Graphical analysis also facilitates identification of erroneous findings. When data are plotted on the graph, a characteristic pattern becomes evident. If an individual finding deviates from this typical pattern, it may indicate that it is erroneous and unreliable.

Although the primary purpose of graphical analysis is simply the visual representation of accommodative and binocular data (2), various guidelines for analyzing these findings have developed over the years. The most popular of these guidelines has been Sheard's criterion. Sheard (3,4) postulated that for an individual to be comfortable, the fusional reserve should be

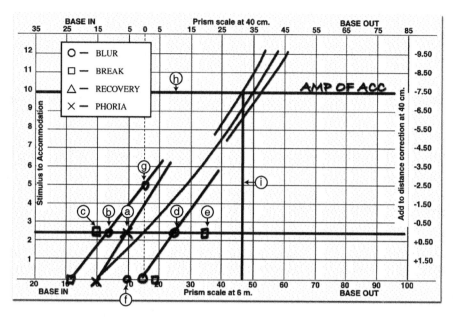

FIG. 2.1. Sample graphical analysis worksheet showing the test findings that are commonly plotted: **(A)** the dissociated phoria; **(B)** base-in to blur; **(C)** base-in to break; **(D)** base-out to blur; **(E)** base-out to break; **(F)** NRA; **(G)** PRA; **(H)** amplitude of accommodation; **(I)** near point of convergence.

twice the demand (phoria). For example, in the case of a 10 Δ exophoria, the positive fusional convergence should be 20 Δ to meet Sheard's criterion. This postulate also can be used to determine the amount of prism necessary to make the patient comfortable or to determine whether lenses or vision therapy will be appropriate.

Disadvantages

The system does have shortcomings, however, which, for the most part, have relegated graphical analysis to the classroom.

- The graphical system fails to identify some binocular vision, accommodation, and oculomotor problems. When using the graphical analysis approach, important data such as accommodative facility, fusion facility, fixation disparity, and Monocular Estimation Method (MEM) retinoscopy findings are not included in the analysis. This is significant because, of the 15 most common accommodative, ocular motor, and binocular vision anomalies discussed in later chapters, five (accommodative excess, accommodative infacility, ill-sustained accommodation, fusional vergence dysfunction, and ocular motor dysfunction) could not be identified using graphical analysis. For example, an individual with a condition called accommodative infacility may have a normal amplitude of accommodation, NRA, and PRA. When the data are plotted according to established graphical analysis guidelines and analyzed according to Sheard's criterion, the result is a normal graph and failure to identify a problem. Accommodative infacility can only be diagnosed when facility testing is performed and analyzed. This type of information, however, is not part of the routine in the graphical system. A condition such as accommodative infacility would, therefore, not be diagnosed using a traditional graphical analysis approach.

- Graphical analysis relies heavily upon criteria—such as those by Sheard (3,4) and by Percival (5)—to determine if a problem exists. These criteria, however, can only be considered guidelines. Although Sheard's criterion has been readily accepted by optometry since its introduction, there has been little research evidence, until recently, to support its validity. A study by Dalziel (6) found that a vision therapy program that was effective in improving fusional vergence to meet Sheard's criterion was effective in relieving symptoms. Sheedy and Saladin (7,8) studied the relationship between asthenopia and various clinical analysis measures of oculomotor balance. The objective was to determine which measures would best discriminate symptomatic from asymptomatic patients. Sheard's criterion was found to be the best for the entire population and exophoria, but the slope of the fixation disparity curve was found to be best for esophores. Worrell et al. (9) evaluated patient acceptance of prism prescribed by Sheard's criterion. They prescribed two pair of glasses for each subject. The glasses were identical in every way accept that one contained a prism based on Sheard's criterion. The results of this study showed that patients with esophoria preferred the glasses with the prism, while those with exophoria preferred the glasses without the prism.

Although these studies are somewhat supportive of Sheard's criterion, there are certainly suggestions that, in some cases, it fails to identify patients who are symptomatic and may not always be the most effective method for determining appropriate management.

- Another shortcoming of graphical analysis is that it may be too precise a method for clinical purposes and is cumbersome to use. Although most optometry students begin their study of case analysis with a presentation of graphical analysis, few continue to graph data throughout their careers. The actual mechanics of plotting the data are cumbersome and time consuming. An experienced clinician rarely needs to actually plot optometric data to reach a decision about diagnosis and management.

Analytical Analysis

Description

The second case analysis approach is referred to as the Analytical Analysis System. Developed by the OEP, this approach has several rigid requirements and steps (10).

- Administration of a 21-point (tests) examination using precise instructional sets
- Checking (comparison of data to a table of expecteds)
- Chaining (grouping the data)
- Case typing (identifying the condition)

In the analytical analysis approach, the specific 21 tests (points) as described by OEP must be used and the instructional sets must be precisely followed. Any deviation from the suggested routine invalidates the results and the analytical system.

Results of the examination must then be compared to a table of expecteds developed by OEP (Table 2.1). This is followed by a procedure referred to as "chaining" or grouping of the data. Chaining simply means that those findings found to be high are entered above a horizontal line, while data that are low are placed below the horizontal line. The data are also grouped together according to specific rules. An example of chaining is illustrated below:

7(5) 14-16A-19
(9-11-16B) 15A 17A-20

TABLE 2.1. *Optometric Extension Program expecteds*

Test	Expected finding
Distance lateral phoria	ortho −0.5 exophoria
Near lateral phoria	6.0 exophoria
Base-out (distance)	blur: 7
	break: 19
	recovery: 10
Base-in (distance)	break: 9
	recovery: 5
Base-out (near)	blur: 15
	break: 21
	recovery: 15
Base-in (near)	blur: 14
	break: 22
	recovery: 18
Negative relative accommodation	+2.00
Positive relative accommodation	−2.25
Fused X-cylinder	+0.50

The results of this "chaining" or grouping of all the high and low data are then analyzed. This process is referred to as case typing. Two basic types or classifications exist in the OEP System, the "B-type" (accommodative problem) and the "C-type" (convergence problem). The "B-type" case is further divided into seven stages or subtypes.

Advantages

Analytical analysis incorporates several unique concepts into its system that are derived from the underlying philosophy of vision of the OEP. Two examples are described below:

• Concept 1: The status of the visual system can deteriorate over time.

OEP stresses the concept that vision problems develop over time and that the deterioration occurs as an adaptation to a stressful condition (e.g., excessive reading or near work) (11). Analytical analysis allows one to evaluate the current stage or deterioration of the vision problem and the therapy prescribed depends upon this determination. If this treatment using lenses or vision therapy is not instituted, continued reading can be expected to result in adaptations that take the form of fusional vergence and accommodative problems, refractive error, and strabismus. This concept is dramatically different from traditional thinking, which suggests that vision disorders occur as random variations or as a failure in development (12).

• Concept 2: Vision problems can be prevented.

OEP philosophy postulates that vision problems develop as an adaptation to near point demands (11). Since analysis of the data can indicate the current stage of development of a vision problem, subtle changes can be detected early. With appropriate intervention using lenses, prism, and vision therapy, many vision problems can be prevented, according to OEP philosophy.

Disadvantages

The analytical approach is mainly used by members of the OEP and has not gained widespread use for several reasons.

- A major problem with this system is that the student or practitioner must be familiar with specific OEP testing protocols. Unless these protocols are precisely followed, the system becomes unusable. Since most schools of optometry do not teach this system of testing, students are generally unfamiliar with the instructional sets.
- An understanding and acceptance of OEP philosophy is a basic requirement.

The OEP is primarily a postgraduate education organization. Students at the various schools and colleges of optometry generally receive only introductory information about the OEP. It is not difficult to understand, therefore, why so few students feel comfortable with this approach.

- The OEP literature is written using a basic language that is often very different from the "classical optometric language" taught in optometry schools. Basic definitions of terms such as accommodation, convergence, blur, break, recovery, and phoria are all significantly different. For example, Manas (13) defines exophoria as:
  A developmental relationship within the visual behavior pattern, between areas of that pattern, operationally active to preserve the integrity of performance of the convergence pattern.

If an optometrist wants to use analytical analysis, it requires a period of time learning this new language. For a student or practitioner who has just spent several years learning one optometric language, the additional effort required is an obstacle that must be overcome before involvement with the OEP analysis system is possible.

Morgan's System of Clinical Analysis (Normative Analysis)

Description

Morgan's system is based on his study, in 1944, in which he presented the concept that it is important to analyze the results of groups of data (14). In Morgan's approach, little significance is attributed to variation from the norm on any one given test. Morgan found that he was able to divide all data into groups based on the direction in which the tests tend to vary. To analyze optometric data using Morgan's analytical approach, one must first compare findings to Morgan's Table of Expecteds (Table 2.2) and then look for a trend in the group A and group B findings (Table 2.3). The important concept in this system is that no single finding is considered significant by itself. However, when a group as a whole varies in a given direction, it is considered clinically significant. If the group A findings are high while the group B data are low, a convergence problem is present. If the group B data are high while the group A findings are low, an accommodative fatigue problem is indicated (15). The data in group C are used to suggest whether lenses, prism, or vision therapy should be recommended as treatment.

Morgan's approach, therefore, is an attempt to present an analytical system that is easily applied and that does not go beyond the exactness and significance of the data involved (15).

Advantages

- The primary advantage of this approach is the concept that it is important to look at groups of findings rather than individual data. Morgan (15) stresses that if one finding falls outside the "normal range" it does not necessarily indicate that the patient has

TABLE 2.2. *Morgan's table of expecteds*

Test	Expected finding	Standard deviation
Distance lateral phoria	1 exophoria	± 2Δ
Near lateral phoria	3 exophoria	± 3Δ
AC/A ratio	4:1	± 2Δ
Base-out (distance)	blur: 9	± 4Δ
	break: 19	± 8Δ
	recovery: 10	± 4Δ
Base-in (distance)	break: 7	± 3Δ
	recovery: 4	± 2Δ
Base-out (near)	blur: 17	± 5Δ
	break: 21	± 6Δ
	recovery: 11	± 7Δ
Base-in (near)	blur: 13	± 4Δ
	break: 21	± 4Δ
	recovery: 13	± 5Δ
Amplitude of accommodation		
Push-up	18–1/3 age	± 2.00 D
Fused X-cylinder	+ 0.50	± 0.50 D
Negative relative accommodation	+ 2.00	± 0.50 D
Positive relative accommodation	− 2.37	± 1.00 D

a problem. He states that "statistical data applies to populations and not necessarily to individuals."

- Another advantage of this system is its flexibility and ease of use, compared to the complexity and rigidity that is associated with graphical and analytical analysis.

Disadvantages

- The primary limitation of Morgan's approach is that the groups developed by Morgan in the 1940s have not been updated to include some of the more recent optometric tests that have been shown to be important clinical findings. As a result, it fails to identify some binocular vision, accommodation, and oculomotor problems. When using Morgan's analysis, approach important data, such as accommodative facility, fusion facility, fixation disparity, MEM retinoscopy, and ocular motility findings, are not included in the analysis.

TABLE 2.3. *Morgan's three groups*

Group A data
Negative fusional vergence at distance—break
Negative fusional vergence at near—blur
Negative fusional vergence at near-break
Positive relative accommodation
Amplitude
Group B data
Positive fusional vergence at distance—blur and break
Positive fusional vergence at distance—blur and break
Binocular cross-cylinder
Monocular cross-cylinder
Near retinoscopy
Negative relative accommodation
Group C data
Phoria
AC/A ratio

Fixation Disparity Analysis

Description

Fixation disparity is a small misalignment of the eyes under binocular conditions (16). This misalignment from exact bifoveal fixation is very small, with a magnitude of only a few minutes of arc. Several clinical methods have been developed to evaluate fixation disparity including the Mallett unit, American Optical vectographic slide, the Bernell lantern slide, the Wesson card, and the Disparometer (17). The associated phoria, or the amount of prism necessary to neutralize the fixation disparity, is determined using the Mallett unit, American Optical vectographic slide, and the Bernell lantern slide. The Wesson card and the Disparometer permit a more complete analysis of the fixation disparity. Using these instruments a fixation disparity curve can be generated and four diagnostic characteristics of the curve can be analyzed. These four characteristics include the type, slope, x-intercept, and y-intercept. Chapter 14 presents an in-depth discussion of fixation disparity.

The use of fixation disparity data has been suggested as a useful method for the analysis and diagnosis of problems of the oculomotor system (16–19). The primary advantage of fixation disparity analysis is that the assessment takes place under binocular and, therefore, more natural conditions. Studies have indicated that analyzing binocular vision using fixation disparity is useful in determining those patients that are likely to have symptoms (18). Some authors (16–19) have suggested that fixation disparity data may be the most effective method for determining the amount of prism to prescribe for binocular vision disorders.

Advantages

- The primary advantage of fixation disparity analysis is that the data is gathered under binocular vision conditions. Other analytical systems depend on phoria vergence testing performed under dissociated conditions that may not truly reflect the way the system operates under binocular conditions. For example, in about one third of patients, a condition referred to as paradoxical fixation disparity is present (19). This is a condition in which the fixation disparity is in the opposite direction to the phoria.
- Studies have shown that fixation disparity provides the most effective method of determining the amount of prism necessary for the treatment of certain binocular vision disorders (7,8).

Disadvantages

Fixation disparity testing is a technique for evaluating binocular vision and does not provide direct information about accommodation or ocular motor disorders.

All of the systems described above have failed to gain widespread acceptance by the profession because of the limitations described. The rest of this chapter is devoted to the presentation of the case analysis system that will be utilized throughout this text. This approach draws from the major contributions of the four systems described above, while it attempts to eliminate most of their disadvantages. Its use allows the optometrist to operate with much more flexibility than available with strict adherence to any of the other approaches.

Integrative Analysis Approach

The integrative analysis approach is an analysis system that attempts to make use of the most positive aspects of other case analysis approaches while avoiding the problems associated with these other systems.

It requires three distinct steps:

Comparing the individual tests to a table of expecteds
Grouping the findings that deviate from expecteds
Identifying the syndrome based on steps 1 and 2

This format uses the concepts of the OEP analytical analysis system: checking, chaining, and typing. However, the primary disadvantages of analytical analysis—that is, the rigidity of the 21-point examination and the OEP language problems, are avoided. The integrative analysis approach also makes use of the following important characteristics of other systems:

1. Some of the unique concepts of the OEP system are utilized, including the following:
   - The status of the visual system can deteriorate over time.
   - Vision problems can be prevented.
2. Morgan's suggestion that it is important to look at groups of findings rather than individual data is a key element in the integrative analysis approach.
3. The inclusion of fixation disparity data performed under binocular conditions.
4. The integrative analysis approach includes an analysis of ocular motor, accommodative facility, vergence facility, MEM retinoscopy, and fixation disparity data. No other analysis system makes use of all of this data.

Specifics

To utilize this case analysis system, the optometrist must be knowledgeable about:

- Expected findings for each optometric test administered
- The relationship of one finding to another or how to group the data that is gathered
- A classification system that categorizes the most commonly encountered vision problems or syndromes

Expected Findings for Optometric Tests

Tables 1.2, 1.4, 1.5, 1.9, and 1.11 list various commonly administered optometric tests and expected findings. These tables are a compilation of data from Morgan's Table of Expecteds, along with newer data for accommodative facility, ocular motor, vergence facility, step vergence, MEM retinoscopy, and fixation disparity testing.

Grouping Optometric Data

The concept of the importance of looking for trends comes from both the OEP analytical analysis and Morgan's system. The integrative analysis approach is simply an expansion of this concept and divides optometric data into six groups, rather than the three proposed by Morgan (Table 2.3). Tests or data are placed in a group if they directly or indirectly evaluate the same function.

Tests Evaluating Positive Fusional Vergence Group

- Positive fusional vergence (PFV)—smooth vergence testing
- PFV—step vergence testing
- PFV—vergence facility testing
- Near point of convergence
- NRA

- Binocular accommodative facility with plus lenses
- MEM retinoscopy and fused cross-cylinder

Tests Evaluating Negative Fusional Vergence Group

- Negative fusional vergence (NFV)—smooth vergence testing
- NFV—step vergence testing
- NFV—vergence facility testing
- PRA
- Binocular accommodative facility with minus lenses
- MEM retinoscopy and fused cross-cylinder

Tests Evaluating the Accommodative System Group

- Monocular accommodative amplitude
- Monocular accommodative facility
- MEM retinoscopy
- Fused cross-cylinder
- NRA/PRA
- Binocular accommodative facility testing
- Binocular accommodative amplitude

Tests Evaluating the Ocular Motor System

- Subjective assessment of saccades using grading scales
- Developmental Eye Movement (DEM) test
- Visagraph
- Subjective assessment of pursuits using grading scales

Tests Evaluating Vertical Fusional Vergence Group

- Supravergence/infravergence
- Fixation disparity

Motor Alignment and Interaction Tests Group (MAIT)

- Cover test at distance
- Cover test at near
- Phoria at distance
- Phoria at near
- Fixation disparity
- AC/A ratio
- CA/C ratio

KNOWLEDGE OF CLASSIFICATION SYSTEM OF COMMON ACCOMMODATIVE AND NONSTRABISMIC BINOCULAR VISION PROBLEMS

Once the test findings are grouped and a trend is identified, the specific syndrome can be selected from the list of the 15 common accommodative, ocular motility, and binocular vision problems listed below. This classification is a modification of the well-known Duane-White classification (20) suggested by Wick (18). The rationale for this classification is described in detail later in this chapter.

Binocular Anomalies

Heterophoria with Low AC/A Ratio

- Orthophoria at distance and exophoria at near-convergence insufficiency
- Exophoria at distance, greater exophoria at near-convergence insufficiency
- Esophoria at distance, orthophoria at near-divergence insufficiency

Heterophoria with Normal AC/A Ratio

- Orthophoria at distance, orthophoria at near-fusional vergence dysfunction
- Esophoria at distance, same degree of esophoria at near-basic esophoria
- Exophoria at distance, same degree of exophoria at near-basic exophoria

Heterophoria with High AC/A Ratio

- Orthophoria at distance and esophoria at near-convergence excess
- Esophoria at distance, greater esophoria at near-convergence excess
- Exophoria at distance, less exophoria at near-divergence excess

Vertical Heterophoria

- Right or left hyperphoria

Accommodative Anomalies

- Accommodative insufficiency
- Ill-sustained accommodation
- Accommodative excess
- Accommodative infacility

Ocular Motor Problems

- Ocular motor dysfunction

ANALYSIS OF SPECIFIC GROUPS

Positive Fusional Vergence Group Data

Optometric data that can be used to determine the status of a patient's PFV are included in this category. These include all data that directly or indirectly assess PFV at both distance and near.

Positive Fusional Vergence—Smooth Vergence Testing

As base-out prism is added, the patient is instructed to keep the target single and clear as long as possible and to report when the target blurs or becomes double. This requires the patient to converge to maintain bifoveal fixation and maintain accommodation at a given level (either distance or near). It is also important to realize that as prism is added and the patient converges, the accommodative response gradually increases due to increased vergence accommodation. The amount of vergence accommodation stimulated depends on the CA/C ratio. The patient must relax accommodation to counterbalance this increased vergence accommodation. When the patient can no longer do this, a blur occurs (the CA/C ratio is discussed in depth in Chapter 15). As more base-out prism is added beyond the blur limit, diplopia occurs when fusion is no longer possible.

An important aspect of this test is that the prism is added in a slow gradual manner. Since the technique requires the patient to maintain accommodation at a given level, accommodative convergence cannot be used to assist convergence. The patient must, therefore, use PFV. If the patient attempts to use accommodative convergence, he or she will report a blur.

Positive Fusional Vergence—Step Vergence Testing

This test is similar to smooth vergence testing described above, except it is performed outside the phoropter with a prism bar. Because a prism bar is used instead of Risley prisms, the actual prismatic demand is presented in a steplike manner. This is in contrast to the smooth demand introduced using Risley prism. A recent study suggested that the expected findings for this test are different from smooth fusional vergence testing for children (21,22).

Positive Fusional Vergence—Vergence Facility Testing

The patient is instructed to keep a vertical line of 20/30 letters single and clear as base-out prism is suddenly introduced (12 base-out and 3 base-in). In order to accomplish this, the patient must maintain his accommodative level at 2.50 D, using 12 Δ of positive fusional vergence to restore bifoveal fixation. Because of the lag of accommodation, the actual accommodative response will generally be less than 2.50 D. The usual accommodative response for a 2.50 D accommodative stimulus is about 1.75 to 2.00 D. If sufficient fusional vergence is available, the response will be a single clear image. A report of diplopia indicates that the patient cannot restore binocularity using PFV. Another possible response is a single but blurred target, suggesting the use of accommodative convergence to compensate for the inability to use the fusional vergence mechanism to restore bifoveal fixation.

The important differentiation between vergence facility testing and standard testing of PFV is that prism is introduced in large increments and over a longer period of time. A patient is forced to make rapid changes in fusional vergence and be able to sustain these changes over time. A patient having adequate smooth fusional vergence ranges may experience difficulty on the vergence facility test.

Negative Relative Accommodation

This test evaluates PFV in an indirect manner. The NRA is comparable to the assessment of smooth fusional vergence ranges, since lenses are introduced in a slow gradual manner. However, with the NRA, the patient is being asked to maintain convergence at a particular level, while changing the accommodative response. As plus lenses are added in +0.25 D increments, the patient is instructed to keep the target *single* and *clear*. To accomplish this, he or she must relax accommodation. However, any relaxation of accommodation is accompanied by a decrease in accommodative convergence. The amount of accommodative convergence change depends on the AC/A ratio.

If the patient allows his or her eyes to diverge as accommodation is relaxed, he or she will report diplopia. To counteract this decrease in accommodative convergence, the patient must use an appropriate amount of PFV. Thus, the result obtained during the NRA test can depend upon the status of the PFV system. Of course, the endpoint in the NRA also can be limited by the patient's ability to relax accommodation as plus lenses are introduced.

To determine which factor—accommodation or PFV—is causing the blur, the patient's accommodative status can be tested monocularly. If he or she can clear +2.50 monocularly, but only +1.50 binocularly, PFV is the causative factor. Another way to differentiate is simply to cover one eye after the patient reports blur on the NRA test. If the target clears under monocular conditions, the fusional vergence system is at fault.

Binocular Accommodative Facility with Plus Lenses

This test is similar to the NRA, since it requires maintenance of convergence at a specific level while the accommodative response changes. As +2.00 lenses are introduced binocularly, the patient is instructed to maintain single and clear binocular vision.

To accomplish this, he must relax about 2.00 D of accommodation to keep the target clear (the actual accommodative response will be about 10% less than the stimulus). The relaxation of 2 D of accommodation, however, causes a reflex decrease in accommodative convergence. The amount of divergence will be directly related to the AC/A ratio. Assuming a 5:1 AC/A ratio, if the patient relaxes 2 D of accommodation, his or her eyes will tend to diverge by 10 Δ. If this occurs, the patient will see two images.

Since the instructions require the patient to maintain single clear vision, he or she must use 10 Δ of PFV to compensate for the decrease in accommodative convergence. The endpoint of this test can be caused by one of two factors. Either the patient has inadequate PFV or is unable to relax his or her accommodative system. To differentiate, one simply needs to cover one eye. If the print clears under monocular conditions, the limiting factor is the fusional vergence system.

Near Point of Convergence

The patient is asked to maintain single vision as a target is moved toward his or her nose. To accomplish this, the patient can use a combination of various types of convergence, including: accommodative convergence, PFV, and proximal convergence. If PFV is deficient, it may affect the patient's ability to achieve the expected finding on this test. A receded near point of convergence is, therefore, an indirect measure of PFV.

Monocular Estimation Method Retinoscopy and Fused Cross-cylinder

Both tests are performed under binocular conditions and are designed to assess the accommodative response. The normal finding is approximately +0.25 to +0.50 for MEM retinoscopy and +0.50 to +0.75 for the fused cross-cylinder. However, when a patient presents with exophoria and low PFV group findings, the MEM and fused cross-cylinder tests often yield less plus than expected.

Decreased plus on these tests is interpreted as overaccommodation for the particular stimulus. This is a common response in a patient with exophoria and reduced PFV. The individual is substituting accommodative convergence for the lack of PFV. By overaccommodating, the patient has additional accommodative convergence available to help overcome the exophoria.

Summary

These seven tests comprise the PFV group and—in the presence of exophoria and symptoms—the data in the PFV group will generally be lower than expected and MEM and the fused cross-cylinder tend to show overaccommodation (less plus than expected). All of the findings in this group provide information about the patient's PFV system and the ability to compensate for exophoria. Occasionally only the *facility* findings will be low, while the amplitude findings are normal. This would be the type of situation missed with the graphical analysis approach.

Negative Fusional Vergence Group Data

This group includes optometric data that reflect the status of a patient's NFV. It includes tests that directly or indirectly assess NFV at both distance and near.

Negative Fusional Vergence—Smooth Vergence Testing

As base-in prism is gradually added, the patient is instructed to keep the target single and clear as long as possible and to report if the target blurs or becomes double.

The test requires the patient to diverge to maintain bifoveal fixation and maintain accommodation at a given level. It is also important to realize that as prism is added and the patient diverges, the accommodative response gradually decreases, due to decreased vergence accommodation. The amount of decrease in vergence accommodation depends on the CA/C ratio. The patient must stimulate accommodation to counterbalance this decreased vergence accommodation. When the patient can no longer do this, a blur occurs. By requiring clarity, we are forcing the patient to use NFV to compensate for the base-in prism.

An important aspect of this test is that the prism is added in a slow gradual manner.

Negative Fusional Vergence—Step Vergence Testing

Although the introduction of the prism demand is different from smooth vergence testing, the instructional set and the explanation of the requirements of the test are similar to that described for smooth vergence testing.

Negative Fusional Vergence—Vergence Facility Testing

The patient is instructed to keep a vertical line of 20/30 letters *single* and *clear* as 12 Δ base-out and 3 Δ base-in prism is abruptly introduced. In order to accomplish this, the patient must maintain his or her accommodative level at 2.50, while using 3 Δ of NFV to restore bifoveal fixation. If sufficient fusional vergence is available, the response will be a single clear image. A report of diplopia would indicate that the patient could not restore binocularity using NFV. A report of a single blurred target indicates the use of a decrease in accommodative convergence to aid the fusional vergence mechanism.

Since this procedure is repeated several times and prism is introduced in large increments, it is an excellent method to evaluate a patient's stamina or ability to make a large number of rapid repetitive fusional vergence changes.

Positive Relative Accommodation

This test evaluates NFV in an indirect manner. Lenses are introduced slowly in 0.25 increments, making this procedure comparable to smooth vergence testing. However, with the PRA, the patient must maintain convergence at a particular level, while changing the accommodative response. As minus lenses are added, the patient must maintain single and clear vision. To accomplish this, he or she must stimulate accommodation. This stimulation of accommodation is accompanied by an increase in accommodative convergence. The amount of additional accommodative convergence involved depends upon the AC/A ratio.

The patient is faced with a dilemma. He or she must accommodate to maintain clarity, but the accommodation automatically causes additional convergence. This additional convergence, however, will result in diplopia because the target remains at 40 cm. To prevent diplopia, the patient must resort to use of NFV to offset the accommodative convergence. The amount of NFV required is related, again, to the AC/A ratio.

The PRA procedure, therefore, is not only an indication of the patient's ability to stimulate accommodation. It also reflects the status of NFV. The endpoint of the procedure is either an inability to stimulate additional accommodation or reduced NFV.

When the endpoint is reached, a differentiation of the causative factor can be made by occluding one eye. If the print now clears, it indicates that the causative factor was reduced NFV.

Binocular Accommodative Facility with Minus Lenses

This procedure is similar to the PRA, since it requires maintenance of convergence at a specific level while the accommodative response changes. As −2.00 lenses are introduced binocularly, the patient is instructed to maintain *single* and *clear* vision. He or she must, therefore, stimulate 2 D of accommodation to restore clarity. This 2 D stimulation, however, causes a reflex increase in accommodative convergence. The amount of additional convergence is directly related to the AC/A ratio. Given a 5:1 AC/A ratio, if the patient stimulates 2 D of accommodation, his or her eyes will converge 10 Δ. If the patient permits this to occur, he or she will see two targets. Since the instructions require that the target be both single and clear, the patient must use 10 Δ of fusional divergence to compensate for the increase in accommodative convergence.

The endpoint of this test can be caused by one of two factors. Either the patient has inadequate NFV or is unable to stimulate 2 D of accommodation. To differentiate, simply cover one eye. If the print remains blurred, the difficulty is the ACC. If it clears, the limiting factor was NFV.

Monocular Estimation Method Retinoscopy and Fused Cross-cylinder

Both MEM retinoscopy and the fused cross-cylinder tend to show more plus than normally expected when NFV is low. This type of response indicates an attempt by the patient to use as little accommodation as possible in order to maintain binocular vision. By decreasing the accommodative response, the demand on NFV is reduced.

Summary

Given a patient presenting with near asthenopic symptoms and esophoria, the NFV group findings tend to be lower than expected, while the fused cross-cylinder and MEM show underaccommodation (more plus than expected). Occasionally, only the facility findings will be low, while the measures of amplitude are normal.

All of the findings in this group provide information about the status of the NFV system and the patient's ability to compensate for esophoria.

Accommodative System Group Data

Two factors must be kept in mind when evaluating the accommodative system. First, we can best assess accommodation under monocular conditions. This eliminates any contamination of test results due to the influence of binocular vision disorders. Some of the testing procedures that were included in the PFV and NFV groups are administered under binocular conditions. Several of these procedures also can yield information about the accommodative system. It is important, however, to realize that they are only indicative of the status of accommodation if the binocular system is unaffected. Tests in this category include: NRA, PRA, binocular accommodative facility, MEM retinoscopy, and the fused cross-cylinder test.

For instance, a low PRA finding can be indicative of an accommodative insufficiency or a problem with esophoria and low NFV. Accommodative insufficiency would only be indicated, however, if other testing revealed adequate NFV. As discussed previously, the endpoint for the PRA can either be an inability to stimulate accommodation or insufficient NFV.

The second important factor is that both the inhibition and stimulation of accommodation should be evaluated and the results interpreted individually.

Monocular Accommodative Amplitude

This procedure is comparable to measures of fusional vergence using the smooth vergence testing technique. It tells us the total amount of accommodation available. Standard procedure calls for one measurement of the accommodative amplitude for each eye. Under these conditions we have little indication of how efficiently the patient is able to use the accommodative amplitude or if he or she can sustain over a reasonable period of time.

To increase the diagnostic significance of this procedure, one needs to repeat the measurement 3 to 4 times or repeat the test at the end of the examination. Both of these variations in procedure will yield information about sustaining ability.

A finding of a lower than expected amplitude of accommodation in a pre-presbyope is indicative of accommodative insufficiency. In such a case, all testing that requires the patient to stimulate accommodation would tend to be lower than expected. This includes the monocular accommodative facility test with minus lenses, binocular accommodative facility with minus lenses, and the PRA.

An adequate amplitude of accommodation does not eliminate the possibility of an accommodative anomaly. A facility problem, sustaining problem, or an inability to relax accommodation could coexist with a normal accommodative amplitude. As a result, additional testing is necessary.

Monocular Accommodative Facility with Plus and Minus Lenses

This procedure requires the patient to make rapid large changes in the accommodative response. The stimulus to accommodation is changed from +2.00 D to −2.00 D with each fixation.

When a patient who presents with near point symptoms is tested, the procedure should be continued for 1 minute. The number of cycles performed in 1 minute can then be compared to the table of expecteds. This permits evaluation of the individual's ability to make rapid and large changes in accommodative level and to sustain over a long period of time.

There are four possible results:

- Adequate performance with both plus and minus lenses.
- Inadequate performance with both plus and minus lenses. This response is indicative of accommodative infacility. Other evidence would be lower than expected findings on the binocular accommodative facility test with both plus and minus lenses and a low PRA and NRA.
- Adequate performance with minus, inadequate with plus. Such a response is indicative of overaccommodation, accommodative spasm, or accommodative excess. The problem can be an isolated accommodative anomaly. However, often a binocular vision anomaly is the underlying cause.

  For example, a patient with a high exophoria, a receded near point of convergence, and reduced PFV will tend to overaccommodate and use accommodative convergence to assist his deficient PFV system. This allows the individual to compensate for the high exophoria. Constant overaccommodation may lead to an accommodative spasm and secondary myopia.
- Adequate performance with plus lenses, inadequate with minus. This patient has difficulty stimulating accommodation and will often have a reduced amplitude of accommodation. This is the response of an individual presenting with an accommodative insufficiency or ill-sustained accommodation problem. Other findings that confirm this diagnosis include a low PRA, high MEM, and fused cross-cylinder findings.

Monocular Estimation Method Retinoscopy

This procedure serves as an objective assessment of a patient's accommodative response. Other optometric procedures used to assess accommodation and binocularity fail to monitor the actual accommodative response.

We typically present a target at 40 cm that represents a 2.50 D accommodative stimulus. Expected findings for MEM retinoscopy are +0.25 to +0.50 D when viewing such a stimulus. The information obtained can be used to confirm the presence of an accommodative and/or a binocular anomaly. A finding of more plus than expected tends to substantiate a diagnosis of accommodative insufficiency. Other relevant findings would include: a low PRA, a high fused cross-cylinder, and difficulty with accommodative facility with minus lenses.

Less plus on MEM or the fused cross-cylinder than expected would indicate an accommodative spasm or accommodative excess. Other relevant findings would include: a low NRA and difficulty with monocular accommodative facility with plus lenses.

Fused Cross-cylinder

More plus than expected indicates underaccommodation that occurs with accommodative insufficiency. Less plus is interpreted as overaccommodation and can be indicative of accommodative spasm or excess.

Binocular Accommodative Facility

If a patient has normal binocular findings (phoria, PFV, NFV), the results from tests such as the NRA, PRA, and binocular accommodative facility can be useful in confirming the presence of an accommodative anomaly and problems with interactions between accommodation and vergence.

For instance, if a normal phoria is present and NFV is adequate, the endpoint of the PRA procedure will generally be determined by the patient's ability to stimulate accommodation. The information obtained in such a case could be utilized—along with the results of other accommodative tests—to determine the nature of the accommodative anomaly.

Summary

When evaluating the accommodative system, it is important to administer monocular tests. Given a patient, however, with adequate positive and NFV, one can use the information obtained from other procedures in order to assess the accommodative system.

In terms of identifying accommodative anomalies, tests that assess a patient's ability to make rapid large changes in accommodative level and sustain over time, are most sensitive. They provide the clinician with test conditions that more closely resemble the normal use of the ACC and may correlate better with reports of near point asthenopia.

Vertical Fusional Vergence Data

Optometric data that can be used to determine the status of a patient's vertical fusional vergence (VFV) are included in this category. Unlike the previous groups that contain tests that directly and indirectly assess the function being evaluated, there are only direct tests of vertical vergence.

Supravergence and Infravergence

Right infravergence is the compensatory fusional vergence for a right hyperdeviation, while right supravergence is the compensatory fusional vergence for a right hypodeviation. When right supravergence is measured, base-down prism is added in front of the right eye as the patient is instructed to keep the target single as long as possible and to report when the target becomes double. This test measures the patient's ability to maintain bifoveal alignment as base-down prism is slowly added. When diplopia occurs, this is recorded as the break finding and then the prism is reduced until a recovery point is determined. Right infravergence is measured by adding base-up prism in front of the right eye.

Vertical Fixation Disparity Testing

In contrast to horizontal fixation disparity testing, forced vergence testing is not necessary. Rather, the amount of prism that reduces the associated phoria to zero is considered to be the most accurate and readily accepted method of prism correction for vertical deviations (23).

Ocular Motor Data

Optometric data that can be used to determine the status of a patient's ocular motor skills are included in this category. Unlike the previous groups that contain tests that directly and indirectly assess the function being evaluated, there are only direct tests of fixation, saccades, and pursuits.

Fixation Status

This is simply a test in which the patient is asked to maintain fixation for at least 10 seconds. The clinician subjectively evaluates the quality of fixation over this 10-second time period.

Saccadic Ability

The most common method for evaluating saccadic ability is to use the NSUCO Oculomotor Test described in Chapter 1 (Table 1.8). When a problem is suspected from this test or from the history, it is best to administer the DEM. This test provides quantification of saccadic ability, along with expected findings by age and grade level.

Pursuit Ability

The most common method for evaluating pursuit ability is to use the NSUCO Oculomotor Test described in Chapter 1 (Table 1.10).

Motor Alignment and Tests of Accommodative Convergence Interaction

Tests that Assess the Direction and Magnitude of the Phoria

Tests such as the cover test and various methods of phoria testing are important because they represent the initial entry point—in this case, analysis approach. Examples of such tests are the distance and near phorias assessed using the Maddox rod, the modified Thorington test or the von Graefe technique and the cover test at distance and near.

The two important pieces of information gained from this testing are the direction of the phoria and the magnitude at both distance and near. The classification system used in this text depends heavily on the distance and near phoria information. Most common binocular vision anomalies that will be considered in this book are all partially defined by this near-to-distance relationship. The distance phoria is a reflection of tonic vergence and is measured when the patient is fixating on a distant object with fusion prevented, accommodation relaxed, and the refractive error corrected. Tonic vergence is the vergence response from some undeterminable divergent position of anatomic rest that is maintained by extraocular muscle tonus. The near phoria is based on the AC/A ratio.

Another important relationship that must be considered is that of the phoria to the compensating fusional vergence. The tendency of the eyes to deviate from bifoveal fixation (phoria) is controlled by fusional vergence. If there is an exophoria, the compensating vergence is PFV. In the presence of esophoria, the NFV is the compensating vergence. For a right hyperdeviation, right infravergence is the compensatory reserve.

When dealing with a patient with a heterophoria, we must consider not only the direct measure but the indirect data as well. The direct and indirect measures form the groups listed above. Thus, for example, with exophoria and asthenopic symptoms, we expect all or most of the findings in the PFV group to be lower than expected.

The presence of a significant exophoria on cover testing should direct initial attention to the PFV group findings; significant esophoria suggests a close examination of the NFV group data. In the absence of a significant phoria at distance or near, the optometrist would then direct his or her attention to the ACC group findings.

Fixation Disparity

The primary advantage of fixation disparity analysis is that the assessment takes place under binocular and, therefore, more natural conditions. Phoria/vergence testing that is performed under dissociated conditions may not truly reflect the way the system operates under binocular conditions. Studies have indicated that analyzing binocular vision using fixation disparity is useful in determining those patients that are likely to have symptoms (8).

Fixation disparity has its most significant value when other testing fails to reveal a basis for a patient's complaints. Fixation disparity may provide an understanding of the patient's problem in such cases (Chapter 14).

AC/A Ratio

The relationship between the distance and near deviations is an important part of case analysis. Since the AC/A ratio is a critical determinant of this relationship, it is a vital part of case analysis. The AC/A ratio is also the major factor that determines the *sequence* of management decisions in patients with heterophoria. This will be discussed in detail in later chapters.

CLASSIFICATION OF THE VISION DISORDER AND IDENTIFICATION OF THE SYNDROME

As optometrists, we are confronted by a finite number of accommodative, ocular motor, and nonstrabismic binocular vision anomalies in clinical care, and a number of classification systems are available to help categorize these disorders. Perhaps the most common is Duane's classification (20):

- Convergence insufficiency
- Convergence excess
- Divergence insufficiency
- Divergence excess

This classification, originally developed by Duane for strabismus, was later extended to nonstrabismic binocular vision anomalies by Tait (24).

This is a descriptive classification and does not necessarily imply etiology. Binocular problems are described according to the type of heterophoria measured at distance and at near. Duane's classification has limitations, however. As illustrated in the list above, only four possible classifications are available. Clinically, however, we find that many other possible combinations exist that do not fit into Duane's classification. For example, one problem with this classification, described by Wick (18), is that it does not have a category for a deviation in which the exo- or esodeviations are equal at distance and near. Another condition that is not included in Duane's classification is fusional vergence dysfunction (25). This is a condition in which there is no significant phoria at either distance or near, but the horizontal fusional vergence ranges are reduced in both base-in and base-out directions.

Because of these and several other limitations, Wick (18) described an alternative classification system for binocular anomalies that represents an expansion of Duane's classification and is based on consideration of the distance phoria (tonic vergence) and the AC/A ratio. This classification takes all possible combinations into consideration and is the system we will use in this text for binocular vision disorders. In this system, there are nine possible diagnoses, rather than the four suggested by Duane.

The nine possible diagnoses can be divided into three main categories of binocular vision problems based on the AC/A ratio. The three categories are low AC/A ratio, normal AC/A ratio, and high AC/A ratio. Within each of these three categories there are three possible

TABLE 2.4. *Classification of binocular, accommodative, and ocular motor anomalies*

Binocular Anomalies
Low AC/A Ratio
1. Orthophoria at distance—convergence insufficiency
2. Exophoria at distance—convergence insufficiency
3. Esophoria at distance—divergence insufficiency
Normal AC/A Ratio
1. Orthophoria at distance—fusional vergence dysfunction
2. Exophoria at distance—basic exophoria
3. Esophoria at distance—basic esophoria
High AC/A Ratio
1. Orthophoria at distance—convergence excess
2. Esophoria at distance—convergence excess
3. Exophoria at distance—divergence excess
Vertical Anomalies
1. Right or left hyperphoria
Accommodative Anomalies
1. Accommodative insufficiency
2. Ill-sustained accommodation
3. Accommodative excess
4. Accommodative infacility
Ocular Motor Anomalies
1. Ocular motor dysfunction

combinations: exophoria, orthophoria, or esophoria at distance (Table 2.4). Convergence excess and insufficiency and divergence excess and insufficiency are included, but a major difference is that our classification has two types of convergence excess and convergence insufficiency. In addition, fusional vergence dysfunction and basic esophoria and exophoria are possible diagnoses. Since the treatment differs for each of these various classifications, we feel that it is desirable to be as specific as possible when classifying binocular and accommodative disorders.

The nine binocular vision anomalies described above are all horizontal heterophoria problems. Vertical heterophoria can also occur. Vertical heterophoria problems are either classified as right or left hyperphoria.

The accommodative classification system used in this text originated with Donders (26), was expanded by Duke-Elder and Abrams (27), and has been popularized by optometric authors (28–30). It includes the categories of accommodative insufficiency, ill-sustained accommodation, accommodative excess, and accommodative infacility (Table 2.4).

In regard to ocular motor anomalies, we will use only one diagnostic category, ocular motor dysfunction. This diagnosis refers to a condition in which there are problems with fixation, saccades, and pursuits.

By becoming knowledgeable about this classification system and the different possible syndromes, the knowledge base necessary for analysis of optometric data becomes complete.

BINOCULAR VISION, ACCOMMODATIVE, AND OCULAR MOTOR ANOMALIES

The characteristics of each of the 15 binocular, ocular motility, and accommodative disorders is briefly described below. In addition, in Chapters 8 through 12, these conditions are discussed in detail, including characteristics, differential diagnosis, and optometric management of each condition.

CLASSIFICATION OF BINOCULAR VISION DISORDERS

Category 1: Binocular Vision Disorders with a Low AC/A Ratio

Orthophoria at Distance—Convergence Insufficiency

This is a patient that has orthophoria at distance (normal tonic vergence), a low AC/A ratio, and moderate to high exophoria at near.

Characteristics

1. **Symptoms** All of the following are associated with reading or other near tasks.
   - Asthenopia and headaches
   - Intermittent blur
   - Intermittent diplopia
   - Symptoms worse at end of day
   - Burning and tearing
   - Inability to sustain and concentrate
   - Words move on the page
   - Sleepiness when reading
   - Decreased reading comprehension over time
   - Slow reading
2. **Signs**
   - Moderate to high exophoria or intermittent exotropia at near
   - Reduced PFV at near
   - Reduced vergence facility at near with base-out prism
   - Intermittent suppression at near
   - Receded near point of convergence
   - Low AC/A ratio
   - Fails binocular accommodative facility testing with +2.00
   - Low MEM and fused cross-cylinder findings
   - Low NRA
   - Exofixation disparity

Exophoria at Distance—Convergence Insufficiency

This is a patient that has exophoria at distance (low tonic vergence) and low AC/A ratio, and thus the near phoria will be significantly greater than the distance phoria. This patient differs from the previous type of exophoria in which the phoria at distance is ortho.

Characteristics

1. **Symptoms** All of the following are associated with reading or other near tasks.
   - Asthenopia and headaches
   - Intermittent blur
   - Intermittent diplopia
   - Symptoms worse at end of day
   - Burning and tearing
   - Inability to sustain and concentrate
   - Words move on the page

TABLE 2.5. *Common accommodative and non-strabismic binocular vision disorders summary of diagnostic findings*

Condition	Cover test	AC/A ratio	NPC	Vergence amplitude	Vergence facility	Stereopsis	Accommodative amplitude	Binocular accommodative facility	Monocular accommodative facility	Negative relative accommodation (NRA)/Positive relative accommodation (PRA)	Monocular estimation method
Accommodative insufficiency	No predictable pattern	Normal	Normal	BO blur at near may be low	Normal	Normal	Low	Fails −	Fails −	Low PRA	High
Ill-sustained accommodation	No predictable pattern	Normal	Normal	BO blur at near may be low	Normal	Normal	Normal	Fails −	Fails −	Low PRA	High
Accommodative excess	No predictable pattern	Normal	Normal	BI blur at near may be low	Normal	Normal	Normal	Fails +	Fails +	Low NRA	Low
Accommodative infacility	No predictable pattern	Normal	Normal	BO and BI blur at near may be low	Normal	Normal	Normal	Fails +/−	Fails +/−	Low NRA and PRA	Normal
Convergence insufficiency	Exo >N	Low	Receded	Low BO	Low BO	Normal	Normal	Fails +	Normal	Low NRA	Low
Convergence excess	Eso >N	High	Normal	Low BI	Low BI	Normal	Normal	Fails −	Normal	Low PRA	High
Fusional vergence dysfunction	Low eso or low exo	Normal	Normal	Low BO and BI	Low BO and BI	Normal	Normal	Fails +/−	Normal	Low NRA and PRA	Normal
Divergence insufficiency	Eso >D	Low	Normal	Low BI at D	Low BI at D	Normal	Normal	Normal	Normal	Normal	Normal
Divergence excess	Exo >D	High	Normal	Low BO at D Low BI at N	Low BO at D Low BI at N	Normal	Normal	Normal	Normal	Normal	Normal
Basic exophoria	Equal exo at D and N	Normal	Normal	Low BO at D and N	Low BO at D and N	Normal	Normal	Fails +	Normal	Low NRA	Low
Basic esophoria	Equal eso at D and N	Normal	Normal	Low BI at D and N	Low BI at D and N	Normal	Normal	Fails −	Normal	Low PRA	High

Cycloplegic Refraction

Static retinoscopy and a dry subjective refraction are sufficient to determine the refractive error in most cases. When esophoria is present or latent hyperopia is suspected, a cycloplegic refraction may be helpful. For children below the age of 3 years, 1 gtt of 0.5% cyclopentalate hydrochloride repeated in 5 minutes is the recommended concentration and dosage. For children age 3 years and older, the dosage is the same as for younger children, while the recommended concentration is 1.0%. After waiting approximately 40 minutes, retinoscopy is performed. To determine the final refractive correction, the following issues must be considered:

- Tonus of the ciliary muscle: If full cycloplegia is achieved, then the normal tonus of the ciliary muscle will also be relaxed. Thus, more plus will be found than can be prescribed. If we know that complete cycloplegia has been achieved, about 3/4 D should be subtracted from the net finding.
- Type of refractive error: In myopes, it is usually not necessary to subtract the 3/4 D of plus, whereas in hyperopia it is necessary.
- Binocular status: If esophoria or intermittent esotropia is present, maximum plus should be considered.

Insignificant Degrees of Refractive Error

There is far less agreement about the management of small amounts of refractive error. This would be defined as a refractive error less than the values listed in Table 3.1. An example would be a patient presenting with a history of eyestrain associated with reading, and the refraction is:

OD: $+0.25 - 0.50 \times 90$
OS: $+0.25 - 0.50 \times 90$

The question the clinician must answer is whether such a refractive error could be the cause of the patient's discomfort. This decision should be based on additional testing and analysis of accommodative and binocular data. There are two scenarios that generally could occur. First, the patient may also present with significant accommodative and binocular problems.

Assume this patient also had a near point of convergence of 6 in./12 in., orthophoria at distance, 12 exophoria at near, and the PFV group of data strongly suggested decreased PFV. In the presence of this additional data, the low refractive error becomes significant only if the clear retinal images achieved through refractive correction will improve fusion and assist in management.

Another possible situation would be a patient with the low refractive error listed above and all accommodative and binocular testing within the expected values. In this case, the clinician may be left with no other possible visual basis for the patient's discomfort and must make a decision about prescribing for the low refractive error. It is wise, in such a situation, to ask additional questions about the nature of the symptoms to clarify whether there truly appears to be a relationship between the use of the eyes and the discomfort. If based on this additional questioning there seems to be a relationship, prescription for the low refractive error may sometimes be helpful—especially if small astigmatism corrections against the rule or oblique axis are present.

In our experience, however, there is often an accommodative, ocular motor, or binocular vision disorder present in addition to the low refractive error. It is very unusual to find a low refractive error in isolation that accounts for the significant symptoms.

Other authors have addressed the issue of prescribing for low refractive errors (3–6). Blume (6) reported that low refractive error-induced symptoms include slightly blurred vision, headaches, and ocular discomfort associated with activities such as reading and other near work. There have been case reports (3–6) demonstrating the positive effect of prescribing for low refractive errors. A critical analysis of these case reports, however, indicates that an assessment of accommodation and binocular vision either was not performed or not reported in the majority of cases. This lack of data about accommodative and binocular function makes it difficult to interpret these reports.

Managing Anisometropia and Aniseikonia in Nonstrabismic Binocular Vision Disorders

Anisometropia is defined as a condition in which the refractive status of one eye differs from that of the other. A difference of 1 D or more in the sphere or cylinder is considered clinically significant. The critical underlying concept that should be considered when deciding about correction of anisometropia is that clear retinal images facilitate fusion. The general rule, therefore, is to fully correct the anisometropia. If the patient is amblyopic, the underlying cause of the amblyopia is the uncorrected refractive error. Unless the refractive error is corrected, there is little reason to expect maximal improvement in acuity, accommodative response, and binocular skills. A possible exception is a patient who might become more symptomatic if corrected. An example is an elderly patient who requires a large increase in cylindrical correction in one eye. For such patients, consider reducing the prescription. In all other cases, fully correct the anisometropia.

There are two additional concerns that one must take into consideration when prescribing for anisometropia. The first issue is the possibility of inducing aniseikonia. Aniseikonia is defined as a condition in which the ocular images are unequal in size and/or shape. The different image sizes induced by the prescription can cause symptoms and affect sensory fusion. This topic is covered in depth in Chapter 18. Although aniseikonia may occur occasionally in clinical practice, it affects only a small percentage of patients with anisometropia. The decision that must be made is whether to prescribe spectacle lenses or contact lenses. Knapp's law provides guidelines and suggests prescribing eyeglasses for aniseikonia secondary to axial length differences and contact lenses for anisometropia due to refractive differences. Since most anisometropia is due to axial length differences, eyeglasses would be the method of choice, according to Knapp's Law.

Clinically, however, we find that this is not the case. The reason for this is the second problem associated with the correction of anisometropia. An anisometropic prescription will always cause prismatic differences for the patient as he or she looks from one position of gaze to another. The greater the degree of anisometropia, the larger the prismatic differences. This creates a motor fusion problem, placing a demand on horizontal and vertical fusional vergence (VFV). Whereas aniseikonia only occurs in a small percentage of patients, this motor problem affects all anisometropes after correction with eyeglasses. As a result, contact lenses should be considered the treatment method of choice in cases of anisometropia.

ADDED LENS POWER (MINUS AND PLUS)

The other primary use of lenses in the treatment of accommodative and binocular disorders is to alter the demand on either the accommodative or binocular systems. The important clinical data that are used to determine whether such an approach will be effective are listed in Tables 3.2 and 3.3. The idea that optometric case analysis should be based on groups of data (Chapter 2) applies to decision making about the possible effectiveness of additional lenses as well. Table 3.2 lists the eight findings that should be considered when trying to

TABLE 3.2. *Consideration for prescribing added plus lenses*

Test	Consider the use of added plus	Added plus not indicated
AC/A ratio	High	Low
Refractive error	Hyperopia	Myopia
Near phoria	Esophoria	Exophoria
Negative relative accommodation (NRA)/ positive relative accommodation (PRA)	Low PRA	Low NRA
Base-out at near	Normal to high	Low
Monocular estimation method retinoscopy	High	Low
Amplitude of accommodation	Low	Normal
Accommodative facility testing	Fails minus sign	Fails plus sign

determine whether added plus lenses should be prescribed, and Table 3.3 lists the findings that should be considered when trying to determine whether added minus lenses should be prescribed.

The primary test finding that helps determine the effectiveness of added lenses is the magnitude of the AC/A ratio. If the AC/A ratio is greater than expected, the use of added lenses will generally be an effective approach. A high AC/A ratio suggests that a very large change in binocular alignment can be achieved with a small addition of lenses. A low AC/A ratio indicates that the use of lenses will have little desirable effect. When the AC/A ratio is in the normal range of 3:1 to 7:1, the other data in Tables 3.2 and 3.3 must be taken into consideration before determining the potential value of prescribing added lenses. It is important to understand the effect that plus or minus lenses will have on all examination findings. Tables 3.4 and 3.5 provide examples of these effects.

If one keeps in mind the effect that a prescription of additional plus or minus will have on all of the different diagnostic tests, it becomes easier to make decisions about appropriate treatment for any particular patient.

The most common example of the effectiveness of the use of lenses in the absence of refractive error is convergence excess. In such a case, the patient will generally have no significant phoria at distance and a moderate to high degree of esophoria at near. The findings in the negative fusional vergence (NFV) group will be low, suggesting decreased NFV, and the AC/A ratio is typically high. These findings suggest that a significant change could be achieved in the amount of esophoria at near simply by prescribing plus lenses for near. If the patient has 12 Δ of esophoria at near, for example, with base-in at near of 4/6/2 and an AC/A ratio

TABLE 3.3. *Consideration for prescribing added minus lenses*

Test	Consider the use of added minus	Added minus not indicated
AC/A ratio	High	Low
CA/C ratio	High	Low
Phoria	Exophoria	Esophoria
Base-in at near	Normal to high	Low
Amplitude of accommodation	Normal	Low
Accommodative facility Testing	Fails plus sign	Fails minus sign
Age	Below age 6	Age 9 or above

TABLE 3.4. *Example of the effect of plus lenses on test results*

Given: AC/A ratio = 8:1; if a + 1.00 add is prescribed, it would be expected to lead to the following changes

Test	Expected change with +1.00
Near phoria	About 8 Δ less esophoria
Negative relative accommodation	Decrease of about 1.00 D
Positive relative accommodation	Increase of about 1.00 D
Base-out (near)	Decrease of about 8 Δ
Base-in (near)	Increase of about 8 Δ
Monocular estimation method retinoscopy	Decrease in plus sign
Amplitude of accommodation	Increase of about 1.00 D
Accommodative facility testing	Better performance with −2.00

of 10:1, an add of +1.00 would be expected to have a considerable beneficial effect. In this case, the add would result in a near point phoria of about 2 esophoria, and the base-in range measured through this add would be expected to increase as well. If, however, the clinical data is somewhat different and the patient has the moderate esophoria at near with a low AC/A ratio, then the use of added lenses may not be sufficient to lead to a resolution of the patient's complaints.

The classic example of the ineffectiveness of the use of lenses in the absence of refractive error is convergence insufficiency. In such a case, the distance phoria is insignificant, while a moderate to large exophoria may be present at near along with a low AC/A ratio, a receded near point of convergence, and low PFV group data. The use of lenses—in this case, to achieve a desirable change in the near phoria—would not be expected to be helpful. For instance, one might consider the use of additional minus at near. If the patient has 12 exophoria at near with an AC/A ratio of 2:1 and base-out at near of 2/4/−2, the use of −1.00 or even −2.00 at near would have little effect on the exophoria or base-out relationship. Thus, because of the low AC/A, the use of lenses in this situation would not be an effective strategy.

The use of added plus or minus lenses is particularly helpful for the conditions listed in Table 3.6. Prescription guidelines for prescribing added plus lenses are based on the information in Table 3.2. This table lists all of the findings from the optometric evaluation that contribute to the final decision about prescribing added plus. The concept, stressed in Chapter 2, that groups of data should be analyzed rather than a single isolated finding, applies to the issue of added plus lenses. Although all of the data points do not have to agree, there will generally be a trend suggesting the amount of plus that should be prescribed. Cases 1, 2, and 3 in Chapter 9 provide specific examples about determining the amount of added plus to prescribe.

TABLE 3.5. *Example of the effect of minus lenses on test results*

Given: AC/A ratio = 8/1; if a −1.00 add is prescribed, it would be expected to lead to the following changes

Test	Expected change with −1.00
Near phoria	About 8 Δ less exophoria
Negative relative accommodation	Increase of about 1.00 D
Positive relative accommodation	Decrease of about 1.00 D
Base-out (near)	Increase of about 8 Δ
Base-in (near)	Decrease of about 8 Δ
Monocular estimation method retinoscopy	Increase in +
Amplitude of accommodation	Decrease of about 1.00 D
Accommodative facility testing	Better performance with +2.00

TABLE 3.6. *Conditions responding favorably to added lenses*

Added plus lenses	Added minus lenses
Convergence excess	High exophoria
Basic esophoria	Divergence excess
Accommodative insufficiency	
Ill-sustained accommodation	

When prescribing added plus lenses, a bifocal prescription is almost always preferable. With children below the age of about 10 years, we recommend setting the segment height at about the lower pupil margin to ensure that the child reads through the segment. A flat-top 28-mm segment works well with young children. In older children and adults, the segment height can be set at the lower lid margin.

Added minus lenses should also be considered in certain cases. Added minus lenses are used for high exophores or exotropes. In such cases, the lenses are used to reduce the angle of deviation using accommodative convergence to supplement fusional vergence. These lenses can be prescribed as training lenses to be used only during active vision therapy or for general wear. When used as a training device, large amounts of minus can be prescribed. For a constant exotrope, it would not be unusual to prescribe 6 or 7 D of additional minus. To determine the prescription, the clinician would find the least amount of minus that allows the patient to fuse. The power of the lenses would gradually be reduced as therapy progresses and the patient's ability to fuse improves.

Added minus lenses can also be prescribed for full-time wear. This would be done to reduce the percentage of time that an intermittent exotropia occurs or to provide more comfortable fusion in high exophoria. When prescribed for this purpose, smaller amounts of minus (i.e., 1.00 to 2.00 D) are used. In such cases, the AC/A ratio is not the critical factor in determining the amount of minus to prescribe. The objective of the added minus is to create a stimulus to convergence. Once this is accomplished, the patient is able to maintain fusion using fusional vergence.

PRISM

The use of prism to treat binocular anomalies should be a consideration in all cases. Generally there are five situations in which the use of prism may be helpful. These include:

- Horizontal relieving prism
- Vertical relieving prism
- Prism as an aid to begin vision therapy
- Prism used when vision therapy is inappropriate or impractical
- Prism used at the end of vision therapy

Horizontal Relieving Prism

If a large lateral heterophoria or an intermittent strabismus is present, it may be helpful to prescribe prism to decrease the demand on fusional vergence. Prism is most often effective in cases of high tonic vergence or esophoria at distance along with a normal to low AC/A ratio. Prism can be prescribed as a temporary measure until a vision therapy program has been completed or it can be prescribed as an attempt to eliminate the patient's symptoms without vision therapy. Although the use of prism to treat heterophoria has been recommended by numerous authors (7–15), there is surprisingly limited research support for its effectiveness. A study by Worrell (14) investigated the effectiveness of prism prescribed, based on Sheard's criterion. They found that prism was only preferred by patients in cases of distance esophoria. For exophoria and esophoria at near, the authors did not find any preference for prism glasses. Payne et al. (15) did a similar study prescribing prism based on fixation disparity testing. They prescribed two pairs of glasses that were identical in every way, except one had prism and one had none. After wearing each pair of glasses for 2 weeks, the subjects were asked to choose the ones they preferred. All of the ten subjects chose the glasses with the prism. The studies that have been done have reported the results of prism in small numbers of subjects. Nevertheless, the use of relieving prism appears to be rather well accepted by most authors (7–13).

The approaches used most often to prescribe prism are fixation disparity analysis, Sheard's criterion, and Percival's criterion.

Fixation Disparity Analysis

Fixation disparity (see Chapter 14) is generally the most desirable method of prescribing horizontal relieving prism. The amount of prism can be based on one of three criteria: the associated phoria, the center of symmetry, or the flat portion of the curve. The criterion used depends on the nature of the forced vergence fixation disparity curve. If the fixation disparity curve is steep, the associated phoria works well. The center of symmetry is most useful when there is a moderate flat portion on the curve. When the curve has a large flat portion, enough prism is prescribed to move the flat portion of the curve to the y-axis. These topics are discussed in detail in Chapter 14.

Sheard's Criterion

Sheard (16) suggested that for a patient to be comfortable, the compensating fusional vergence should be twice the phoria. For exophoria, the compensating vergence is base-out or PFV and for esophoria, the compensating vergence is base-in or NFV. Sheard suggests that prism can be prescribed if this criterion is not met. Although this criterion can be applied to any type of heterophoria, research suggests that Sheard's criterion works best with exophores (17). Clinically the following formula can be used to determine the amount of prism to prescribe to meet Sheard's criterion:

Prism needed = 2/3 phoria − 1/3 compensating fusional vergence.

EXAMPLE 1:

For example, if a patient has 10 Δ of exophoria and the base-out to blur finding is 10 Δ, the amount of prism needed would be:

$$P = 2/3(10) - 1/3(10)$$

$$P = 6.67 - 3.33$$

$$P = 3.34 \, \Delta$$

In this case, to meet Sheard's criterion, one would have to prescribe about 3 Δ base-in. Base-in is used in this example because the deviation is exophoria.

Percival's Criterion

Like Sheard, Percival developed a guideline for the prescription of prism (18). There has also been little clinical research to support this criterion, although recent studies suggest that Percival's criterion is most effective with esophoria (17).

According to Percival, the patient should be operating in the middle third of the vergence range. This is independent of the phoria and can be described by the following formula:

$$P = 1/3\,G - 2/3\,L$$

Where P = prism to be prescribed
      G = greater of the two lateral limits (base-in or base-out)
      L = lesser of the two lateral limits (base-in or base-out)

If P is a positive number, it represents the amount of prism to be prescribed. If the number is zero or a negative number, prism is not required.

EXAMPLE 1:

Phoria: 12 exophoria
Base-out vergence: 6/9/6
Base-in vergence: 18/24/21

$$P = 1/3G - 2/3L$$
$$P = 1/3\,(18) - 2/3\,(6)$$
$$P = 6 - 2$$
$$P = 4$$

4 $\triangle$ base-in would be required in this case because the deviation is exophoria.

EXAMPLE 2:

Phoria: 4 exophoria
Base-out vergence: 21/24/18
Base-in vergence: 18/24/21

$$P = 1/3\,G - 2/3\,L$$
$$P = 1/3\,(21) - 2/3\,(18)$$
$$P = 7 - 12$$
$$P = -5$$

Prism is not necessary in this case because the result is a negative number.

Of the ten nonstrabismic binocular vision anomalies discussed in Chapter 2, prism tends to be most effective for divergence insufficiency, basic esophoria, and vertical heterophoria and, to a substantially lesser extent, convergence insufficiency and basic exophoria (7). An important characteristic shared by the four horizontal binocular vision conditions is a low to

TABLE 3.7. *Recommended treatment approach by diagnosis*

Diagnosis	Primary recommended treatment approach	Secondary treatment recommendations
Ocular motor dysfunction	Vision therapy	Added +
Accommodative insufficiency	Added +	Vision therapy
Ill-sustained accommodation	Added +	Vision therapy
Accommodative excess	Vision therapy	
Accommodative infacility	Vision therapy	
Low AC/A conditions		
Convergence insufficiency	Vision therapy	Prism
Divergence insufficiency	Prism	Vision therapy
High AC/A conditions		
Convergence excess	Added lenses	Vision therapy
Divergence excess	Vision therapy	Added lenses
Normal AC/A conditions		
Basic esophoria	Vision therapy and added lenses	Prism
Basic exophoria	Vision therapy	Added lenses
		Prism
Fusional vergence dysfunction	Vision therapy	
Vertical disorders		
Vertical phoria	Prism	Vision therapy

normal AC/A ratio. Prism tends to be less effective than lenses in conditions with high AC/A ratios such as divergence excess and convergence excess.

Given the high success rates of vision therapy for most nonstrabismic binocular vision problems (19–22) and the limited research on the efficacy of prism therapy, relieving prisms should be used primarily when there is high tonic vergence (esophoria) at distance or other situations in which vision therapy is unlikely to achieve good results. Table 3.7 lists the cases in which prism would be most likely to be effective. We generally reserve the use of relieving prism for those cases that do not respond successfully to vision therapy or for those people who do not accept the recommendation of vision therapy because of financial or other concerns.

Vertical Relieving Prism

London and Wick (23) have reported that correction of a vertical fixation disparity may have a beneficial effect on the horizontal deviation. Based on this finding, they suggest that when a vertical and horizontal deviation are both present, the clinician should first consider prism correction of the vertical component. Wick (8) does not feel that vertical prism needs to be prescribed in all cases, however. He suggests that vertical prism should be prescribed when it results in improved visual performance, such as decreased suppression and increased fusion ranges. When management of a horizontal heterophoria is not proceeding well, it is worthwhile to recheck for a small vertical component that may have not been detected initially. As little as 1/2 Δ of vertical prism may be beneficial for fusion.

The most accepted criterion for determining the amount of vertical prism to prescribe is the associated phoria measurement (8,9). This is determined using a fixation disparity device, as described in Chapter 14. In vertical heterophoria, prescribe the prism that reduces the fixation disparity to zero. Another method that has been described is Sheard's criterion. Enough vertical prism is prescribed to establish a situation in which the vertical vergence is twice the vertical phoria. There is sufficient evidence in the literature, however, demonstrating that the use of the associated phoria is preferable to Sheard's criterion (17).

Prism Used as an Aid to Begin Vision Therapy

With very high degrees of heterophoria or when an intermittent strabismus is present, prism is sometimes helpful in the initial phase of vision therapy. Prism is used in such a case to decrease the overall demand on the binocular system. For example, base-out prism would be used to reduce the demand on NFV. This enables the clinician to more easily find a starting point for vision therapy. When prescribed for this purpose, prism glasses are generally used primarily during office or home therapy.

Prism Used When Vision Therapy Is Inappropriate or Impractical

Although vision therapy may be indicated for a particular patient, there are factors that may limit the prognosis for vision therapy. Such factors include cooperation, motivation, the age of the patient, scheduling issues, and finances. If a child is too young to be able to communicate or cooperate, if an elderly patient is unable or unwilling to perform vision therapy, if there is simply a lack of time or money for vision therapy, then prism becomes an option that should be considered.

Prism Used at the Conclusion of Vision Therapy

If the patient's symptoms persist after the conclusion of a vision therapy program, prism should be considered. In such cases, prism is prescribed as a relieving prism to reduce the demand of the fusional vergence system. Criteria for prescribing are identical to those described for horizontal and vertical relieving prism.

OCCLUSION

Occlusion is a commonly used treatment option in the management of strabismus and its associated conditions: amblyopia, eccentric fixation, suppression, and anomalous correspondence. There are also instances in which occlusion is necessary in the treatment of patients with heterophoria and it must be included as part of the sequential considerations in the management of nonstrabismic binocular anomalies.

Occlusion is used when heterophoria is associated with anisometropic amblyopia. This topic is discussed in depth in Chapter 16. The length of occlusion is important in anisometropic amblyopia. There have been reports in the literature of strabismus caused by the use of full-time occlusion (24). Full-time occlusion generally refers to the use of an occluder for 8 hours or more per day. We, therefore, recommend direct total occlusion for 2 to 3 hours per day, with a maximum of 4 to 6 hours. There are exceptions to this rule, however. We suggest more aggressive occlusion in anisometropia of greater than 7 D and cases of high unilateral myopia. In these cases, minimal occlusion is not always effective and longer periods of occlusion may be necessary. Even in such cases, it is prudent to begin with short amounts of occlusion. If acuity does not improve, the number of hours of occlusion can be increased gradually, until a treatment effect occurs.

Another type of occlusion that should be considered in heterophoria is the use of regional occlusion of a lens. This is particularly useful when a strabismus is present at one distance or one direction of gaze, while a heterophoria exists at other distances or positions of gaze. An example is a patient with a 25 Δ constant right exotropia at distance and a 5 Δ exophoria at near. An appropriate treatment option would be occlusion of the upper portion of the lens of the right eye, with the lower portion of the lens clear. This setup permits reinforcement of binocularity at near, while preventing suppression and other adaptations at distance.

VISION TRAINING

A significant percentage of patients with binocular vision and accommodative problems cannot be successfully treated with lenses and/or prism alone. Of the 15 different accommodative, ocular motor, and binocular disorders discussed in Chapter 2, for instance, only accommodative insufficiency, divergence insufficiency, convergence excess, basic esophoria, and vertical heterophoria are readily treated with lenses or prism alone. Prism is generally most effective for divergence insufficiency (Table 3.7). Analysis of the data for the other conditions indicates that the use of optics and prism would not be expected to be totally effective. The goal of a lens and/or prism prescription for many of these cases, however, is to maximally increase binocularity optically. This can then be reinforced with vision therapy management.

Vision therapy is the treatment of choice for convergence insufficiency, divergence excess, fusional vergence dysfunction, basic exophoria, accommodative excess, accommodative infacility, and ocular motor dysfunction. It can also be used successfully, either alone or in conjunction with lenses or prism, to treat accommodative insufficiency, convergence excess, basic esophoria, and vertical heterophoria.

Vision therapy has been shown to be effective for accomplishing the following in accommodative, ocular motor, and nonstrabismic binocular vision disorders (19,20):

- Increase amplitude of accommodation
- Increase accommodative facility
- Eliminate accommodative spasm
- Increase fusional vergence amplitudes
- Increase fusional vergence facility
- Eliminate suppression
- Improve stereopsis
- Improve the accuracy of saccades and pursuits
- Improve stability of fixation

Determining the Necessity of Vision Therapy

The decision to recommend vision therapy should be based on a careful analysis of the following factors:

- Age and intelligence of the patient
- Analysis of data
- Determination of prognosis for the particular patient and the specific problem
- Financial issues
- Motivation
- Relationship between the chief visual complaint and optometric findings
- Time course of therapy

Age and Intelligence of the Patient

Vision therapy involves a learning process and therefore requires a certain level of maturity and intelligence. Although vision therapy is a viable option with infants and very young children (25), this treatment tends to be used in the treatment of strabismic and amblyopic patients at this age. It is, of necessity, rather passive and involves very short therapy sessions with as little communication as possible. Vision therapy for heterophoria patients, as described in this text, involves the need for good attention and the ability to concentrate for significant periods of time. Communication of feelings and an ability to follow instructions and work independently are all important characteristics of the successful vision therapy patient.

Age is one factor affecting the success of a vision therapy program. As a general rule, vision therapy programs are seldom initiated before the age of 6 years old for heterophoria patients. And, children who are immature or have limited intelligence may not be good candidates even at older ages. On the other hand, children as young as 3 or 4 years old are often ready for vision therapy when the problem is strabismus or amblyopia. In such cases, the therapy tends to be more passive than that necessary for heterophoria.

Thus, the decision to recommend vision therapy requires some experience and clinical judgment about the child's age, level of maturity, intelligence, and the clinical diagnosis.

While a lower age or maturity limit exists, there is no real upper limit. As long as a patient is motivated and can communicate and interact with the therapist, vision therapy can be successful. Studies have demonstrated that the success rates of vision therapy to treat binocular vision disorders in presbyopes are excellent (26–28). Many clinicians who are involved with vision therapy actually prefer the adult patient because of the ease with which therapy generally progresses, due to the motivation and understanding of the adult patient. Of course, some elderly patients may not be able or willing to participate in a vision therapy program. Lack of desire, inability to attend and concentrate, as well as financial and transportation problems may also interfere with vision therapy.

Analysis of Data

Depending on analysis of the data in the various groups described in Chapter 2, one or more treatment alternatives may be present. Table 3.7 lists the treatment options available by diagnosis. It is important to understand that while vision therapy is a viable option in all 15 common accommodative and binocular vision disorders, added lenses and prism are only options for some diagnoses. Prism is very useful for divergence insufficiency and vertical deviations, helpful with basic esophoria, and of occasional value in cases of convergence insufficiency and basic exophoria. The use of added lenses is a viable option for 4 of the 12 diagnoses: accommodative insufficiency, convergence excess, basic esophoria, and divergence excess. To make these decisions, it is helpful to refer to Tables 3.2 and 3.3, which describe the criteria for determining whether added plus lenses will be useful. Table 3.6 lists the binocular and accommodative conditions that respond well to added plus and minus lenses.

Determination of Prognosis for the Particular Patient and the Specific Problem

For each patient, a determination must be made about the prognosis for successful treatment using vision therapy. The prognosis for all accommodative and nonstrabismic binocular vision problems is excellent, with the exception of divergence insufficiency (19–22). In recent years, there have been several studies that have reviewed success rates for various types of accommodative and binocular disorders. These studies clearly demonstrate the efficacy of vision therapy for these conditions.

Studies investigating the clinical efficacy of vision therapy for accommodative dysfunction have shown success in approximately 9 of 10 cases. Daum (29), in a retrospective study of 96 patients, found partial or total relief of both objective and subjective difficulties in 96% of the subjects studied. Hoffman et al. (30) reported a vision therapy success rate of 87.5% in a sample of 80 patients with accommodative problems.

Other studies, using objective assessment techniques, have investigated the actual physiological changes that occur due to vision therapy. Both Liu et al. (31) and Bobier and Sivak

(32) found that the dynamics of the accommodative response were significantly changed after therapy. Liu et al. found that the latency of the accommodative response was decreased and the velocity of the response was increased. Bobier and Sivak were able to show a decrease in symptoms along with objective changes in accommodative dynamics.

Numerous investigators have shown that vision therapy for nonstrabismic binocular vision disorders leads to improved fusional vergence ranges. Most studies have investigated the use of vision therapy to treat convergence insufficiency and other nonstrabismics problems associated with exophoria.

In both prospective (33) and retrospective studies (34), Daum showed that relatively short periods of vision therapy can provide long-lasting increases in fusional vergence. Other studies (35–38) have used both experimental and control groups to demonstrate the efficacy of binocular vision therapy. Daum (35) investigated the effectiveness of vision therapy for improving PFV using a double blind placebo controlled experimental design. He found statistically significant changes in vergence in the experimental group, with no changes in the control group. Vaegan (36) also found large and stable improvement in vergence ranges in his experimental group, with no changes in the control group. Cooper et al. (37) studied patients with convergence insufficiency using a matched subjects control group crossover design to reduce placebo effects. They found a significant reduction in asthenopia and a significant increase in fusional vergence after the treatment. During the control phase, significant changes in symptoms and vergence were not found.

In recent years, there have been several studies that have also investigated the use of vision therapy as a treatment option for convergence excess (39–41). Gallaway and Scheiman (41) reviewed the records of 83 patients with convergence excess that had completed vision therapy and found that 84% reported total elimination of symptoms. They found significant increases in NFV. Other investigators have also reported reduction in symptoms (39,40) and increases in NFV (40).

Clinical studies have also been performed to investigate the efficacy of treating oculomotor dysfunction. Wold et al. (42) reported on a sample of 100 patients who had completed a vision therapy program for a variety of problems including accommodation, binocular vision, pursuits, and saccades. Saccadic and pursuit function was determined using subjective clinical performance scales like those described in Chapter 1. Vision therapy consisted of three 1-hour visits per week. The number of visits ranged from 22 to 53. It is important to understand that these patients did not only have eye movement disorders. Almost all patients had accommodative and binocular vision problems as well. Pre- and posttesting revealed statistically significant changes in both saccadic and pursuit function.

In a more recent clinical study, Rounds et al. (43) used a Visagraph Eye-Movement Recording System to assess reading eye movements before and after vision therapy. This investigation is one of the few to specifically study eye movement therapy alone. They used 19 adults with reading problems and assigned 12 to the experimental group and 9 to a control group. The experimental group received 4 weeks (12 hours) of exclusively oculomotor skill enhancement vision therapy. The therapy consisted of three 20-minute office sessions and six 20-minute home sessions per week for 4 weeks. The control group received no intervention of any kind. Although no statistically significant changes were found, the experimental group showed trends toward improving reading eye movement efficiency (less regressions and number of fixations and increased span of recognition) compared to the control group.

Young et al. (44) also used an objective eye movement recording instrument (Eye Trac) to assess reading eye movements before and after therapy. They studied 13 school children who had failed a vision screening. The children each had three 5-minute vision therapy sessions per day for 6 weeks. They received a total of 6 hours of eye movement vision therapy. Posttesting revealed significant decrease in number of fixations, an increase in reading speed, and a decrease in fixation duration.

Fujimoto et al. (45) investigated the potential for using vision therapy procedures prerecorded on videocassettes for eye movement vision therapy. They had three groups of subjects. The first group of nine subjects received standard eye movement vision therapy. The second group received videocassette-based eye movement therapy, while the third group received no treatment. The results showed that both standard eye movement vision therapy and videocassette-based therapy were equally effective in improving saccadic ability.

Punnett and Steinhauer (46) studied two different approaches for eye movement therapy. They compared the effectiveness of vision therapy for eye movements using feedback versus no feedback. They used the Eye Trac to monitor eye movements and studied nine subjects. They found that the use of verbal feedback and reinforcement during vision therapy led to better treatment results.

In a recent study (47), oculomotor-based auditory biofeedback was used to improve saccadic ability and reading efficiency in fifteen subjects ranging in age from 18 to 38 years old. Eleven of the 12 subjects exhibited varying degrees of improvement in overall reading efficiency. There was a decrease in the number of saccades and regressions when reading, a decreased number of saccades per return sweep, and an increased reading rate. The authors concluded that oculomotor-based auditory biofeedback can be an effective training tool, especially in low–normal readers.

Although the success rates are excellent for all cases of binocular, ocular motility, and accommodative disorders, all patients with these problems may not be good candidates for vision therapy. Issues such as motivation, age, ability to communicate, and financial factors must all be taken into consideration before a recommendation is made for vision therapy.

Financial Issues

Finances must be a consideration as well. An intelligent, cooperative, and highly motivated patient may not be enough to guarantee a successful vision therapy program. If the cost of vision therapy creates a burden for a family, compliance and consistency will be problems leading to less than adequate results. Financial issues must be discussed with the patient when various options are being considered. It is therefore important for the optometrist to have an understanding of insurance reimbursement for vision therapy. These issues are addressed in detail in Chapter 22.

Motivation

The importance of motivation should not be underestimated. Any optometrist who practices vision therapy has experienced dramatic and surprising success in cases with apparently poor prognoses. Conversely, simple cases of convergence insufficiency with excellent prognoses, based on findings alone, can be failures in the absence of motivation. It is not always easy to judge the patient's level of motivation. When dealing with an adult, it is generally easier to decide whether sufficient motivation exists. A discussion of the patient's symptoms and the effects of the vision problem on performance can usually lead to a good understanding of the patient's desires. With a child, this decision is not always as simple. Children may be reluctant, unable, or unwilling to discuss their feelings and symptoms. In such cases, the clinician must then look to the parents for their understanding and motivation and hope that the parent can motivate the child.

We recommend that the issue of motivation be considered a key factor in determining the advisability of vision therapy. With a highly motivated patient, vision therapy should at least be attempted, even if the prognosis is poor.

Relationship Between the Chief Visual Complaint and Optometric Findings

Although vision therapy has been shown to be an extremely effective treatment approach for nonstrabismic binocular disorders, accommodative dysfunction, and ocular motor dysfunction, there are situations in which vision therapy may not be appropriate. Most clinicians look very carefully at the relationship between the patient's symptoms and clinical findings. When an apparent relationship can be established, treatment is generally recommended. An example of a match between symptoms and findings is a patient presenting with complaints of intermittent diplopia and eyestrain related to reading, and findings that include a receded near point of convergence, high exophoria at near, and reduced PFV. A patient could, however, be asymptomatic with the identical findings just described. It becomes a matter of clinical judgment to determine whether vision therapy should be prescribed in such a case. An astute clinician will inquire about whether the patient simply avoids reading or other near work. Often, once the clinician begins probing, it becomes apparent that the patient is not reading or has avoided certain situations because the activity may lead to discomfort. A classic example is the child with learning difficulties. Children with such problems do not read for long periods of time and, therefore, do not complain of the symptoms typically associated with accommodative and binocular vision problems. Thus, the absence of symptoms does not mean that the child is not being adversely affected by the vision anomaly. Treatment of the underlying vision disorder should still be considered in such cases.

In addition to avoidance, another explanation for a lack of symptoms—in the presence of a significant binocular disorder—is suppression. For example, a patient with a severe convergence insufficiency, in which an intermittent exotropia is present at near, may suppress. Suppression eliminates the need to overcome the deviation and thereby decreases or eliminates asthenopia. In either a case of avoidance or suppression, a recommendation of vision therapy may be still be appropriate.

In most situations, if an accommodative, ocular motor, or binocular problem is present and the patient is asymptomatic, an explanation such as those just described will be found. It is, therefore, important to recognize that it is necessary to try and establish a relationship between findings and symptoms, as well as to investigate issues such as avoidance and suppression.

Time Course of Therapy

Once a diagnosis of an accommodative, ocular motor, or binocular problem is reached, the next objective is to select appropriate treatment alternatives. The treatment alternatives are those that have been described in this chapter: optical correction of ametropia, added lenses, prism, occlusion, vision therapy, and surgery. When there is more than one viable treatment option, one factor that should be considered is the time frame for eliminating symptoms. Intuitively it makes some sense to select a treatment approach that will eliminate a patient's problem as quickly and as easily as possible. Thus, if analysis of the data suggests that lenses or prism may be effective, these treatment options should be considered initially. If lenses and prism appear to be reasonable treatment approaches, the beneficial effects of these options occur almost immediately. Weeks of vision therapy may be required before a patient begins to experience beneficial changes.

There are clinical situations in which the time course of the various treatment options is very important to a patient. Examples include busy professionals and college- and graduate-level students who may need positive results as quickly as possible.

In most instances, however, the time course, although important, is not the most significant issue. The long-term effect of the treatment option may be the most critical factor. Although the use of lenses and prism may be desirable because of the short time course, it is important to remember that the long-term effect of lenses and prism is to permit the patient to perform comfortably in spite of the presence of an underlying dysfunction. The patient must continue to wear the prescription to maintain this comfort. The long-term effect of vision therapy, however, is to develop normal motor and sensory fusion and accommodative skills to overcome the binocular, ocular motor, or accommodative dysfunction. This is an important distinction that should be considered and discussed when various treatment options are considered.

SURGERY

Although the need to recommend surgery for the treatment of nonstrabismic binocular vision anomalies is highly unusual, it must at least be considered a management option. The one situation in which a clinician may need to consider surgery is in the presence of a very large phoria. If the magnitude of the horizontal deviation exceeds 30 Δ, the prognosis for success with vision therapy alone decreases (48). Occasionally, after all of the nonsurgical options listed above have been attempted, a patient may complain of discomfort or blurred vision late in the day. In such instances, the original phoria may have been very large and, in spite of improvement in accommodative and convergence findings, the patient remains uncomfortable. Gallaway et al. (49) and Frantz (50) recently reported cases of an intermittent exotropia treated with vision therapy. The patient in the former study required surgical intervention because blur and asthenopia continued after vision therapy, while the patient in the latter required surgery because of poor compliance with lenses, prism, and vision therapy.

It is important to emphasize the unlikelihood of a recommendation of surgery for a nonstrabismic binocular vision anomaly. Hermann (51) reported on a large sample of convergence insufficiency patients in his ophthalmological practice. He reviewed records from 10 years of practice and found that of approximately 1,200 patients treated with orthoptics over that time span, 14 (or 1%) still complained of discomfort and required surgery.

The efficacy of surgical intervention for nonstrabismic binocular anomalies is equivocal. Very few cases have been reported in the literature. The few reports available have studied the effectiveness of surgery for convergence insufficiency. Reports by von Noorden (52) and Hermann (51) indicate that surgery is an effective approach for relieving the symptoms of these patients. Haldi (53), however, found that five of the six patients in her sample demonstrated a recurrence of the exodeviation and no relief of symptoms.

In summary, a recommendation of surgery for a nonstrabismic binocular vision anomaly is highly unlikely. In addition, there is no definitive study suggesting that surgery in such cases is an effective treatment strategy. However, the optometrist may find, in some cases of very high magnitude phorias or intermittent strabismus, that vision therapy alone may leave the patient with residual symptoms. In such cases, a recommendation of surgery should be considered.

SUMMARY

Treatment of accommodative, ocular motor, and nonstrabismic binocular vision disorders is one of the more rewarding aspects of optometric care. The success rates using the treatment approach we have presented are outstanding. Patients often come to our offices after previous unsuccessful attempts to find help for their discomfort. If we are able to eliminate their symptoms and resolve the underlying vision disorders, patient satisfaction is extremely high.

A primary objective of the model we presented in this chapter was to emphasize the significance of considering all treatment options for every accommodative, ocular motor, and binocular vision disorder encountered. This approach will ensure that no management option will be ignored and should lead to more frequent and rapid success.

STUDY QUESTIONS

1. Explain why correction of refractive error is an important first step when treating binocular and accommodative problems.

2. Describe a situation in which correction of refractive error may have a negative effect on a coexisting binocular vision problem.

3. Name the tests that you would use to determine if an add is appropriate for a given patient and present the expected findings for the above tests that suggest an add is appropriate.

4. Name the one key finding that generally helps determine if plus will be an effective treatment approach.

5. Describe clinical situations in which prescription of prism may be appropriate.

6. Name those binocular vision (BV) conditions that respond best to prism. What is the common factor for these conditions that makes prism effective?

7. Describe three clinical procedures for determining the amount of prism to prescribe for BV problems.

8. A patient has a near phoria of 12 exophoria. His PFV is 4/8/2 and his NFV is 12/20/14. How much prism would you prescribe based on Sheard's criterion?

9. A patient has a near phoria of 12 exophoria. His PFV is 4/8/2 and his NFV is 12/20/14. How much prism would you prescribe based on Percival's criterion?

10. What factors should be considered when deciding if vision therapy is an appropriate treatment approach for any given patient?

REFERENCES

1. Blum HL, et al. Vision screening for elementary schools: the Orinda study. Berkeley: University of California Press, 1958.
2. Dwyer P, Wick B. The influence of refractive correction upon disorders of vergence and accommodation. *Optom Vis Sci* 1995;72:224–232.
3. White JA. The practical value of low grade cylinders in some of asthenopia. *Trans Am Ophthalmol Soc* 1894;12:153–168.
4. Cholerton M. Low refractive errors. *Br J Physiol Opt* 1955;12:82–86.
5. Nathan J. Small errors of refraction. *Br J Physiol Opt* 1957;14:204–209.
6. Blume AJ. Low power lenses. In: Amos JF, ed. *Diagnosis and management in vision care*. Boston: Butterworth-Heineman, 1987:239–246.
7. Carter DB. Fixation disparity and heterophoria following prolonged wearing of prisms. *Am J Optom Physiol Opt* 1965;42:141–152.
8. Wick B. Horizontal deviations. In: Amos JF, ed. *Diagnosis and management in vision care*. Boston: Butterworth-Heineman, 1987:461–513.
9. London R. Fixation disparity and heterophoria. In: Barresi BJ, ed. *Ocular assessment: the manual of diagnosis for office practice*. Boston: Butterworth-Heineman, 1984:141–150.
10. Sheedy JE. Fixation disparity analysis of oculomotor imbalance. *Am J Optom Physiol Opt* 1980;57:632–639.
11. Borish IM. *Clinical refraction,* 3rd ed. Chicago: Professional Press, 1975:1285–1286.
12. Griffin J. *Binocular anomalies: procedures for vision therapy*, 2nd ed. Chicago: Professional Press, 1982.

13. Hofstetter HW. *Graphical analysis in vergence eye movements*. In: Schor C, Cuiffreda KJ, eds. Vergence eye movements: basic and clinical aspects. Boston: Butterworth-Heineman, 439–464.
14. Worrell BE, Hirsch MJ, Morgan MW. An evaluation of prism prescribed by Sheard's criterion. *Am J Optom Physiol Opt* 1971;48:373–376.
15. Payne CR, Grisham JD, Thomas KL. A clinical evaluation of fixation disparity. *Am J Optom Physiol Opt* 1974;51:90–93.
16. Sheard C. Zones of ocular comfort. *Am J Optom* 1930;7:9–25.
17. Sheedy JE, Saladin JJ. Association of symptoms with measures of oculomotor deficiencies. *Am J Optom Physiol Opt* 1978;55:670–676.
18. Percival AS. *The prescribing of spectacles*, 3rd ed. Bristol, UK: John Wright & Sons, 1928:125.
19. The efficacy of optometric vision therapy. The 1986/1987 AOA Future of Visual Development/Performance Task Force. *J Am Optom Assoc* 1988;59:95–105.
20. Suchoff IB, Petitio GT. The efficacy of visual therapy. *J Am Optom Assoc* 1986;57:119–125.
21. Grisham JD. Visual therapy results for convergence insufficiency: a literature review. *Am J Optom Physiol Opt* 1988;65:448–454.
22. Griffin JR. Efficacy of vision therapy for non-strabismic vergence anomalies. *Am J Optom Physiol Opt* 1987;64:11–14.
23. London RF, Wick B. The effect of correction of vertical fixation disparity on the horizontal forced vergence fixation disparity curve. *Am J Optom Physiol Opt* 1987;64:653–656.
24. Crewther DR, Crewther SG, Mitchell DE. The efficacy of brief periods of reverse occlusion in promoting recovery from the physiological effects of monocular deprivation in kittens. *Invest Ophthalmol Vis Sci* 1981;21:357–362.
25. Wick B. Vision therapy for infants, toddlers and preschool children, in pediatric optometry. In: Scheiman M, ed. *Problems in optometry*. Philadelphia: JB Lippincott, 1990.
26. Wick B. Vision therapy for presbyopic nonstrabismic patients. *Am J Optom Physiol Opt* 1977;54:244–247.
27. Cohen AH, Soden R. Effectiveness of visual therapy for convergence insufficiencies for an adult population. *J Am Optom Assoc* 1984;55:491–494.
28. Birnbaum MH, Soden R, Cohen AH. Efficacy of vision therapy for convergence insufficiency in an adult male population. *J Am Optom Assoc* 1999;70:225–232.
29. Daum K. Accommodative insufficiency. *Am J Optom Physiol Opt* 1983;60:352–359.
30. Hoffman L, Cohen A, Feuer G. Effectiveness of non-strabismic optometric vision training in a private practice. *Am J Optom Arch Am Acad Optom* 1973;50:813–816.
31. Liu JS, Lee M, Jang J, et al. Objective assessment of accommodative orthoptics. I. dynamic insufficiency. *Am J Optom Physiol Opt* 1979;56:285–291.
32. Bobier WR, Sivak JG. Orthoptic treatment of subjects showing slow accommodative responses. *Am J Optom Physiol Opt* 1983;60:678–687.
33. Daum K. The course and effect of visual training on the vergence system. *Am J Optom Physiol Opt* 1982;59:223–227.
34. Daum K. Convergence insufficiency. *Am J Optom Physiol Opt* 1984;61:16–22.
35. Daum K. Double blind placebo-controlled examination of timing effects in the training of positive vergences. *Am J Optom Physiol Opt* 1986;63:807–812.
36. Vaegan JL. Convergence and divergence show longer and sustained improvement after short isometric exercise. *Am J Optom Physiol Opt* 1979;56:23–33.
37. Cooper J, Selenow A, Ciuffreda KJ, et al. Reduction of asthenopia in patients with convergence insufficiency after fusional vergence training. *Am J Optom Physiol Opt* 1983;60:982–989.
38. Daum K. A comparison of results of tonic and phasic training on the vergence system. *Am J Optom Physiol Opt* 1983;60:769–775.
39. Shorter AD, Hatch SW. Vision therapy for convergence excess. *N Engl J Optom* 1993;45:51–53.
40. Ficarra AP, Berman J, Rosenfield M, et al. Vision training: predictive factors for success in visual therapy for patients with convergence excess. *J Optom Vis Dev* 1996;27:213–219.
41. Gallaway M, Scheiman M. The efficacy of vision therapy for convergence excess. *J Am Optom Assoc* 1997;68:81–86.
42. Wold RM, Pierce JR, Keddington J. Effectiveness of optometric vision therapy. *J Am Optom Assoc* 1978;49:1047–1053.
43. Rounds BB, Manley CW, Norris RH. The effect of oculomotor training on reading efficiency. *J Am Optom Assoc* 1991;6:92–99.
44. Young BS, Pollard T, Paynter S, et al. Effect of eye exercises in improving control of eye movements during reading. *J Optom Vis Dev* 1982;13:4–7.
45. Fujimoto DH, Christensen EA, Griffin JR. An investigation in use of videocassette techniques for enhancement of saccadic movements. *J Am Optom Assoc* 1985;56:304–308.
46. Punnett AF, Steinhauer GD. Relationship between reinforcement and eye movements during ocular motor training with learning disabled children. *J Learn Disabil* 1984;17:16–19.
47. Fayos B, Ciuffreda KJ. Oculomotor auditory biofeedback training to improve reading efficiency. *J Behav Optom* 1998;9:143–152.

48. Ludlam W. Orthoptic treatment of strabismus. *Am J Optom Arch Am Acad Optom* 1961;38:369–388.
49. Gallaway M, Vaxmonsky T, Scheiman M. Surgery for intermittent exotropia. *J Am Optom Assoc* 1989;60:428–434.
50. Frantz K. The importance of multiple treatment modalities in a case of divergence excess. *J Am Optom Assoc* 1990;61:457–462.
51. Hermann JS. Surgical therapy for convergence insufficiency. *J Pediatr Ophthalmol Strab* 1981;18:28–31.
52. von Noorden GK. Resection of both medial rectus muscles in organic convergence insufficiency. *Am J Ophthalmol* 1976;81:223–226.
53. Haldi BA. Surgical management of convergence insufficiency. *Am J Orthopt* 1978;28:106–109.

PART II

Vision Therapy Procedures and Instrumentation

4

Introduction and General Concepts

This chapter provides detailed information and guidelines for vision therapy, and Chapters 5 to 7 describe a select group of vision therapy procedures for the treatment of vergence, accommodative, and ocular motility disorders. There are hundreds of vision therapy techniques in use by optometrists, and manuals are available describing a wide variety of instrumentation and procedures (1,2). In our opinion, presentation of a vast array of procedures tends to make vision therapy appear overly complicated. We believe that this may discourage optometrists from becoming involved in vision therapy.

In Chapters 5 to 7, we present a select group of procedures and instruments. Our primary emphasis is on presentation of the principles underlying the vision therapy techniques we have selected. An understanding of this small group of vision therapy procedures will enable an optometrist to successfully treat the vast majority of accommodative, ocular motility, and non-strabismic binocular vision disorders and achieve success rates consistent with those discussed in the literature (3,4). In addition, the principles discussed for these vision therapy techniques are common to all procedures. Therefore, an appreciation of the key issues and principles in this chapter will allow the clinician to understand almost any other procedure and will permit growth as the practitioner gains experience and confidence.

It is not unusual for us to hear students and clinicians unfamiliar with vision therapy ask the question, "What do I do with it?" regarding vision therapy equipment. Therefore, one of the primary objectives of the following four chapters is to provide a detailed description of how to actually use the vision therapy equipment described. We have provided a detailed sequence of therapy procedures to perform with the specific instruments described. We are well aware that there are other ways to use this instrumentation, but our goal is to present a starting point for clinicians who then can expand their utilization of this equipment as they gain experience in the area of vision therapy.

CATEGORIZATION OF VISION THERAPY INSTRUMENTATION AND PROCEDURES

Binocular vision therapy procedures have traditionally been subdivided into two broad categories. The first category, referred to as "instrument training," includes all techniques in which the patient is required to look directly into an instrument. With instrument training, movement of the patient is restricted, and it may be difficult to see the patient's eyes. These conditions are generally described as being less natural or more artificial than other forms of therapy. The most common example of instrument training is the use of a stereoscopic-type device.

The second category, called free space training, refers to techniques in which the patient is in a less restricted environment, more movement is possible, and it is easier to observe the patient's eyes. This type of vision therapy more closely approximates normal seeing conditions and is considered less artificial than "instrument" training.

Upon careful analysis of this division, several problems become apparent. The first difficulty is the lack of precise criteria for placing a particular procedure in either category. For example, while the Aperture Rule, illustrated in Fig. 4.1, is generally considered to be a "free space"

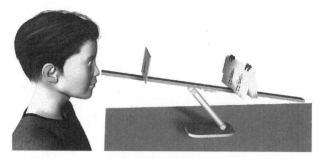

FIG. 4.1. The Aperture Rule.

technique, a patient using this device clearly has to position him- or herself directly against the device and look into the "instrument." The same is true of the double mirror stereoscope shown in Fig. 4.2. Although these two devices do not use lenses or prism, they clearly resemble "instrument" devices, such as the stereoscopes shown in Fig. 4.3. Another problem is how to categorize anaglyphic and Polaroid filter procedures. Are these techniques truly "free space," or do the filters constitute an interference and alteration of the normal visual environment?

We believe that the "free space" versus "instrument" dichotomy is an artificial division that leaves too many devices and procedures without a clear fit into either category. We recommend a classification of vision therapy instrumentation and techniques that is based to a greater extent on the type of equipment being used. This classification includes:

1. Anaglyphs and Polaroid filters
2. Lenses, prisms, and mirrors
3. Septums and apertures
4. Paper, pencil, and miscellaneous tasks
5. Stereoscopes
6. Afterimages, entoptic phenomena, and electrophysiological techniques

This classification system will be used throughout Chapters 5 to 7 as common vision therapy techniques are described. Table 4.1 lists many of the various instruments and procedures that fall into these six different categories.

The concept of natural versus artificial training conditions, however, is a useful one that we will emphasize throughout this text. There is a general consensus that vision therapy procedures

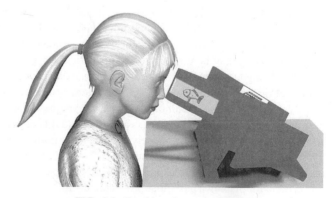

FIG. 4.2. Double mirror stereoscope.

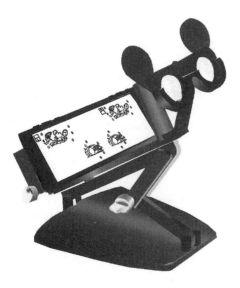

FIG. 4.3. Bernell-O-Scope stereoscope.

that approximate normal seeing conditions tend to be more effective in achieving the desired objectives of vision therapy.

CATEGORY ONE: ANAGLYPHS AND POLAROID FILTERS

Anaglyphs and Polaroids are filters that block out light from a portion of the target being viewed so that one part is visible by one eye and one part is visible by the other eye. These techniques are widely used for heterophoria patients.

TABLE 4.1. *Classification of vision therapy instrumentation and procedures*

1. **Stereoscopes**
   Brewster stereoscopes
   Wheatstone stereoscopes
   Haploscopes
   Cheiroscopes
2. **Anaglyphs and Polaroid filters**
   Tranaglyphs
   Vectograms
   Bar readers
   TV trainer
   Computer programs using red/blue
      or red/green glasses
3. **Lenses, prisms, and mirrors**
   Flip lenses
   Loose lenses
   Flip prisms
   Loose prisms
   Prism bars
   Hand-held mirrors
4. **Septums and apertures**
   Aperture rule
   Remy separator
   Tasks based on Turville test
5. **Paper, pencil, and miscellaneous tasks**
   Lifesaver cards
   Free space cards
   Eccentric circles
   Barrel card, three-dot card
   Brock string
   Computer techniques
   Hart chart and other miscellaneous charts
   Letter tracking
   Tracing
6. **Afterimages, entoptic phenomena,
   and electrophysiological techniques**
   Devices for creating after images
   Maxwell's spot
   Haidinger's brush
   Auditory biofeedback

Advantages

Anaglyphs (red/green targets) and Polaroids allow good control of stimulus parameters. A wide variety of targets including second degree, third degree, central, peripheral, accommodative, and nonaccommodative targets are available. These techniques work well with shallow to moderate suppression and they can be used to train both jump (phasic) or smooth (tonic) vergence. Because the patient does not have to look into an instrument, these procedures more closely resemble normal seeing conditions than instrument type devices.

Disadvantages

Young children may lose interest, and it is important to use a variety of these targets to maintain interest. The primary disadvantage of Polaroid techniques is high expense. They are approximately 10 times as expensive as anaglyphs. Another problem associated with Polaroids is that if the patient tilts his or her head, both targets can be seen by one eye. This would allow the patient to see both targets even if he or she is suppressing. Although anaglyphs are less expensive, these filters (particularly the red) are darker than Polaroids and may precipitate suppression (1). A potential disadvantage associated with both anaglyphs and Polaroids is that if there is rapid alternate suppression it may be difficult to determine if suppression is present.

CATEGORY TWO: LENSES, PRISMS, AND MIRRORS PROCEDURES

Lenses change the accommodative and vergence demand, while prisms and mirrors change the direction of light. Lenses, prisms, and mirrors are often used in conjunction with anaglyphs and Polaroids and are among the most widely used procedures for heterophoria patients. These procedures are useful for antisuppression training, fusional vergence, as well as accommodative and ocular motility therapy.

Advantages

Lenses are very effective for accommodative therapy. These devices also allow the clinician to increase or decrease the level of demand of all binocular and accommodative techniques. They can be used to train both smooth (tonic) and jump (phasic) vergence.

Disadvantages

Young children may lose interest and it is important to use a variety of targets to maintain interest.

CATEGORY THREE: SEPTUMS AND APERTURES

A septum is a dividing wall that separates the view of each eye in normal space so that one eye sees one portion of a target while the other eye sees another. An example is the Remy separator (Fig. 4.4). An aperture is an opening or window that separates the views of each eye so that one eye sees one portion of the target while the other sees another part. The Aperture Rule (Fig. 4.1) is a popular vision therapy technique based on the use of an aperture.

Advantages

A moderate variety of targets are available, and more targets can be made by the clinician. Apertures and septums work well to treat patients with shallow to moderate suppression.

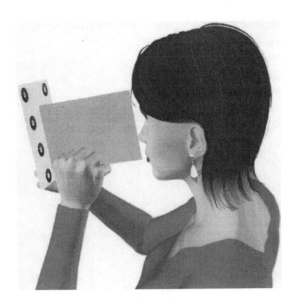

FIG. 4.4. Remy separator.

Disadvantages

It is sometimes difficult to keep a young child's interest with these techniques. Head position is also important with apertures and septums, and the child must sit still and maintain the prescribed head position. The demand of the target cannot be set at zero, forcing the patient to make an initial fusional vergence movement. Because of this, apertures and septums are generally used after anaglyphs, Polaroids, and lenses, prisms, and mirrors.

CATEGORY FOUR: PAPER, PENCIL, AND MISCELLANEOUS TASKS

This category includes training techniques that are printed on paper and designed to train vergence, accommodation, and accurate eye movements. Many of the eye movement tasks are

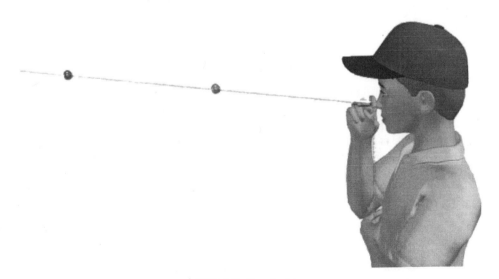

FIG. 4.5. Brock string.

also useful for suppression training when combined with anaglyphs. Another type of technique included in this category is the Brock String (Fig. 4.5). This is a string with beads that is used to take advantage of physiological diplopia.

Advantages

These techniques are generally the least expensive therapy procedures. A sufficient variety of targets are available, and these techniques work well with shallow to moderate suppression. These techniques work especially well for convergence therapy.

Disadvantages

It is difficult to maintain interest in young children.

CATEGORY FIVE: STEREOSCOPES

Stereoscopes are designed on the principle of dividing physical space into two separate areas of visual space, each of which is visible to only one eye. This is accomplished by dissociating the eyes mechanically with a septum (Brewster stereoscopes, Fig. 4.3) or by using two separate viewing tubes or mirrors (Wheatstone stereoscopes, Fig. 4.2). In addition, stereoscopes use lenses and prisms (Brewster stereoscopes) or mirrors (Wheatstone stereoscopes) to allow one to test and train at different simulated distances. In most cases, vision therapy for heterophoric patients can be successfully completed without the use of stereoscopes. Instrument training is useful, however, under the following circumstances:

1. If a patient is experiencing difficulty fusing with techniques from other categories Some patients respond better initially to instrument training techniques that present stimuli under less natural seeing conditions. Although this is unusual and not totally predictable, it is worthwhile to try stereoscopic procedures when a patient is not responding well to free space techniques.

2. After a patient has successfully completed the nonstereoscopic techniques described in Chapters 5 to 7 that are more natural, it is often useful to perform some training with stereoscopes Such training allows considerable flexibility with the type of target used and the distance at which therapy can occur. With conditions such as divergence excess, the most difficult task is a first-degree target at a distance setting. Stereoscopes are well designed to deliver this type of stimulus.

3. Variety is an important consideration in vision therapy The use of stereoscopes is another way to improve fusional ranges and facility. A particularly useful technique, only available with stereoscopes, is called tromboning. Tromboning can be performed with Brewster-type stereoscopes. It is a procedure in which a target is moved toward and then away from the patient. The unique aspect of this technique is that as the target is moved toward the patient, he or she must accommodate to maintain clarity and diverge to maintain fusion. As a target is moved away, the patient must relax accommodation and converge. This, of course, is opposite to that which occurs in the normal seeing environment and is why this procedure is valuable.

Advantages

The primary strengths of this approach for nonstrabismic binocular anomalies are the ability to present a large variety of targets at distance and intermediate settings and the ability to select first, second, and third-degree targets. Stereoscopes can be effective, even in cases of deep suppression.

Disadvantages

The artificial nature of the tasks involved in instrument training is a disadvantage of this approach. Questions have been raised about the transfer of improvements in binocular vision, from the instrument to situations outside the instrument (1).

Stereoscopes are the most expensive vision therapy techniques and they can be heavy and bulky. As a result, many varieties are more appropriate for office therapy than home therapy.

CATEGORY SIX: AFTERIMAGES, ENTOPTIC PHENOMENA, AND ELECTROPHYSIOLOGICAL TECHNIQUES

Techniques in this category are used in the treatment of amblyopia, eccentric fixation, anomalous correspondence, constant strabismus, and nystagmus. Because these topics fall outside the scope of this text, we will not describe the majority of these procedures. Examples of therapy techniques included in this category are devices for creating afterimages, Maxwell's spot, Haidinger's brush, and auditory biofeedback. Afterimages are used occasionally in the treatment of ocular motor dysfunction, and we will describe these procedures.

GENERAL PRINCIPLES AND GUIDELINES FOR VISION THERAPY

Before describing the various categories of vision therapy procedures, it is important to understand that there are general principles and guidelines that apply to all vision therapy techniques and specific principles and guidelines for binocular vision, ocular motility, and accommodative techniques. Vision therapy is similar in many ways to other types of therapy that involve learning and education. If we look at other types of learning, it becomes clear that there are specific guidelines to facilitate learning and success. Since vision therapy can be considered to be a form of learning and education, similar principles and guidelines must be used to achieve success. The following guidelines have been derived from basic learning theory.

General Principles and Guidelines for Vision Therapy

Before beginning vision therapy, follow sequential management considerations (Chapter 3).

When developing the vision therapy program, always consider amblyopia and suppression therapy before beginning fusional vergence therapy.

- Determine a level at which the patient can perform easily.
- Be aware of frustration level.
- Use positive reinforcement.
- Maintain an effective training level.
- Emphasize to the patient that changes must occur within his or her own visual system.
- Make the patient aware of the goals of vision therapy.
- Use vision therapy techniques that provide feedback to the patient.

1. Determine a level at which the patient can perform easily Working on this level makes it easier for the patient to become aware of the important feedback cues, strategies, and objectives involved in vision therapy and also builds confidence and motivation.

2. Be aware of frustration level Signs of frustration include: general nervous and muscular tension, hesitating performance, and possibly a desire to avoid the task.

3. Use positive reinforcement The patient should be rewarded for attempting a task, even if it is not successfully completed. Reinforcers can be verbal praise, tokens that can be exchanged for prizes, or participating in a task that the patient enjoys. Feldman (5) has described, in detail, the various principles of behavior modification applied to optometric vision therapy. It is a valuable reference for clinicians involved with vision therapy.

4. Maintain an effective training level Start at the initial level at which the task is easy and gradually increase the level of difficulty, being very careful to watch for signs of frustration. Vision training should be success oriented; that is, build on what the patient can do successfully, as opposed to giving tasks that are too difficult.

5. Emphasize to the patient that changes must occur within his or her own visual system Birnbaum (6), in defining some of the critical concepts of which the vision therapist must be aware, goes beyond *what* should be done and concentrates on *how* vision therapy should be performed and the role of the vision therapist. This role, according to Birnbaum, is to carefully arrange conditions for learning to occur. His view parallels ours, stressing the use of learning theory principles.

More importantly, and perhaps the key to vision therapy, is teaching the patient to internalize changes in visual function, as opposed to just achieving certain criteria for specific techniques. Often, as patients go through a vision therapy program, they gain the impression that it is the instrumentation, lenses, or prism that affect the change in their visual system. Unless told otherwise, a patient may believe that these external items are the keys to their success in vision therapy.

Birnbaum (6) stresses that "the patient must be made aware that the changes actually occur internally, within the visual system, and not externally in the instruments and paraphernalia utilized in vision therapy." To accomplish this objective, the language used in communication between the optometrist and patient is critical. Birnbaum provides several excellent examples, including the following scenario. When performing a fusional vergence technique, the clinician might say "try and keep the picture single." The problem with this instructional set is that while the patient is asked to try, the instructions are given in terms of what happens to the targets rather than what changes the patient must make internally to achieve the desired result. Birnbaum suggests the following as being a preferable instructional set.

Explain to the patient that if the picture is double, it is because he or she is looking too far or too close in space. In order to make it single, the patient needs to look nearer or farther; the patient needs to make adjustments in him- or herself, in where he or she is pointing his or her eyes in space, and then the picture will become single.

The underlying important concept is that it is not just the specific technique that leads to success in vision therapy. Rather, the key factor is to get the patient to take responsibility for creating internal change.

6. Make the patient aware of the goals of vision therapy The patient must know why he or she is in vision therapy. The patient should be able to explain what his or her problem is, how it affects performance, and the goals of vision therapy. This is true for children as well as adults. Even with a young child, the therapist should try to establish some understanding on the part of the child about what is wrong with his or her eyes and why vision therapy is necessary. For each therapy technique, the child should be able to explain what he or she needs to do to accomplish the desired task.

7. Set realistic therapy objectives and maintain flexibility with these objectives or endpoints With all therapy techniques, there are certain general objectives that we expect to achieve before we proceed to the next procedure. In this text, we call these objectives "endpoints." For instance, in Chapter 5, we recommend ending the Tranaglyph procedure when the patient can fuse to about 30 base-out, and ending accommodative facility when the patient can complete 12 cpm of accommodative facility with +2.00/2.00 lenses using a 20/30 target.

It is important to understand that these endpoints are only guidelines and that flexibility and clinical judgment are ultimately just as important in deciding when to move on to another procedure. The objective of vision therapy is to solve the patient's problems as quickly as possible. If a patient can only achieve 25 base-out with the Tranaglyph procedure, in spite of sufficient effort, it makes sense to move on and try another technique.

8. Use vision therapy techniques that provide feedback to the patient All therapy and teaching progresses more effectively when feedback about performance is available to the student or patient. The various feedback mechanisms used in vision therapy include:

1. Diplopia
2. Blur
3. Suppression
4. Luster
5. Kinesthetic awareness
6. Small In, Large Out (SILO)
7. Float
8. Localization
9. Parallax

Description of Feedback Mechanisms Used in Vision Therapy

Diplopia

Diplopia is a powerful feedback cue and relatively easy to explain to a patient. If a patient experiences diplopia during a therapy procedure, he or she receives immediate feedback that he or she is not aligning his or her eyes appropriately. It is important to try and provide the patient with methods of overcoming diplopia. These methods are discussed below.

Blur

Explain to the patient that blur represents feedback that the focusing system is either overfocusing or underfocusing. As the patient gains control over the accommodative system, he or she should be able to make the necessary changes in accommodation to overcome blur.

Suppression

Suppression is also an easy feedback mechanism to demonstrate and explain to patients. Virtually all binocular vision therapy procedures contain elements in the targets that can be used to monitor suppression. For example, there is often a letter "R" and a letter "L" printed on vergence therapy techniques. The "R" is seen only by the right eye and the "L" only by the left eye. If one of these letters is not seen by the patient, he or she receives feedback about suppression. Other techniques use different stimuli, such as a dot, cross, or a vertical or horizontal line, to help monitor suppression. In all cases, the clinician should identify what the suppression cues are for a given therapy technique and utilize these cues to make the patient aware of suppression.

Luster

Luster is the perception of the combination of colors seen when the patient is asked to fuse targets of different colors. Sometimes patients also report a shimmering effect when they fuse targets of different colors. Vision therapy procedures using red and green targets lead to this perception of luster. The clinician should make the patient aware that the fused image is a mixture of the two colors. The absence of luster is clinically significant. For example, if the patient sees only red or only green, it is one indication that he or she may be suppressing.

Kinesthetic Awareness

A common theme throughout all vision therapy techniques for accommodation and binocular vision is stressing an awareness of the sensation of accommodating or converging. We want the patient to be able to feel the difference between stimulating and relaxing accommodation and the difference between converging and diverging. When performing any technique, ask the patient to explain what he or she is feeling. "Does it feel like you are straining or relaxing your eyes? Does it feel like you are looking close and crossing your eyes or looking far and relaxing your eyes?" Therapy will often progress considerably faster if the patient is able to develop this awareness.

"Small In Large Out" Response

"Small In Large Out" Response Associated with Vergence

The term SILO is an acronym for **S**mall **I**n **L**arge **O**ut. It refers to the fact that as a patient is asked to maintain fusion while divergence or convergence demand is varied, he or she will experience perceptual changes. Specifically, as the convergence demand is increased and the patient maintains fusion, the target may appear to become smaller and move closer or in toward the patient. This is the "SI" of the acronym SILO and stands for **S**mall and **I**n. Conversely, as the divergence demand is increased and the patient maintains fusion, the target may appear to become larger and move farther away or out. This is the "LO" of the acronym SILO and stands for **L**arge and **O**ut.

The underlying basis for the SILO phenomenon is size constancy. Leibowitz et al. (7) and Leibowitz and Moore (8) studied the role of accommodation and convergence in the size constancy phenomenon and their findings offer one explanation for the SILO phenomenon. The authors noted that as one's gaze shifts from a far to a near object, accommodative and convergence changes must occur for the observer to maintain clear single vision. They found that the initiation of these accommodative and convergence movements is coupled with an expectation that this action will be accompanied by an alteration in retinal image size. Anticipating such a change, the patient corrects for it and thereby maintains size constancy.

According to this theory, when an observer accommodates and converges as an object approaches, the retinal image size increases. The perceptual system, therefore, must make a correction to maintain size constancy and shrink the size of the image. As an object is moved farther away, the retinal image size decreases and the perceptual system must expand the image. With vision therapy techniques under consideration here, the important difference is that the retinal image size is never changing while accommodative and convergence changes occur. Therefore, the shrinkage adjustment of the perceptual size constancy system normally associated with convergence and accommodation leads to a perception that the object is becoming smaller. Similarly, the normal expansion adjustment associated with a relaxation

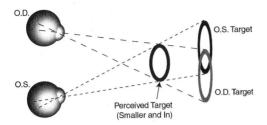

FIG. 4.6. Geometric explanation for the "Small In, Large Out" phenomenon. The illustration demonstrates that the fused target would appear to be smaller and closer than either of the real targets during a base-out fusion technique.

of accommodation leads to a perception that the object is becoming larger with divergence techniques. Thus, the perceived size change is directly related to accommodative and vergence changes.

In regard to the apparent distance changes, subjects give variable responses. Some report that the object becomes smaller as it moves closer (SILO). Others report that the image becomes smaller and moves farther away or out (SOLI) (Small Out Large In). These different responses can be explained, if we assume that individuals use different cues for distance perception. The first possibility is that an individual uses vergence as a cue for his perception of distance. This person perceives the object to be moving closer because he or she is converging and he or she "knows," from previous experience, that when he or she converges, it means he or she is looking at an object moving closer. Conversely, when the person diverges, he or she "knows," from prior experience, that the object must be moving away.

Those that do not use vergence as a cue to perceive distance probably use apparent size as a cue. An individual using apparent size as a cue would be expected to report SOLI. For example, as the person converges using a vectogram target, he or she will perceive the target becoming smaller, based on Leibowitz's study. Since the target is becoming smaller, the person perceives the target as moving out or farther away. The person perceives things this way because, from previous experience, as a target becomes smaller, it generally means it is moving away.

There is also a geometric explanation for the SILO phenomenon. Figures 4.4 and 4.5 illustrate the expected response for a convergence and divergence demand in fusional vergence therapy technique. In Fig. 4.6, the right eye is viewing the left target and the left eye is viewing the right target. The visual axes cross between the patient's eyes and the targets and represent the location in space at which the patient perceives the fused target. Thus, the target will appear to move closer or in. The illustration also demonstrates that the fused target would appear to be smaller than either of the real targets. Figure 4.7 is a geometric explanation for a patient's perception of larger and out during a divergence task. In this illustration, the right eye is viewing the right target and the left eye, the left target. The fused image is perceived where the visual axes cross, which is beyond the plane of the targets. The fused target is, therefore, perceived as farther away and as Fig. 4.7 illustrates, larger.

"Small In Large Out" Response Associated with Lenses

When an individual accommodates through plus or minus lenses, perceptual changes in the apparent size and distance of the object occur similar to those described above. The reasons for these perceived changes, however, must be different because with lenses, the retinal image size *does* change, whereas with vergence, the retinal image size remains constant. Minus lenses cause minification of the retinal image and plus lenses cause magnification.

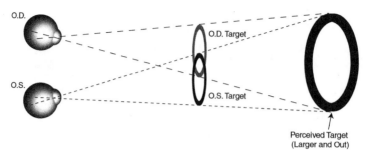

O.D.

O.D. Target

O.S.

O.S. Target

Perceived Target
(Larger and Out)

FIG. 4.7. Geometric explanation for the "Small In, Large Out" phenomenon. The illustration demonstrates that the fused target would appear to be larger and farther away during a base in fusion technique.

A possible explanation for perceptual changes that occur with lenses is that minus lenses minify the retinal image and cause the response of "smaller," while plus lenses magnify the retinal image and lead to the response of "larger." Based on the perceived change in size, the patient says "the target is smaller, therefore, it must be farther away" with minus lenses and "the target is larger, therefore, it must be closer." This would be a SOLI response and is actually the expected finding with lenses.

Clinical Relevance of "Small In Large Out" Response

It is apparent from the literature and clinical experience that SILO is not the only normal or expected response to vergence or accommodative techniques. This is particularly true with lenses.

A response of SOLI is not necessarily an indication of a binocular or accommodative problem. Rather, it is a reflection of the individual's perceptual style and attention to visual stimuli. While the appreciation of the object becoming smaller with convergence demand and minus and larger with divergence and plus seems to be almost universal, the perception of the distance change is by no means predictable. From clinical experience, we have found that adults are more likely to respond with SOLI than SILO. A possible explanation for this is that adults are more likely to respond with "what they know" should occur as a target becomes smaller and to report that the object must be moving away from them. Children tend to be less rigid in their perceptions and will respond with "what they see"; the object is becoming smaller and moving closer.

It is important to remember that the main value of the SILO phenomenon is to provide feedback to the patient about his or her performance. As long as a consistent pattern can be established, the feedback is useful. Thus, if a patient consistently feels that with increasing convergence demand the target appears to become smaller and move away, this will still represent a useful feedback technique for this patient.

It is desirable, however, to spend some time initially with the patient to try and make him or her more aware of "what he or she is seeing" and try and elicit a SILO response. The reason for the desirability of a SILO response is that it helps the therapist create an awareness on the part of the patient of what is occurring during the therapy procedure. For example, if we are performing a convergence technique, it is helpful to be able to establish that the patient must cross his or her eyes and look closer as the targets are separated. If the patient perceives that the target is becoming smaller and moving closer, this reinforces the concept of looking closer and crossing the eyes. If a patient experiences SILO, the therapist can say the following.

Do you see how the target appears to become closer and smaller as we separate the targets? This is feedback for you about what your eyes are doing during this task. The target looks like it is moving closer to you because you are looking closer as the task becomes more difficult.

If a SILO response cannot be elicited, the clinician has to use other feedback cues to establish the concept of looking close.

Float

Float refers to the perception that a target is "floating closer or farther away" as the demand is changed from convergence to divergence during vergence therapy. With convergence, the target should appear to float closer and with divergence, farther away. This perception is actually part of the SILO phenomenon. As discussed previously, not all patients see the target moving closer with convergence or farther with divergence. If this response can be elicited, it becomes a very helpful feedback cue that can be used by the therapist to establish the concept of looking closer during convergence and farther during divergence therapy.

Localization

Localization is one of the more valuable feedback cues available for vergence therapy. It refers to the ability of the patient to point to where the target appears to be when fusion occurs and is based on the concept of physiological diplopia. Figure 4.6 illustrates the concept of localization. In Fig. 4.8, the patient is working with a Quoit Vectogram and is fusing with a convergence demand. The visual axes cross before the targets and the patient should perceive the target as smaller and closer. The patient is now asked to pick up a pointer and point to where he or she sees the target "floating." The objective is for the patient to point to the target and perceive one target and one pointer.

If the patient places the pointer in the general area of where his or her visual axes cross, he or she will perceive one target and one pointer. If the patient points closer or farther away than the intersection of his or her visual axes, he or she will report diplopia of either the target or the pointer. The importance of localization is that it allows the patient to develop an understanding of what changes must occur within his or her visual system to accomplish the therapy task. If the patient can localize the target, he or she will begin to understand that, when the targets are separated to create a convergence demand, he or she must look closer and cross his or her eyes to maintain single vision and fusion. We cannot overemphasize the importance of the patient

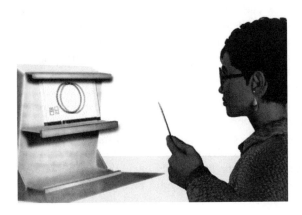

FIG. 4.8. Patient working with a Quoit Vectogram is fusing with a convergence demand. Patient points to where she sees the target.

developing this understanding of what changes he or she must make to accomplish a particular task.

Often when a patient is first asked to try and localize during convergence therapy, he or she experiences difficulty. At first, the patient may tend to point to the actual plane of the target, rather than the intersection of the visual axes. It is useful to state:

We both know that the targets are back there, but what I want you to do is to try and get the feeling of where you are looking and where the target is floating.

If the patient continues to have problems localizing, the next step is to make him or her aware of the concept of physiological diplopia and to use this phenomenon to get the patient started. The explanation we use with patients is as follows.

"The way the visual system works is that whatever object we are directly viewing is seen as one, while all other objects are seen as double." It is then useful to demonstrate this by having the patient look at a pointer while you hold another object in the background. Have the patient experiment with this concept for several minutes until he or she is comfortable with this idea and is satisfied that he or she can experience physiological diplopia. Demonstrate that when the more distant object (seen as two) is moved closer to the fixation object, it will also be seen singly when it is in approximately the same position in space. If the patient now understands the concept that we experience single vision if we point to where the eyes are looking, the idea can be applied to vision therapy techniques. For example, assume the patient is fusing a Quoit Vectogram using positive fusional vergence. We ask the patient to localize and point to where he perceives the Quoit. The patient, however, points too far away and experiences diplopia. If the patient understands the concept of physiological diplopia, we would say the following:

This time I want you to hold the pointer at the slides and look directly at the pointer. Do not try to keep the ropes single. If you look at the pointer, while you do so, you will see two ropes in the background. Now slowly move the pointer toward yourself, always looking directly at the pointer and being aware of the two ropes. As you do this, you will notice that, as you move the pointer toward yourself, the two ropes appear to move closer to one another. Continue moving the pointer toward yourself very slowly and you will notice that, at some distance, you will see one pointer and one set of ropes. This is where you must look to accomplish this task. Do you feel yourself looking closer? Try and get the feeling of where you have to look. Can you now understand where you have to look to see one rope? Can you see that the rope is floating closer?

Generally the patient continues to be unable to simply pick up the pointer and immediately localize correctly. However, with repetition, most patients will soon understand what they must do visually during convergence therapy. Once they grasp this concept, the rest of therapy is simplified.

Localization is a very powerful feedback cue for convergence therapy. With divergence therapy, it is more difficult to use, but it can still be an important aid to therapy. The primary difficulty with divergence is that as the fusional vergence demand increases, the object floats farther away from the patient and the patient can no longer point to it because it is too far away to physically reach with a pointer. Another problem is that depending on the target being used, the patient must visualize an object moving farther away, passing through an opaque background. For example, if we are using a vectogram such as Quoits, with the Polachrome Illuminated Trainer (Fig. 4.9), the patient would be asked to visualize the rope floating behind the white stand. The ability of people to visualize varies greatly, and an inability to do so interferes with the use of localization for divergence therapy.

This second problem is rather simple to overcome and merely involves selecting targets that are printed on clear plastic, such as Vectograms, Tranaglyphs, Free Space Circles, and

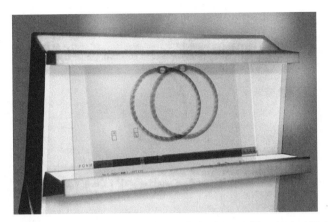

FIG. 4.9. Quoit Vectogram setup in the Polachrome Illuminated Trainer.

Eccentric Circles (Fig. 4.10). In addition, if the targets are to be placed in a holder, the holder should also be transparent, like the one illustrated in Fig. 4.10.

The first problem, not being able to point to the target as the divergence demand increases, can also be overcome. The following divergence therapy procedure is a very powerful training technique and, in most instances, will lead to excellent progress with divergence therapy. The patient is asked to stand several feet in front of a ball that has been suspended from the ceiling (Fig. 4.11A,B). The height of this ball should be adjustable to permit the therapist to change the height so that it is at eye level for any given patient. A Quoit Vectogram is placed in a clear holder, and the patient is instructed to hold the target at arm's length so that he or she can see the ball in the background, directly in the center of the Quoit. As the Quoit targets are slowly separated to create a divergence demand, the patient is asked to maintain fusion and describe where the target is floating. At this point, the therapist pushes the ball to create motion in an arc moving toward and away from the patient. The patient should perceive that the ball is moving in front and behind the Quoit, which itself appears to be floating behind the plane of the actual Vectogram targets. As the targets are separated, the patient will have to continue moving backward to keep the Quoit floating out at the point at which the ball just swings in front of and behind the Quoit. Once appreciated, this is quite a startling experience for the patient and provides the feedback necessary for him or her to understand that, when fusing during divergence therapy, he or she has to relax his or her eyes as if something is moving farther away.

Parallax

Parallax refers to the appreciation of movement of the fused target as the patient moves. Specifically, if a patient is fusing a target set for convergence and moves to the right, he or she should see the target move to the right. With a convergence demand, the target moves in the same direction as the patient. With divergence, the target should appear to move in the direction opposite to the patient's movement. Thus, if a patient is working in the divergence direction and moves to the left, the target should appear to move to the right. If the same patient moves away from the target by taking two steps backward, the target should appear to move away from him or her.

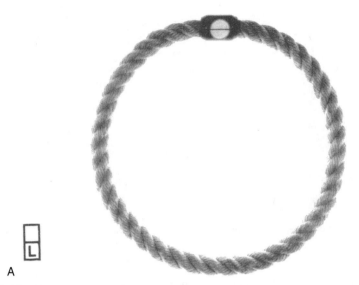

A

FIG. 4.10. Selected targets that are printed on clear plastic: **(A)** Quoit Vectogram; **(B)** Tranaglyph; **(C)** Free Space Fusion Cards and Lifesaver Cards; **(D)** Eccentric Circles.

Knowledge of parallax can be used by the therapist as an aid to monitoring the responses of a young child. The therapist can periodically ask the child to move right to left and back and forth and question the child about movement of the target. For the older patient, parallax becomes another feedback cue that can be used to provide information about whether the patient is accomplishing the desired task.

BINOCULAR VISION THERAPY: UNDERLYING CONCEPTS

There are several basic underlying concepts shared by all binocular vision therapy techniques. To increase fusional vergence ranges, a technique must do one of two things—either maintain accommodation at the plane of regard and change the stimulus to the vergence system or maintain vergence at the plane of regard and change the stimulus to accommodation. The most common approach used in binocular vision therapy techniques is to maintain accommodation at the plane of regard, which is generally 40 cm from the patient. While the patient keeps the target clear, the vergence demand is altered. With convergence, the plane of vergence is moved toward the patient and with divergence, the plane of vergence is moved beyond the plane of accommodation. The greater the separation between the plane of accommodation and the plane of vergence, the greater the demand on the fusional vergence system.

These concepts are illustrated in Figs. 4.12 and 4.13. An example of this type of procedure would be to ask a patient to fixate on a 20/30 letter held at 40 cm and maintain clear and single vision while you gradually increase the convergence demand. To maintain clarity, the patient must maintain accommodation at 40 cm. To maintain single binocular vision, the patient must converge as the base-out prism is added. The only way to converge while accommodation is held constant is to use positive fusional vergence (PFV). The important concept to remember is that by forcing the patient to hold accommodation steady, accommodative convergence is also inhibited and the patient must use fusional vergence or will experience diplopia. Forcing the use of fusional vergence by controlling accommodation is the basis of many binocular vision therapy techniques.

Endpoint

Discontinue this therapy technique when the patient is able to successfully achieve clear single binocular vision with all 12 cards with convergence, and card 6 with divergence.

Modified Remy Separator

Objective

The objectives of the modified Remy separator are identical to those listed for the Aperture Rule.

Equipment Needed

1. Septum made from cardboard.
2. Lifesaver cards,[c] Free Space Fusion Cards A,[a] or B or stereograms.[a,c]

Construction and Description

The modified Remy separator is based on the principle of a Remy separator. The Remy separator is a vision therapy device that uses a septum. Because of the physical setup of the instrument, its primary value is for divergence therapy. Unless auxiliary base-out prism is used, Remy separator-type instruments only present a divergence demand. The amount of divergence demand can be calculated, based on the formula presented earlier in this chapter, for the Aperture Rule. For example, if the targets are separated by 40 mm, the divergence demand is 10 base-in (4 mm = 1 Δ at 40 cm). The base-in demand is increased by separating the targets and decreased by moving them closer together. The two principal companies that manufacture vision therapy equipment in the United States do not currently produce a Remy separator. This instrument can be purchased from European companies.

It is possible, however, to easily make a Remy separator by using stereogram targets or Free Space Fusion Cards A and B or Lifesaver cards (Fig. 5.14), along with a septum. Simply cut a septum from cardboard, making sure that the length of the septum is 40 cm, and place the septum against the stereogram or other target.

Therapy Procedures with the Modified Remy Separator

The modified Remy separator is used for divergence therapy. Because the patient must make a step vergence change, this technique is more difficult than variable Tranaglyphs or Vectograms. For some patients, it may be easier than working with Eccentric Circles or Free Space Fusion Cards B. The main difference between the modified Remy separator and Eccentric Circles or Free Space Fusion Cards A is that the septum eliminates the annoying two side images that are perceived with the Eccentric Circles and Free Space Fusion Cards.

This technique is useful for home therapy after the patient has already made some progress in vision therapy and has successfully begun to use the Aperture Rule for divergence therapy. If the patient experiences any difficulty, plus lenses are helpful to get started. Have the patient attempt to fuse the targets and hold fusion for 10 seconds, then look away and regain fusion.

As the patient progresses, reduce the amount of plus. The divergence demand can also be increased by separating the targets, adding minus lenses, or base-in prism. The divergence

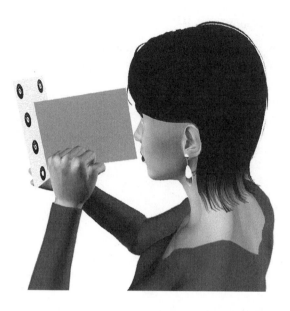

FIG. 5.14. Modified Remy separator using a septum and Lifesaver Card.

demand can be decreased by moving the targets together, using plus lenses, and base-out prism.

Endpoint

Discontinue this technique when the patient can achieve fusion with a divergence demand of about 15 base-in.

FUSIONAL VERGENCE PROCEDURES (PAPER, PENCIL, AND MISCELLANEOUS TASKS)

Eccentric Circles[c]/Free Space Fusion Cards[a]

Objective

The objectives of Eccentric Circles and Free Space Fusion Cards A are identical to those listed on page 176.

Equipment Needed

1. Keystone Opaque Eccentric Circles.[c]
2. Keystone Transparent Eccentric Circles.[c]
3. Bernell Opaque Free Space Fusion Cards A.[a]
4. Bernell Transparent Free Space Fusion Cards A.[a]
5. Flip lenses.[a,b]
6. Flip prism.[a,b]
7. Pointer.

Description and Setup

This is another free space, chiastopic, or orthopic technique. Prisms, lenses, or glasses are not required. Rather, the patient fuses by converging in front of the plane of accommodation

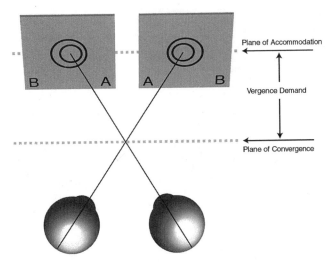

FIG. 5.15. Eccentric Circles setup for convergence therapy, illustrating planes of accommodation and vergence.

(chiastopic) or diverging beyond the plane of accommodation (orthopic). Figure 5.15 illustrates the Eccentric Circle setup and the location of the planes of accommodation and vergence when the patient is converging. During convergence (Fig. 5.15), accommodation is approximately at the cards, while vergence is in front of the cards. With divergence, accommodation is still approximately at the plane of the cards, while vergence is behind the cards. The cards present a third-degree fusion (stereopsis) target. Each card also contains antisuppression cues and accommodative controls.

If one compares this procedure to the Aperture Rule technique, it should be clear that both procedures are based on the same principle. Both are examples of chiastopic/orthopic fusion. When the patient is working with the Eccentric Circles and Free Space Fusion Cards A with convergence, the right eye views the left card and the left eye views the right card. While the right eye fixates the left target, the image of the right card is projected on the nasal retina of the right eye. The right eye, therefore, will perceive two targets. The same is true of the left eye. The left eye fixates the right target and the left card image is projected on the nasal retina of the left eye. When the patient converges to the appropriate plane, the two middle images will overlap and the patient will achieve chiastopic fusion. However, he or she will also perceive two other targets: one to the left and one to the right of the "fused" target. Because of the eccentricity of the inner circles on the cards, retinal disparity will be created and the patient should perceive stereopsis or an impression of depth.

For convergence therapy, the Eccentric Circles and Free Space Fusion Cards A may be more difficult initially than the Aperture Rule for a patient because, when fused properly, the patient sees three sets of circles rather than one set. For divergence therapy, the Eccentric Circles and Free Space Fusion Cards A are usually easier than the Aperture Rule for the patient because they are transparent and allow the patient to look through the target. The only difference between the Aperture Rule and Free Space Fusion Cards A is the single or double aperture, which serves to eliminate the annoying two side images.

One of the more common misconceptions about the Eccentric Circles is that the letters "A" and "B" printed on the bottom of the cards represent the method of changing the task from convergence to divergence. It is incorrect to think that holding the cards with the "A's" together

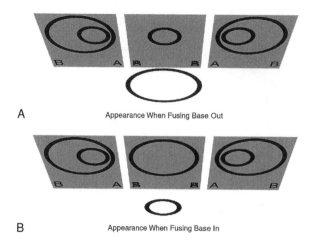

A   Appearance When Fusing Base Out

B   Appearance When Fusing Base In

FIG. 5.16. A: Patient's perception of Eccentric Circles setup with the "A's" during chiastopic fusion. The outer rings appear to be floating closer. **B:** Patient's perception of Eccentric Circles setup with the "A's" during orthopic fusion. The inner rings appear to be floating closer.

is a convergence task and, with the "B's" together, a divergence task. An understanding of the underlying principles of the task dispels this idea. The "A" and "B" markings are simply present to help the therapist monitor the patient's responses. When the cards are held with the "A's" together and the patient is fusing base-out, he or she should perceive the outer circle floating closer (Fig. 5.16A). When fusing with a divergence demand with the "A's" together, the patient will perceive the inner circle floating closer. This perception of stereopsis or float will be exactly the opposite when the cards are held with the "B's" together (Fig. 5.16B). Thus, the target is used for divergence or convergence training. The only variable is what the patient does with his or her eyes.

Unlike the other binocular vision training procedures discussed previously, with the Eccentric Circles and Free Space Fusion Cards A, there is no scale to indicate the prismatic demand. Rather, the therapist must use the formula discussed earlier in this chapter to determine the prismatic demand at a given separation of the cards. The demand at any separation will depend on the working distance and the distance between similar points on the two cards. For example, if the cards are held at a working distance of 40 cm and separated by 12 cm, the demand would be 30Δ (at 40 cm, 4 mm = 1 Δ).

Sequentially, the Eccentric Circles and Free Space Fusion Cards are often used after a patient successfully completes the variable Tranaglyphs, nonvariable Tranaglyphs, and Aperture Rule procedures. There are patients, however, that are able to work with these procedures, even in the early stages of treatment. In fact, many patients find the Eccentric Circles and Free Space Cards easier than the Aperture Rule, particularly with divergence therapy. It is important to be flexible when implementing a vision therapy program. We have proposed a specific sequence, in Chapters 8 to 12, but other sequences may work as well in specific cases. Also, it is important to keep in mind that an objective of vision therapy is to successfully complete the treatment as quickly as possible. Thus, if a patient can easily accomplish one of the procedures in the recommended sequence, it should be skipped. The clinician should use the sequence suggested in this chapter as a guide only. The objective is to empirically find procedures that the patient can barely perform and skip those that are easy.

If the Eccentric Circles and Free Space Fusion Cards A are introduced toward the end of the therapy program, it is usually rather simple to teach the patient to fuse them. By this time, the patient is so familiar with all of the methods used previously to help him or her fuse during convergence and divergence therapy, that he or she is often able to apply these skills to any new technique.

Therapy Procedures with Eccentric Circles/Free Space Fusion Cards A

Either have the patient hold the cards or place them in the Polachrome Illuminated Trainer, the horizontal holder, or any other suitable device. The cards should be held about 40 cm from the patient. Begin with the two cards together, with the "A's" touching. The patient should see two cards at this point. Now ask the patient to try and cross his or her eyes and get the feeling of looking closer. If the patient cannot do this voluntarily, use localization with a pointer to demonstrate the point to which he or she must converge to achieve fusion. Tell the patient that when he or she achieves fusion, he or she will see "three sets of circles." Explain that the patient is to concentrate only on the middle set and is to ignore the two side images. Ask the patient about the middle set of cards. The patient should be able to spontaneously indicate that he or she sees two circles, one larger than the other and that the larger one appears to be floating closer to him or her. In addition, the patient should see the word "clear," in focus. If he or she does not spontaneously respond with this information, ask leading questions to elicit this information. It is important to make the patient aware that this perception of depth is a feedback cue to him or her about his or her performance. If the patient is successfully performing chiastopic fusion with the "A's" together, the larger ring will appear to float closer.

Once the patient can achieve fusion, ask him or her to hold the position for 10 seconds, look away momentarily, and look back at the cards and regain fusion. Instruct the patient to repeat this 10 times and then separate the cards about 1 cm and repeat the entire procedure. Continue until the patient is able to achieve fusion and look away and back with the cards separated about 12 cm.

Another procedure that can be performed with the Eccentric Circles and Free Space Fusion Cards A is to have the patient use two or more sets of the cards. The cards should be placed in different positions of gaze and the patient must alternately look from one position of gaze to another and fuse the cards. You can instruct the patient to first perform orthopic and then chiastopic fusion as he or she changes fixation from one set of cards to the other. The objective of this procedure is to combine vergence training with saccades. This tends to make the task more comparable to real seeing conditions.

The same general procedures are performed for divergence therapy, except that the patient must now diverge behind the plane of the cards. Because it is difficult for some patients to visualize looking behind an opaque object, translucent Eccentric Circle cards are available for divergence therapy. Patients often initially experience some difficulty with this procedure. It is helpful to show them where they must look to achieve orthopic fusion. To accomplish this, tape a pointer to the wall at the patient's eye level. Have the patient stand about 3 to 4 ft away from the wall and hold the translucent Eccentric Circle cards about 25 cm away from his or her eyes. Instruct the patient to look at the pointer on the wall and, while doing so, to be aware of the circles. The patient should be able to see three sets of circles. If the patient cannot, have him or her walk 6 in. closer or farther away, until he or she does appreciate three circles. Tell the patient to concentrate on the middle set and ignore the side images. Once the patient can achieve this, have him or her repeat the same procedures described for convergence therapy. The only difference is that because of the lower physiological limit for divergence, the final separation will be smaller. Fusion with a 6 to 8 cm separation is considered adequate.

The final task is to instruct the patient to achieve clear chiastopic fusion, hold it for 10 seconds, and then switch to clear orthopic fusion and hold it for 10 seconds. Instruct the patient to continue alternating back and forth for several minutes. The objective is for the patient to be able to achieve 20 cpm of alternation with the cards separated to the maximum level possible for the patient. This maximum separation is dependent on the size and direction of the phoria, the AC/A ratio, and the working distance.

Other therapy procedures, important factors to be considered, and methods of increasing and decreasing the demand are similar to those listed in Tables 5.2, 5.3, and 5.4.

Endpoint

Discontinue this therapy technique when the patient is able to:

1. Successfully achieve clear chiastopic fusion with a card separation of 12 cm and clear orthopic fusion with a card separation of 6 cm. These are only guidelines, and it is important to be flexible and realize that the final endpoint for any given patient will be dependent on the size and direction of the phoria, the AC/A ratio, and the working distance.
2. Switch between chiastopic and orthopic fusion with the cards held 6 cm apart, 20 cpm.
3. Maintain chiastopic and orthopic fusion with a card separation of 6 cm, while moving the cards laterally or in a circular fashion.

Lifesaver Cards/Free Space Fusion Cards B

Objective

The objectives of Lifesaver Cards and Free Space Fusion Cards B are the same as those for the Aperture Rule (see p. 164).

Equipment Needed

1. Keystone Opaque Lifesaver Cards.[c]
2. Keystone Transparent Lifesaver Cards.[c]
3. Bernell Opaque Free Space Fusion Cards B.[a]
4. Bernell Transparent Free Space Cards B.[a]
5. Flip lenses.[a,b]
6. Flip prism.[a,b]
7. Pointer.

Description and Setup

Lifesaver Cards and Free Space Fusion Cards B are essentially identical to the Eccentric Circles and Free Space Fusion Cards A. The only significant difference is that instead of altering the demand by increasing the separation of the cards, various target separations are preprinted on the cards (Fig. 5.17).

Therapy Procedure

When performing convergence therapy with the Lifesaver Cards and Free Space Fusion Cards B, the patient is asked to fuse the bottom target, which has the least demand, hold it for 10 seconds, and then jump to the next target and fuse. This is repeated for all of the targets on the card for several minutes at a time. To work with divergence therapy, the clear cards are generally used. If the patient experiences difficulty with either chiastopic or orthopic fusion, use the procedures discussed for the Eccentric Circles and Free Space Fusion Cards A to assist him or her.

Other therapy procedures, important factors to consider, and methods of increasing and decreasing the demand are similar to those listed in Tables 5.2, 5.3, and 5.4.

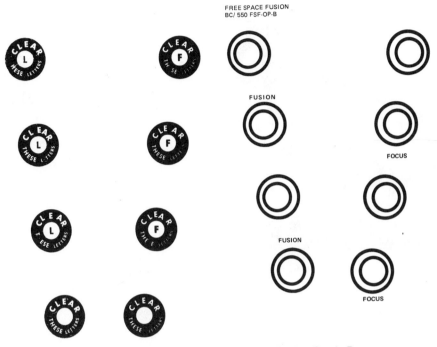

FIG. 5.17. Lifesaver and Free Space Fusion Cards B.

Endpoint

Discontinue this therapy technique when the patient is able to:

1. Successfully achieve clear chiastopic and orthopic fusion with all of the targets on the Lifesaver Cards and Free Space Fusion Cards B.
2. Switch between chiastopic and orthopic fusion with all of the targets on the Lifesaver Cards and Free Space Fusion Cards B.
3. Maintain chiastopic and orthopic fusion with all targets on the Lifesaver Cards and Free Space Fusion Cards B, while moving the cards laterally or in a circular fashion.

FUSIONAL VERGENCE PROCEDURES (STEREOSCOPES) PROCEDURES

Brewster Stereoscopes

Objective

The objectives of Brewster-type stereoscopes are similar to those listed below:

Binocular Vision Therapy Objectives

1. Increase the amplitude of NFV and PFV.
2. Decrease the latency of the fusional vergence response.
3. Increase the velocity of the fusional vergence response.

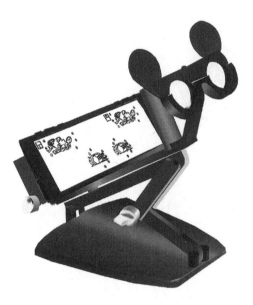

FIG. 5.18. Bernell-O-Scope.

Equipment Needed

1. Keystone stereoscope.[c]
2. Bernell-O-Scope.[a]
3. Bernell Variable Prismatic Trainer.[a]
4. Stereoscopic cards
   (a) Bioptograms.[a]
   (b) Bernell prism base-in/base-out slides.[a]
   (c) Keystone AN Series.[c]
   (d) Keystone BU Series.[c]
   (e) Other.
5. Flip lenses.[a,b]
6. Flip prisms.[a,b]
7. Pointer.

Construction and Description

A Brewster-type stereoscope is a device designed to separate the fields of the two eyes using a septum (Fig. 5.18). The optical system consists of +5.00 D spheres. The optical centers are usually separated by 95 mm, which induces base-out prism because of the wider separation than the average patient interpupillary distance. Stereoscope targets can be placed at varying distances from a distance setting (20 cm if lenses are 5 D) to any near point setting. The therapist, therefore, is able to vary both the accommodative demand and convergence demand.

Different targets are currently produced by Keystone and Bernell (Fig. 5.19). There are numerous series of cards designed to:

Create convergence and divergence therapy demand
Create jump vergence demand
Allow for eye–hand coordination techniques
Permit accommodative training

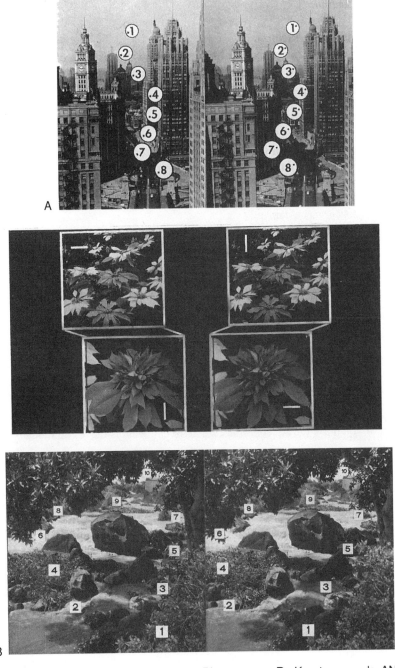

FIG. 5.19. Sample stereograms. **A:** Base-out Bioptograms. **B:** Keystone cards AN 9 and AN 77.

Permit antisuppression training
Present first-, second-, and third-degree fusion targets.

Specific cards are selected, based on the patient's condition and the specific objectives of the therapy program. For instance, in the early stages of therapy for a divergence excess patient, third-degree targets would be selected. As therapy progresses, the objective would be to move from third-degree to second-degree to first-degree cards. The working distance selected is also dependent on the patient's specific problem. With a divergence excess patient, we begin training at a near point setting and move towards a distance setting as therapy progresses.

Determination of Accommodative and Convergence Demands at Different Settings

When using a Brewster-type stereoscope, it is important to be able to determine the accommodative and convergence demands.

Accommodative Demand

Since the power of the stereoscope lenses is known and the distance of the target from the lens plane is known, one can easily calculate the accommodative demand, using the following formula:

$$A = (1/TD) - P$$

where A = accommodation (D)
   TD = distance between target and lens plane (m)
     P = power of stereoscope lenses (D)

Example: You are working with a stereoscope with +5.00 D lenses and a 95 mm lens separation. If you place the stereoscopic card at 20 cm, what is the accommodative demand?
Answer:

$$A = (1/TD) - P$$
$$A = (1/.2) - 5$$
$$A = 5 - 5 = 0$$

At a working distance of 20 cm, there is no accommodative demand. This is the distance setting for this particular stereoscope.
Example: If the target is now moved to a working distance of 13 cm, what is the accommodative demand?
Answer:

$$A = (1/TD) - P$$
$$A = (1/.13) - 5 = 7.6 - 5 = 2.6D$$

At a working distance of 13 cm, the accommodative demand is about 2.6 D.

Convergence Demand

Flax (13) presented formulas that are applicable to any Brewster-type stereoscope and permit rapid calculation of the vergence demand in a manner simple enough for routine clinical application. The formula is also independent of the patient's interpupillary separation.

$$C = (P \times LS) - (TS/TD)$$

C = Vergence demand in prism diopters
P = power of stereoscope lenses
LS = separation of optical centers of stereoscope lenses (cm)
TD = distance of stereogram from stereoscope lenses (m)
TS = separation of corresponding points of the stereogram (cm)

Plus values represent a convergence demand and minus values a divergence demand. One of the reasons this formula is simple to use is because part of the equation, (P × LS), becomes a constant value when using a specific instrument with a fixed lens separation. Thus, as long as you use the same instrument this part of the equation is a given.

Example: You are working with a stereoscope with +5.00 D lenses and a 95 mm lens separation. What is the vergence demand for a 60 mm target set at 20 cm?

Answer:

$$C = (P \times LS) - (TS/TD)$$

$$C = (5 \times 9.5) - (6.0/.2) = 47.5 - 30 = 17.5 \text{ base-out}$$

Example: If you use the same stereoscope as the previous example and the same card now set at a working distance of 13 cm, what is the vergence demand?

Answer:

$$C = (P \times LS) - (TS/TD)$$

$$C = 47.5 - 6.0/.13 = 47.5 - 46.0 = 1.5 \text{ base-out}$$

Therapy Procedures with the Brewster Stereoscope

When training, nonstrabismic binocular vision disorders stereoscopes are generally used only toward the middle to the end of the therapy program. By the time these instruments are introduced, the patient has a good kinesthetic awareness of converging and diverging and has reasonably well-developed fusional vergence ranges. Stereoscopes are used to move the patient to a slightly higher level by challenging him or her with different types of targets in a less natural setting. They are also used to provide a greater variety of techniques and maintain a high level of interest and motivation for the patient.

The specific stereoscope card and working distance are selected, based on the vision disorder being treated and the objectives of therapy. Instruct the patient to look into the stereoscope and to describe what he or she sees. You want the patient to report if the target is clear, single, and to describe any depth he or she sees. Many of the cards have a series of letters or numbers, each of which has a different disparity. Ask the patient to change fixation from one number to another and hold fixation at each number for 5 seconds. Some cards have jump vergence targets, meaning that there are two or more separate targets with different disparities. When using a jump vergence card, instruct the patient to fixate one target for 10 seconds, keeping it single and clear, and then to change fixation to the other. Repeat this several times and then select a card with a slightly greater demand.

Another procedure that is popular with stereoscopes is called tromboning. In this procedure, the patient slowly slides the card from distance to near and tries to maintain single and clear binocular vision. The card can then be moved back to the distance setting.

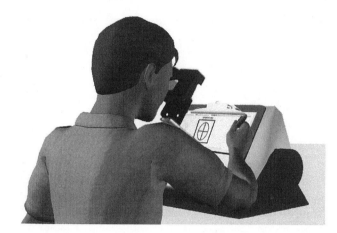

FIG. 5.20. Keystone Correct-Eye-Scope setup for cheiroscopic tracing.

Other therapy procedures that can be performed, along with important considerations and methods of increasing and decreasing the level of difficulty of the task, are similar to those listed in Tables 5.2, 5.3, and 5.4.

Endpoint

Discontinue this therapy technique when the patient is able to successfully achieve clear single binocular vision with the selected cards at the selected distance.

Cheiroscope

Brewster-type instruments have been developed that serve a somewhat different purpose (Keystone Correct-Eye-Scope). This instrument, sometimes referred to as a cheiroscope, can be used as a diagnostic tool to assess binocular stability, binocular alignment, and the presence and extent of suppression. It is used as a training device to improve binocular stability and reduce or eliminate suppression. The instrument is shown in Fig. 5.20.

Diagnostic Procedure

The target used for the cheiroscope is shown in Fig. 5.21. One side of the paper has a target and the other side is blank. The paper is placed on the cheiroscope, at the distance setting, with the blank side in front of the eye that corresponds to the dominant hand. Ask the patient to look into the cheiroscope and trace the target that he or she sees, on the blank paper in front of him or her, with a pencil.

Interpretation

As the patient is tracing, he or she should be asked if either the pencil or any part of the picture appears to be disappearing. When the tracing is complete, measure the separation between corresponding points. A separation of 77 to 80 mm represents an orthophoria response. A separation greater than 80 mm is an exophoria posture and less than 77 mm is an esophoria posture. A vertical phoria can be detected if the tracing is higher or lower than the original. If

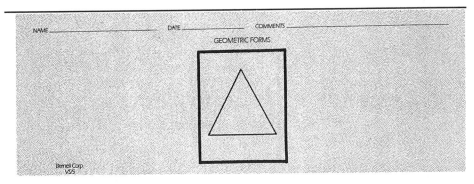

FIG. 5.21. Cheiroscopic tracing forms.

the target was traced with the left hand in front of the left eye and is higher, a left hyperphoria is present.

Binocular instability is indicated if you observe the patient shifting his hand while attempting to trace, or actual drifts in the tracing are evident (Fig. 5.22). Suppression is present if the patient reports parts of the picture or the pencil disappearing. With some patients, suppression is so deep that they are unable to trace the picture. Another problem that occurs with very high esophoria or exophoria is that the object appears to drift so far to the left or right of the paper that the patient is also unable to trace it.

Therapy Procedure with the Cheiroscope

Place a cheiroscopic target on the cheiroscope and set the instrument at the distance setting. Place the target to be traced before the eye corresponding to the nondominant hand. Instruct the patient to look into the instrument and trace the target. If suppression or instability is evident, the following suggestions are generally helpful:

1. If the patient is unable to trace because the image is drifting off the page or too close to the septum, draw the corners of the tracing on the blank side of the paper This provides some structure and support and tends to reduce the instability. Draw the corners so that similar points are about 80 mm apart. If the patient has a high exophoria, draw the corners

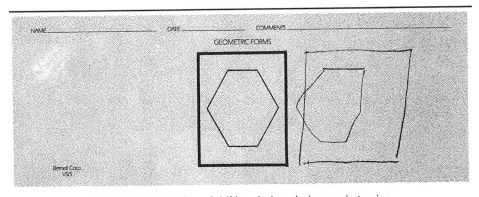

FIG. 5.22. Illustration of drifting during cheiroscopic tracing.

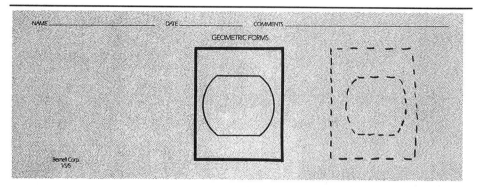

FIG. 5.23. Illustration of the use of short pencil strokes during cheiroscopic tracing.

farther away, at 90 mm or so. Conversely, if the patient has a high esophoria, draw the corners closer together, at about 70 mm. As the patient's abilities improve, eliminate one corner at a time and move the drawings closer to the orthophoria setting of 80 mm.

2. If the patient is intermittently suppressing, it is helpful to suggest that he or she make a short pencil stroke, lift the pencil off the paper, and then make another short pencil stroke. (Fig. 5.23.) Have the patient continue this until the tracing is complete. As the patient's skills improve, he or she can make longer and longer pencil strokes.

3. Another procedure that is sometimes helpful, if the patient is suppressing, is using horizontal scrubbing type strokes of the pencil. (Fig. 5.24.)

Wheatstone Stereoscope

Objective

The objectives of the Wheatstone stereoscope are similar to those listed for the Brewster stereoscopes.

Equipment Needed

1. Bernell Variable Prismatic Stereoscope.[a]
2. Stereoscopic cards.[a,c]

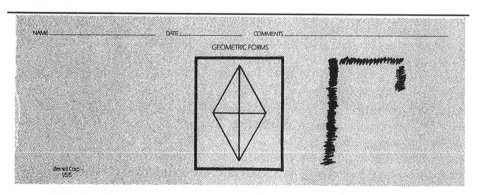

FIG. 5.24. Illustration of the use of scrubbing during cheiroscopic tracing.

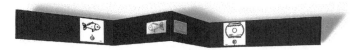

FIG. 5.25. Variable prismatic stereoscope.

3. Flip lenses.[a,b]
4. Flip prisms.[a,b]

Construction and Description

Instead of using the Brewster-type stereoscope design of a septum to separate the two fields, Wheatstone stereoscopes accomplish this by using two tubes with either individual targets or mirrors. The most commonly used Wheatstone stereoscope for the treatment of nonstrabismic binocular vision disorders is the Bernell Variable Prismatic Stereoscope, illustrated in Fig. 5.25.

The major amblyoscope is another Wheatstone-type stereoscope, used primarily for the diagnosis and treatment of strabismus. Although it is an important instrument for the diagnosis and treatment of strabismus, it is rarely used in the treatment of nonstrabismic binocular disorders. We will, therefore, not discuss the major amblyoscope in this text. We will limit our discussion in this chapter to the Bernell Variable Prismatic Stereoscope. The working distance for this instrument is 33 cm and, since there are no lenses, the accommodative demand is 3 D. This can be altered with either plus or minus lenses. The vergence demand is determined by the separation of the stereoscope. The actual prismatic demand can be read directly off the scale of the instrument. As the stereoscope is moved apart, base-in vergence demand is generated; when moved together, base-out vergence is generated.

Therapy Procedures with the Wheatstone Stereoscope

The Bernell Variable Prismatic Stereoscope can be used with nonstrabismics to develop fusional ranges and facility. The primary value of this instrument is to provide some variety to a vision therapy program and maintain a high level of interest and motivation for the patient.

A variety of cards come with this instrument and vary from first- to third-degree fusion targets. The specific cards selected are based on the objective of therapy. Once the cards are selected, they are placed on the right and left sides of the instrument. Ask the patient to place his or her nose against the tip of the instrument and describe what he or she sees (Fig. 5.26). Once it is apparent that the patient has clear single binocular vision, have him or her slowly move the stereoscope in and out to create base-out and base-in demand. Tell the patient to try and maintain clear single vision for as long as he or she can. Another procedure is to have the patient separate the target several centimeters, regain clear single vision, look away momentarily, and look back. Have the patient repeat this several times at each level.

Other therapy procedures, important factors to consider, and methods for increasing and decreasing the level of difficulty of the task are similar to those listed in Tables 5.2, 5.3, and 5.4.

Endpoint

Discontinue this therapy technique when the patient is able to successfully achieve clear single binocular vision with the selected cards to 30 base-out and 15 base-in.

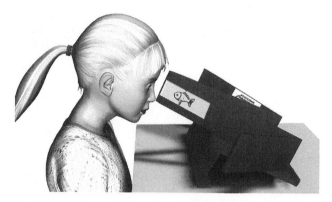

FIG. 5.26. Patient working with variable prismatic stereoscope.

VOLUNTARY CONVERGENCE PROCEDURES

Brock String

Objectives

The objectives of the Brock string are to:

- Develop the kinesthetic awareness of converging and diverging
- Develop the ability to voluntarily converge
- Normalize the near point of convergence

Equipment Needed

1. Brock string.[a]
2. Flip lenses.[a,b]
3. Flip prism.[a,b]
4. Pencil.

Description and Setup

The Brock string is simply a long white cord with three attached wooden beads of different colors. It is used primarily with convergence insufficiency patients to create the feeling and awareness of converging and to normalize the near point of convergence. It can also be used with esophores to teach accuracy of the vergence response. To use the Brock string, one end is tied to a door knob or other convenient secure location, and the patient holds the other end of the string at the bridge of his or her nose (Fig. 5.27A).

Therapy Procedures

Step 1

We recommend using just two beads and about 4 ft of string. Instruct the patient to hold the string taut and against the bridge of his or her nose. Set one bead about 2 ft (red bead) from the patient and the other about 1 ft away (green bead). Ask the patient to look at the closer bead and describe what he or she sees. Because of physiological diplopia, the patient should report that he or she sees one green bead and two red beads (Fig. 5.27B). In addition, the patient

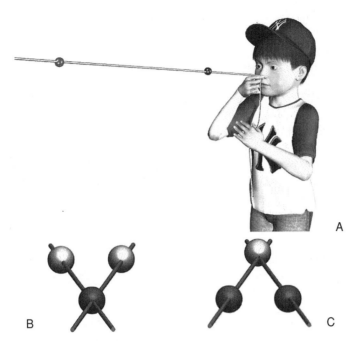

FIG. 5.27. A: Patient working with Brock string. **B,C:** Patient's perception when looking at the near or far bead when using the Brock string.

should perceive two strings crossing at the green bead, with one string extending from his or her right eye and the other appearing to extend from his or her left eye. Ask the patient to fixate the far bead (red) and he or she should now report one red bead with the strings crossing at the red bead (Fig. 5.27C). The patient will also see two green beads. It is important to explain the meaning of all of this to the patient. We suggest the following explanation.

This is a procedure that is designed to teach you how to improve your ability to cross your eyes. The technique is set up to provide you with feedback about what your eyes are doing at all times. The way the visual system works is that wherever your eyes are pointing, you perceive single vision. All other objects in front or behind the object you are looking at will be seen as double. Look at the green bead and you will see one green bead, two red beads behind it, and a string that crosses right at the green bead and forms the letter "X." The strings should look as if they are extensions of your right and left eyes. Where you perceive the two strings cross is actually where your eyes are aimed. Thus, if you are trying to look at the green bead, but the strings appear to cross farther away than the bead, this is an indication that you are looking too far away. Use this information to try and correct your eye position and look closer.

If the patient experiences difficulty accomplishing any of the goals listed above, there are several techniques that the therapist can use to help him or her overcome this obstacle.

1. Have the patient touch the bead that he or she is trying to fuse. This kinesthetic feedback is sometimes enough to help the patient achieve single vision.
2. Use minus lenses to stimulate accommodative convergence.
3. Suggest that the patient try and get the feeling of looking close and crossing his or her eyes.

Once the patient is able to fuse the near and far beads, instruct him or her to hold fixation at the near bead for 5 seconds and then switch fixation to the far bead and hold for 5 seconds.

Have the patient repeat this 3 times and then move the near bead 1 in. closer while always maintaining the far bead at 2 ft. Have the patient repeat the step of alternately fixating the far and near beads for 5 seconds, 3 times. Continue moving the near bead closer, until the patient can successfully converge at a distance of 2 in. from his or her nose.

Step 2

If the patient can now converge within 1 to 2 in. in front of his nose, he or she should have a relatively good sense of what it feels like to converge, look close, or cross his or her eyes. The next step is called "bug on string" and is performed with the same setup described above, except that the beads are removed from the string. The objective of this second step is to continue to develop the ability to converge as some of the structure of the therapy task is eliminated. Instruct the patient to fixate the very end of the string and to try and see that the two strings cross at the end of the string. Now have the patient very slowly fixate closer and closer, until he or she is fixating 1 in. in front of his nose. It is important to emphasize to him or her that the change in fixation from far to near should be very gradual. After the patient can converge all the way to his or her nose, reverse the process and have him gradually diverge to the end of the string. Repeat this procedure for several minutes.

Step 3

The final procedure is to eliminate the use of the string entirely. Instruct the patient to try and get the feeling of looking close and to try and converge his or her eyes voluntarily. This convergence should be very slow and gradual.

Other Therapy Procedures that Can Be Done with the Brock String

The Brock string can be used in several other ways. To make the task more difficult, flip prism can be used to increase the level of difficulty of the task. While the patient is converging to any point on the string, prism can be inserted before his or her eyes, and he or she must maintain fusion as the prism is alternated from base-in to base-out.

The Brock string can also be used for saccadic and pursuit therapy. In the last phase of therapy for ocular motor dysfunction, an important objective is to combine saccades and pursuits with changes in vergence and accommodation.

One common procedure for saccadic therapy is to use multiple Brock strings. Set up three strings, for instance, all having an origin in a different position of gaze. One would be to the patient's right, a second straight ahead, and the third, to the patient's left. Instruct the patient to hold the ends of all three strings against the bridge of his or her nose. Since each string will have two beads, there will be six fixation targets that vary in location, both from left to right and from far to near. Instruct the patient to look from target to target in any given pattern that you specify. The objective for the patient is to quickly regain single binocular vision after each fixation change. To increase the level of difficulty, a metronome can be used. Ask the patient to change fixation every fifth click, for example, of the metronome. The actual origin of the various Brock strings can be varied to include the vertical dimension as well.

A frequently used procedure for pursuit therapy is to tie the end of the string to a pencil and have the patient hold the pencil at arm's length (Fig. 5.28). Instruct the patient to slowly rotate the string in a circular fashion, while he or she maintains fusion at the far or near bead. This setup integrates pursuits with vergence and saccadic changes.

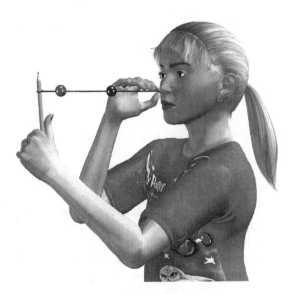

FIG. 5.28. Brock string setup for vergence and pursuits.

Important Factors

When performing this procedure, it is important to emphasize the following issues:

1. The kinesthetic feeling of converging and diverging.
2. The ability to regain fusion binocular vision as quickly as possible.
3. The patient, not the therapist, should manipulate the string and beads.
4. Emphasize that the string and beads are not doing anything, rather the changes are internal, occurring within the patient's own visual system.

Changing the Level of Difficulty of the Task

Decreasing the Level of Difficulty of the Task

Minus lenses and base-in prism decrease the level of difficulty. Another way to decrease the difficulty is to move the beads farther away from the patient.

Increasing the Level of Difficulty of the Task

Plus lenses, base-out prism, and decreasing the working distance increase the level of difficulty.

Endpoint

Discontinue this therapy technique when the patient is able to:

1. Successfully converge to 1 in. from his nose
2. Can appreciate the feelings of converging and diverging
3. Can voluntarily converge
4. Can accurately converge and diverge

Barrel Card

Objective

The objectives of the Barrel card are identical to those for the Brock string.

Equipment Needed

1. Barrel card.[a]

Description and Setup

The barrel card setup is illustrated in Fig. 5.29. It is a white card with three colored barrel-shaped targets on each side of the card. The barrels are red on one side and green on the other. It is used primarily with convergence insufficiency-type patients to create the feeling and awareness of converging and to normalize the near point of convergence. The concept and underlying principles are identical to the Brock string. We generally use the barrel card after the patient has completed the Brock string sequence of activities, or for variety.

Therapy Procedures

Instruct the patient to hold the barrel card against the bridge of his or her nose and to fixate on the barrel farthest away from him or her. The patient should be able to report one barrel that is a mixture of the red and green colors. The other two barrels should be seen as double. The patient then fixates on the middle barrel, holds for 10 seconds, and then fixates on the nearest barrel and holds for 10 seconds. Instruct the patient to continue alternating fixation from one barrel to the other.

Important factors to consider and methods for increasing and decreasing the task are identical to those discussed for the Brock string.

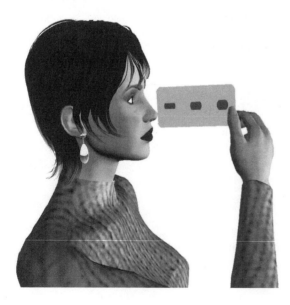

FIG. 5.29. Patient working with barrel card.

Endpoint

Discontinue this therapy technique when the patient is able to:

1. Successfully converge to 1 in. from his or her nose
2. Can appreciate the feelings of converging and diverging
3. Can voluntarily converge

ANTISUPPRESSION PROCEDURES

Bar Reader[a]

Objective

The objectives of the bar reader are to provide a suppression check during BAF training or fusional facility training.

Equipment Needed

1. Red/green bar reader or Polaroid bar reader.[a]
2. Red/green glasses or Polaroid glasses.[a,b]
3. Age-appropriate reading material.
4. Flip lenses.[a,b]
5. Hand-held loose prism.[a,b]
6. Flip prisms.[a,b]

Construction and Description

The bar reader is a piece of plastic with alternating stripes of red and green or Polaroid material (Fig. 5.30). The bar reader can be placed on any working material and, when combined with the patient wearing red/green or Polaroid glasses, provides feedback about suppression. As we stated in Chapter 4, to be effective, all vision therapy procedures must provide feedback to the patient about performance. Whenever a patient is engaged in a binocular task, suppression can occur. If the training technique does not provide feedback to the clinician and patient, it cannot be considered an effective technique.

In Chapter 6, we describe BAF training. This technique is binocular and could be accomplished without a bar reader. If we are working with a patient that does tend to suppress, however, it is important to use a suppression control such as the bar reader.

Therapy Procedures with the Bar Reader

Refer to Chapter 6 for examples of therapy techniques during which the use of a bar reader is helpful. These include:

1. Binocular accommodative facility
2. Loose prism jumps
3. Flip prism

For all three of these procedures, the bar reader can be used to treat suppression, as well as vergence or accommodation.

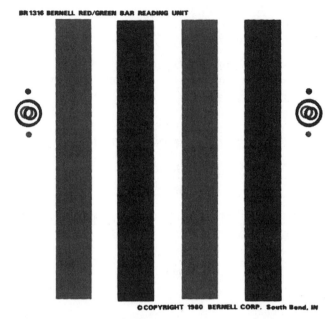

FIG. 5.30. Red/green bar reader (alternating bars are green and red).

TV Trainer[a]

Objective

The objectives of the TV trainer are to decrease the intensity and frequency of suppression.

Equipment Needed

1. TV Trainer.
2. Red/green glasses.
3. Television set.

Construction and Description

The TV trainer is a sheet of plastic with one side all green and the other side all red. This plastic sheet usually comes with two suction cups attached, so that the TV trainer can be easily attached to a television (Fig. 5.31A). The device is attached to the television, and the patient must wear red/green glasses (Fig 5.31B). The eye behind the red filter sees through the red side of the TV trainer, while the eye behind the green filter sees through the green side of the TV trainer. If the patient is suppressing while watching television, one side of the TV trainer will turn black. For instance, if the right eye is suppressing, the television picture behind the red half of the TV trainer will be impossible to see.

TV trainers also are made from Polaroid material. The Polaroid version has one serious drawback that is common to all Polaroid techniques. If the child tilts his or her head to the left or right shoulder, the entire screen can be visible through the TV trainer even if suppression is present. Because the TV trainer is often used for young patients, this problem is very significant. If the child cannot or will not maintain an upright head posture when using the TV trainer, its usefulness diminishes.

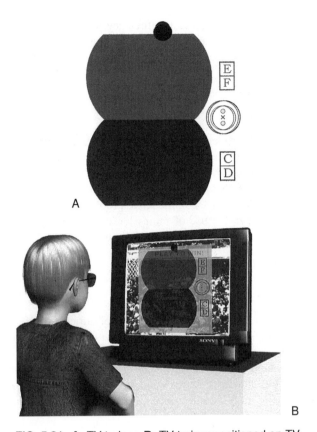

FIG. 5.31. A: TV trainer. **B:** TV trainer positioned on TV.

The TV trainer is a device that provides feedback to the patient about suppression. The patient is encouraged to try and eliminate the suppression by blinking, trying to converge or diverge (based on the underlying diagnosis), or by moving closer or farther away from the television.

Therapy Procedures with the TV Trainer

The TV trainer is considered a passive form of therapy. The patient simply watches television as usual, except that the TV trainer is placed on the television. The patient is encouraged to try and see through both sides of the plastic. Watching television becomes impossible if suppression occurs. This calls attention to suppression and a need for the patient to do something to eliminate the suppression.

Changing the Level of Difficulty of the Task

To increase or decrease the level of difficulty of the task, lenses and prism can be used or the working distance can be increased or decreased.

Varying the Working Distance

Many patients tend to suppress more at one distance than others. For example, a patient with divergence excess will suppress when objects are placed at a distance, but will have normal binocular vision at near. The convergence insufficiency patient will do the opposite. When using the TV trainer with a divergence excess patient, begin with a short working distance initially. If the patient can succeed at short distances, the working distance can be gradually increased.

Lenses

While working with the TV trainer at any particular distance, minus lenses can be used binocularly to increase or decrease the level of difficulty of the task. If the patient is exophoric, minus lenses will generally make fusion and avoidance of suppression easier. If the patient is esophoric, minus lenses will increase the level of difficulty of the task by placing a greater demand on NFV. If an accommodative problem such as accommodative insufficiency or infacility is present, the use of minus lenses may not be effective. Plus lenses have limited value because the TV trainer is generally used at a working distance of 5 ft or greater.

Prism

Prism can also be used to increase or decrease the level of difficulty of the task. Both base-in and base-out prism can be used. Using a flipper with base-out on one side and base-in on the other, fusional facility therapy can be done while the child watches television. In this case, the TV trainer represents a suppression control for the fusional facility technique. Prism is also useful to help the patient eliminate the suppression. If a patient has high exophoria at distance and suppresses while using the TV trainer, base-in prism may facilitate fusion and decrease suppression.

Endpoint

The endpoint for this technique is reached when the patient can maintain single binocular distance without suppression at the distance of concern.

Red/Green Glasses and Penlight

Objective

The objectives of the red/green glasses and penlight are to decrease the intensity and frequency of suppression. Because the patient is dissociated during this procedure, pathological diplopia occurs. This procedure, therefore, should not be used if the patient is strabismic and has anomalous correspondence.

Equipment Needed

1. Red/green glasses.
2. Penlight or transilluminator.
3. 6 Δ loose prism.
4. A rheostat to control room illumination or several sources of room illumination that can be controlled independently.

Construction and Description

To perform this therapy activity, the patient wears red/green glasses and holds a 6 Δ prism base-down before his or her dominant eye while viewing a penlight or transilluminator. The important factor in this procedure is the ability to control room illumination. It is best to perform this technique in a room with a rheostat. As we described in Chapter 4, one of the main issues in suppression therapy is to structure the training environment so that the patient is least likely to suppress. Clinically, we have several ways of modifying the stimulus to decrease the likelihood of suppression. These include:

- Changing target illumination
- Changing target contrast
- Changing target focus
- Moving the target
- Flashing the target

The rheostat allows the clinician to vary the room illumination and reach the level of illumination to achieve the best result. We usually begin suppression therapy in artificial conditions and gradually move toward more natural seeing conditions. Red/green glasses and penlight is an example of a therapy procedure using this progression for antisuppression treatment.

Therapy Procedures

With the patient wearing red/green glasses and holding the 6 Δ prism before one eye, the room illumination is turned down until the only visible target is the light of a transilluminator or penlight. Ask the patient how many lights and what color lights are seen. This is a very artificial environment and will often be sufficient to eliminate suppression. If not, the light can be moved from side-to-side or the clinician can rapidly move an occluder from one eye to the other. Once the patient can maintain diplopia under these conditions, the room illumination can be gradually increased until the patient can maintain diplopia awareness with full room illumination. To make conditions more natural, the red/green glasses are then removed, which generally will result in suppression again. If this occurs, the room illumination is again decreased until the patient experiences diplopia. Room illumination is gradually increased, until the patient can finally appreciate diplopia with full illumination and without red/green filters. This process typically may require 2 to 4 weeks of both in-office and home therapy.

Endpoint

Discontinue this procedure when the patient can maintain diplopia without the red/green glasses in normal room illumination.

Vertical Prism Dissociation

Objective

The objective of vertical prism dissociation is to decrease the patient's tendency to suppress. The vertical prism is used to create diplopia during binocular viewing.

Vertical prism dissociation is used for patients who have moderate to strong suppression. This is common in anisometropia and high degrees of heterophoria or intermittent strabismus. In such cases, the suppression interferes with fusional vergence therapy. If techniques like Vectograms, Tranaglyphs, the Aperture Rule, and the Eccentric Circles or Free Space Cards are used, the patient may be frustrated and unable to progress because of intermittent suppression.

Equipment Needed

1. Penlight or an isolated letter that is within the resolution capacity of the patient
2. 6 to 8 Δ hand-held prism

Description and Setup

When treating suppression, it is important to select room illumination and a target with characteristics that will tend to limit suppression. These concepts were reviewed in Chapter 4.

Usually the procedure begins with low room illumination and a penlight. Place a penlight at a distance of about 5 to 10 ft. Choose the specific distance based on the patient's problem. If the patient's suppression is worse at distance, begin this technique at a close distance. If the suppression is worse at near, begin at a greater distance. The general rule is to begin at a distance at which the patient can succeed and gradually move to the distance at which the patient experiences difficulty.

Ask the patient to look at the target and place a 6 Δ prism base-down before the dominant eye (the dominant eye is the eye that does not tend to suppress). It is best to have the patient hold the prism if he or she is old enough. The patient should now experience diplopia. While the patient maintains diplopia, gradually turn up the illumination in the room. This is most easily accomplished if the illumination is controlled by a rheostat. If not, having several light sources available may be effective. The objective is for the patient to be able to maintain awareness of diplopia as the room illumination changes from low to normal lighting.

It is also possible to combine the use of vertical prism with saccadic and pursuit procedures to increase the level of difficulty of the task. Multiple targets can be used, and the patient must maintain diplopia as he or she makes saccades from one target to another. A commonly used procedure is to use the Hart chart and have the patient call off the first row of letters by viewing the top image and the next row when viewing the bottom image. The patient continues to alternate back and forth between the two images.

A target can also be placed on a rotating device (Chapter 7) and the patient, while maintaining diplopia, alternates between the top and bottom images, trying to maintain accurate fixation of the rotating target.

This antisuppression technique can also be used while working to develop the feelings of convergence and divergence. While the patient experiences diplopia, ask him or her to try and make the images move laterally by converging and diverging. For example, if the patient is exophoric and the bottom image is seen by the right eye, he or she will experience crossed diplopia with the bottom image to the left of the top image.

Ask the patient to try and make the bottom image move to the right of the top image by converging. Once the patient can alternate from crossed diplopia to uncrossed diplopia, it is useful to use a metronome. Instruct the patient to converge and hold for five beats, then try to vertically align the images for five beats, and finally to diverge and hold for five beats of the metronome. This technique can be performed for several minutes.

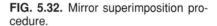

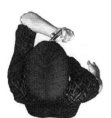

FIG. 5.32. Mirror superimposition procedure.

Endpoint

Discontinue this therapy technique when the patient is able to maintain diplopia under normal room illumination conditions.

Mirror Superimposition

Objective

The objectives of mirror superimposition are to decrease the intensity and frequency of suppression.

Equipment Needed

1. Small mirror (about 2 in. × 2 in.)
2. Variety of fixation targets

Construction and Description

To perform mirror superimposition, the patient holds a small mirror at a 45-degree angle in front of one eye and views a target through the mirror. With the other eye, he or she views another target. The patient must try to superimpose one image on top of the other.

Right Eye Target

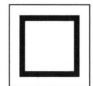
Left Eye Target

Patient's view when
targets are superimposed

FIG. 5.33. First-degree targets used with mirror superimposition.

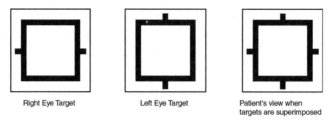

Right Eye Target   Left Eye Target   Patient's view when targets are superimposed

FIG. 5.34. Second-degree target used with mirror superimposition.

This technique is generally only necessary when suppression is intense enough to interfere with binocular vision therapy procedures such as the Tranaglyphs, Vectograms, the Aperture Rule, and the Eccentric Circles or Free Space Cards.

Therapy Procedures with Mirror Superimposition

While the patient fixates a target with one eye, he or she holds the mirror at about a 45-degree angle before the other eye and views another target (Fig 5.32). The objective is for the patient to maintain awareness of both images simultaneously. A variety of targets can be used with mirror superimposition to vary the difficulty of the task. Usually, first- and second-degree targets are used. Samples of each are illustrated in Figs. 5.33 and 5.34.

First-degree targets, also referred to as superimposition, involve the use of two totally different targets. Figure 5.33 shows a typical set of first-degree targets used with mirror superimposition. Using these targets, the patient should report seeing both the circle and the square simultaneously. Such targets are difficult to suppress and are generally used in the early phases of antisuppression therapy.

Second-degree, or flat fusion targets, are identical targets that incorporate suppression checks into their design. An example of a second-degree target is illustrated in Fig. 5.34. When such targets are used for mirror superimposition, the patient sees the square with the vertical and horizontal suppression checks.

Another variable that is important for mirror superimposition is the size of the target. In Chapter 4, we reviewed the various factors that must be considered in antisuppression therapy. One of these factors is the size of the target. We generally begin antisuppression therapy using large peripheral targets and gradually make the targets smaller and more central.

Endpoint

This procedure is usually continued until the patient can maintain awareness of both images, even when small central first-degree targets are used. Another criterion that can be used to decide when to discontinue this technique is the patient's performance on other binocular vision tasks. If the patient can successfully work with Tranaglyphs, Vectograms, the Aperture Rule, and Eccentric Circles or Free Space Cards, mirror superimposition is no longer necessary.

STUDY QUESTIONS

1. List four procedures that can be used to improve convergence. For each procedure, describe how you would set up the technique and a therapy sequence you would follow.
2. How could you make the task easier for a patient who is struggling to fuse with the Brock string (other than moving the beads away from the face)?

3. The Quoit Vectogram targets are separated by 20 mm for a patient seated 40 cm from the target. What is the prismatic demand?
4. How do you create base-out and base-in demand with Vectograms and Tranaglyphs?
5. A patient is fusing the Quoit Vectogram set at 20 base-out. If the target is single and clear, where is the plane of accommodation and the plane of convergence?
6. Describe the differences between the Quoit, Clown, and Spirangle Vectograms.
7. If you increase the working distance you_____the base-out demand and you_____the base-in demand.
8. Describe four ways to increase and decrease the prismatic demand when using Vectograms and Tranaglyphs.
9. Explain how a chiastopic fusion technique works.
10. Explain how an orthopic fusion technique works.
11. Why is the Aperture Rule more difficult than the Vectograms/Tranaglyphs?
12. How do you compute the prismatic demand using the Aperture Rule?
13. If a patient reports clear single vision with card 5, using the double aperture on the Aperture Rule, where is the plane of accommodation and where is the plane of convergence?
14. How can you help a patient who is having difficulty fusing base-out on the Aperture Rule?
15. How can you increase the demand for a patient during base-in fusion on the Aperture Rule?
16. Describe how you would explain to a patient how to fuse base-in with the Eccentric Circles.
17. What is the significance of the letters "A" and "B" on the Eccentric Circles?
18. If a patient reports clear single vision while fusing base-in with the Eccentric Circles, where is the plane of accommodation and where is the plane of convergence?
19. The Eccentric Circles are separated by 5 cm. What is the prismatic demand if the working distance is 20 cm?
20. Name three advantages of the Computer Orthoptics Random Dot Stereopsis Program. What is the most important advantage?

REFERENCES

1. Bogdanovich G, Roth N, Kohl P. Properties of anaglyphic materials that affect the testing and training of binocular vision. *J Am Optom Assoc* 1986;57:899–903.
2. Press LJ. Computers and vision therapy programs. Optometric Extension Program. Santa Ana, CA Curr II, 1987, vol 60(1):29–32.
3. Maino DM. Applications in pediatrics, binocular vision, and perception. In: Maino JH, Maino DM, Davidson DW, eds. *Computer applications in optometry.* Boston: Butterworth-Heineman, 1989:99–112.
4. Cooper J. Review of computerized orthoptics with specific regard to convergence insufficiency. *Am J Optom Physiol Opt* 1988;65:455–463.
5. Cooper J, Feldman J. Operant conditioning of fusional convergence ranges using random dot stereograms. *Am J Optom Physiol Opt* 1980;57:205–213.
6. Daum KM, Rutstein RP, Eskride JB. Efficacy of computerized vergence therapy. *Am J Optom Physiol Opt* 1987;64:83–89.
7. Cooper J, Selenow A, Ciuffreda KJ, et al. Reduction of asthenopia in patients with convergence insufficiency after fusional vergence training. *Am J Optom Physiol Opt* 1983;60:982–989.
8. Cooper J, Feldman J, Selenow A, et al. Reduction of asthenopia after accommodative facility training. *Am J Optom Physiol Opt* 1987;64:430–436.
9. Kertesz AE, Kertesz J. Wide-field fusional stimulation in strabismus. *Am J Optom Physiol Opt* 1986;63:217–222.
10. Somers WW, Happel AW, Phillips JD. Use of a personal microcomputer for orthoptic therapy. *J Am Optom Assoc* 1984;55:262–267.
11. Griffin JR. Efficacy of vision therapy of nonstrabismic vergence anomalies. *Am J Optom Physiol Opt* 1987;64:411–414.
12. Cooper J, Citron M. Microcomputer produced anaglyphs for evaluation and therapy of binocular anomalies. *J Am Optom Assoc* 1983;54:785–788.
13. Flax N. Simple formulas for computation of prism vergence and accommodation stimulation in a Brewster stereoscope. *Am J Optom Physiol Opt* 1976;53(6):297–302.

SOURCES OF EQUIPMENT

(a) Bernell Corporation: 4016 North Home Street, Mishawaka, IN 46545; 800-348-2225.

(b) GTVT: 29425 144th Avenue SE, Kent, WA 98042; 800-848-8897.

(c) Keystone View Company: 2200 Dickerson Road, Reno, NV 89503; 800-806-6569.

(d) RC Instruments: 21444 Hague Road, Noblesville, IN 46060; 800-348-2225.

(e) Computer Assisted Vision Therapy (CAVT). Contact Bernell Corporation.

6
Accommodative Techniques

PROCEDURES

Anaglyphs and Polaroids

Red–red rock

Lenses, Prisms, and Mirrors

Lens sorting
Loose lens rock
Biocular loose lens rock
Binocular accommodative facility

Paper, Pencil, and Miscellaneous Tasks

Hart chart accommodative therapy

ACCOMMODATIVE PROCEDURES (ANAGLYPHS AND POLAROIDS)

Red–red Rock[c]

Objective

This is an example of an anaglyphic procedure whose objectives are to improve accommodative amplitude and facility. Although both eyes are open for this task, the conditions are not truly binocular because central fusion is not possible. This is referred to as a biocular task. Red/green filters are placed before the eyes and, because of the nature of the targets, neither eye can see both targets.

Equipment Needed

1. Cheiroscope, with red–red rock attachment[c]
2. Red–red rock tiles[c]
3. Red and green glasses
4. Halberg-type clips
5. Trial lenses

Description and Setup

The setup for this procedure is illustrated in Fig. 6.1A. The therapist selects white tiles and a matching red transparent slide with black lettering. The tiles and slide are shown in Fig. 6.1B. The red transparent slide with black lettering is attached to the rear-illuminated screen of a cheiroscope. The patient wears red/green glasses with the red lens over his right eye and the green lens over his left. Give the patient a set of white tiles that have words printed on them in red. On the transparent red slide (40 cm in front of the patient), these same words appear in black lettering. The eye with the red lens sees only the words on the red slide, while the words on the white opaque tiles can only be seen by the eye with the green lens. The patient looks at the first white tile and clears the print (eye with green lens) in order to identify the word that must be found on the red slide. He or she then tries to find the matching word on the red slide. To do so, the patient must use his or her right eye with the red filter. Thus, although both eyes are open, central fusion is not possible. Rather, to perform the task, the patient is alternating from the right to the left eye. The addition of clip-on lenses over the red/green glasses introduces the accommodative component to the task. A plus lens is placed before the right eye and a minus lens before the left. As the patient shifts from the tiles to the red slide and back to the next tile, he or she must alternately inhibit and stimulate accommodation. The power of these lenses is increased in small increments, until the patient can perform the task through +2.50 and −6.00.

1. Level One Ask the patient to complete the matching task with no time consideration. The plus and minus lenses can be alternated from visit to visit so that, at times, the right eye is viewing the target through plus lenses and, at other times, through minus lenses.

2. Level Two To increase the level of difficulty of the task, add the variable of time.

Important factors to consider and methods of increasing and decreasing the level of the task are listed in Tables 6.1 and 6.2.

Endpoint

For patients less than 20 years old, discontinue this therapy technique when the patient is able to successfully clear +2.50 and −6.00, 20 cpm. For patients older than 20 years, the endpoint

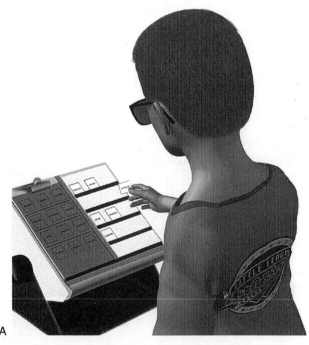

A

FIG. 6.1. A: Cheiroscope with red–red rock therapy procedure (slide on left-hand side). **B:** Close-up of red–red rock tiles and slide.

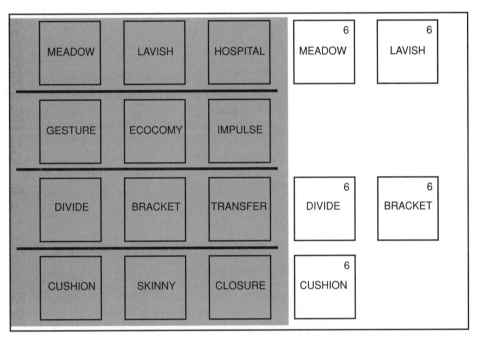

FIG. 6.1. *Continued.*

TABLE 6.1. *Important factors to emphasize when performing accommodative therapy*

- The feeling of stimulating and relaxing accommodation
- The ability to clear the target as quickly as possible when changing lenses
- The patient, not the therapist, should hold and manipulate the lenses
- Changes must occur within the patient's own visual system
- Equalize the performance in the two eyes
- The awareness of diplopia during biocular techniques

depends on the amplitude of accommodation. Discontinue this procedure when the patient can clear minus lenses equal to one half the amplitude of accommodation.

ACCOMMODATIVE PROCEDURES (LENSES, PRISMS, AND MIRRORS)

Lens Sorting (Monocular)

Objective

Lens sorting is a monocular accommodative technique designed to develop an awareness of the ability to relax and stimulate accommodation. A second objective is to teach the patient to voluntarily accommodate or relax accommodation.

Equipment Needed

1. Loose uncut lenses
2. Accommodative Rock Cards[a] (Fig. 6.2) or other age-appropriate reading material in various print sizes from 20/80 to 20/30
3. Eye patch

Description and Setup

The actual lenses used for this procedure depend on the age of the patient. In all instances, be careful to select minus lenses that are less than one half of the patient's amplitude of accommodation. When working with a 30-year-old patient with an amplitude of accommodation equal to 8 D, the highest minus lens used would be 4 D. For the example below, we assume the patient is less than 20 years old. With one eye occluded, the

TABLE 6.2. *Procedures to modify the level of demand of accommodative techniques*

Decreasing the Level of Difficulty of the Task
- Decrease power of lenses
- Increase size of print
- For plus lenses, decrease the working distance
- For minus lenses, increase the working distance

Increasing the Level of Difficulty of the Task
- Increase power of lenses
- Decrease size of print
- For plus lenses, increase the working distance (this is limited to reciprocal of lens power)
- For minus lenses, decrease the working distance

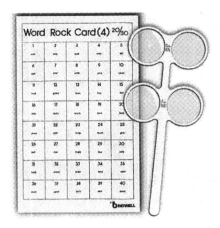

FIG. 6.2. Accommodative Rock Cards can be used as a target for loose lens rock.

patient is instructed to view age-appropriate reading material with about 20/30-size print. A moderate power minus lens (−3.00 to −5.00) is placed before the patient's right eye and he or she is asked to clear the print. The minus lens is removed and is replaced by a low plus lens (+1.00 to +1.50). The patient is again asked to clear the print through the plus lens. After repeating this several times, the patient is asked to describe the differences he or she experiences through the minus and plus lenses. The questions should be open-ended at first. If the patient is unable to describe any differences, ask the following questions:

- With which lens is the print larger or smaller?
- With which lens do you feel more strain or effort?
- Does this lens make you look close or far?

The objective is for the patient to realize that he or she can either stimulate or relax the accommodative system and learn to voluntarily do this. Any other questions that will lead the patient to this objective would be appropriate.

Once the patient can consistently describe that the print becomes smaller with the minus lenses and appears either closer or farther away, the second objective is to help the patient develop a kinesthetic awareness of accommodation. We want the patient to be able to appreciate the difference in feeling between relaxing and stimulating accommodation. Often it is necessary to ask specific questions and spend some time explaining what the patient is experiencing. The following is an example of such an explanation.

Does it feel like you are working harder or straining your eyes now? That is the feeling of focusing. If you cannot see clearly through this lens, try to get the feeling of straining, looking close, or focusing your eyes. (Conversely, with plus lenses you would ask the patient to get the feeling of looking far away, relaxing the eyes, or the sensation of drifting off to sleep.)

Once the patient can appreciate the differences between looking through a plus and minus lens, he or she is ready to begin the actual procedure of lens sorting. The therapist now places six to eight unmarked uncut lenses on the table in front of the patient. The patient is asked to sort the lenses from strongest to weakest—the strongest being the lens that makes him focus the most, the weakest being the lens that causes the greatest relaxation. Begin with large increments, such as +2.50, +1.25, −1.00, −2.00, −3.00, or −4.00. As the patient's ability to feel and distinguish the difference between stimulation and relaxation of accommodation improves, use smaller and smaller increments. Ultimately, the objective is for the patient to be so sensitive that he or she will be able to recognize very small, barely noticeable, differences such as a 0.5 D increment.

Important Factors

When performing this procedure, one must stress the following issues (Table 6.1):

1. The feeling of stimulating and relaxing accommodation
2. The ability to work with smaller and smaller increments
3. The ability to sort the lenses as quickly as possible

Changing the Level of Difficulty of the Task

Decreasing the Level of Difficulty of the Task

Occasionally a patient will be unable to clear the plus lenses or the minus lenses because of an accommodative insufficiency or accommodative excess problem. To overcome this problem, simply use lenses with which the patient can succeed. For example, if the patient has an accommodative excess problem and cannot clear even low levels of plus, use only minus lenses. Here the goal would be for the patient to be able to differentiate between low and high degrees of minus lenses. As therapy proceeds and accommodative ability improves, plus lenses can be gradually introduced. Another way to overcome this obstacle is to use the lenses that the patient has difficulty with, but with larger print size.

For a patient with accommodative infacility and difficulty with both plus and minus lenses, the best method for making the task easier is to use larger print size. The therapist must proceed slowly with this procedure and, as the patient begins to show improvement in accommodative facility, the print size can be made smaller and the standard technique utilized.

Increasing the Level of Difficulty of the Task

To make this task more difficult, the increments can be made as small as 0.25 D. Another approach is to introduce the variable of speed and determine how quickly the patient can sort eight lenses.

Endpoint

Discontinue this therapy technique when the patient is able to successfully sort eight lenses with 0.5 D increments, in order from most minus to most plus.

Loose Lens Rock (Monocular)

Objective

The objectives of the loose lens rock are to restore normal accommodative amplitude and facility. Both the range over which the patient can accommodate and the speed of the accommodative response are considered important in this technique.

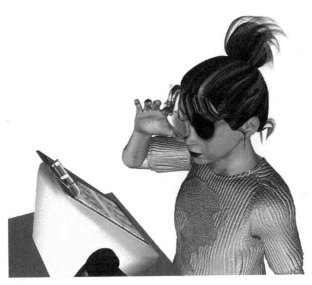

FIG. 6.3. Loose lens rock procedure.

Equipment Needed

1. Age-appropriate reading material of varying print sizes from 20/80 to 20/30
2. Uncut plastic lens blanks from −6.00 to +2.50, in 0.25 D increments
3. Eye patch

Description and Setup

1. Level One The setup for this procedure is illustrated in Fig. 6.3. Occlude the patient's left eye and ask him or her to clear and read print held at 40 cm through plus and minus lenses that are alternately held in front of his or her eye. The initial lenses selected are empirically determined, based upon the results of the diagnostic testing.

In the initial phase of this technique, give the patient as much time as necessary for him or her to clear and read the print. The goal is merely to achieve clear vision, without regard to the time factor. For children and teenagers, once the patient can clear +2.50 to −6.00, speed becomes the next objective. For adults, the strongest minus lens value used should be equal to one half the expected amplitude of accommodation.

2. Level Two Now ask the patient to regain clarity as quickly as possible. Begin with low power lenses and ask him or her to clear the print through +0.50 and −0.50, 20 cpm. When this can be accomplished, increase the power of the lenses until the patient can perform 20 cpm, with +2.00 and −4.00. (For adults, this minus lens value should not exceed one half the expected amplitude of accommodation.)

Important factors that should be considered along with methods of increasing and decreasing the level of difficulty of the task are listed in Tables 6.1 and 6.2.

Endpoint

For patients less than 20 years old, discontinue this therapy technique when the patient is able to successfully clear +2.50 and −6.00, 20 cpm. For patients older than 20 years old, the endpoint depends on the amplitude of accommodation. Discontinue this procedure when the patient can clear minus lenses equal to one half the amplitude of accommodation.

Biocular Loose Lens Rock

Objective

The objectives of this procedure are to restore normal accommodative amplitude and facility while eliminating suppression. Both the range over which the patient can accommodate and the speed of the accommodative response are considered important in this technique. While this procedure is often unnecessary, we do recommend its use when elimination of suppression is a therapy objective.

Equipment Needed

1. Age-appropriate reading material of varying print sizes from 20/80 to 20/30
2. Uncut plastic lens blanks from −6.00 to +2.50 in 0.25 D increments
3. Halberg clips[a]
4. 6 Δ loose prism

Description and Setup

1. Level One The setup for this procedure is essentially identical to that just described for the loose lens rock. The main difference is that both eyes are open, and the patient wears a 6 Δ vertical prism before one eye, to dissociate the two eyes. This can be accomplished using a trial frame or Halberg clips with the patient's current prescription or glasses with plano lenses. Because of the weight of a trial frame, even if the patient does not wear glasses, it is best to have plano training glasses available.

Use 20/20- to 20/30-size print that is appropriate for the patient's reading level. The working distance should be 40 cm. With the vertical prism in place, add low plus lenses before one eye and low minus before the other eye. The patient should report diplopia. Ask him or her to attend to the lower target first and clear the print. After the patient reads one line, he or she should now clear the print on the upper target and read one line. In the initial phase of this technique, give the patient as much time as necessary to clear and read the print. The goal is merely to achieve clear vision without regard to the time factor. Once the patient can clear +2.50 to −6.00, speed becomes the next objective.

2. Level Two Now ask the patient to regain clarity as quickly as possible. Begin with low power lenses and ask him or her to clear the print through +0.50 and −0.50, 20 cpm. When this can be accomplished, increase the power of the lenses until the patient can perform 20 cpm, with +2.00 and −4.00.

Important factors to consider and methods for increasing and decreasing the level of difficulty of this task are listed in Tables 6.1 and 6.2.

Endpoint

For patients less than 20 years old, discontinue this therapy technique when the patient is able to successfully clear +2.50 and −6.00, 20 cpm. For patients older than 20 years, the endpoint depends on the amplitude of accommodation. Discontinue this procedure when the patient can clear minus lenses equal to one half the amplitude of accommodation.

Binocular Accommodative Facility

Objective

The objectives of binocular accommodative facility (BAF) are to decrease the latency and increase the speed of the accommodative response under binocular conditions.

Equipment Needed

1. Flip lenses in various powers: ±0.50, ±0.75, ±1.00, ±1.25, ±1.50, ±1.75, ±2.00, ±2.25, and ±2.50[a,b]
2. Accommodative Rock Cards[a] or other age-appropriate reading material in various print sizes from 20/80 to 20/30
3. Polaroid or red/green bar reader[a,b]
4. Polaroid or red/green glasses[a,b]
5. Any binocular vision target, such as Vectograms,[a] Tranaglyphs,[a] the Aperture Rule,[a] Eccentric Circles,[c] or Free Space Fusion Cards[a]

Description and Setup

Procedure 1

This procedure is illustrated in Fig. 6.4. A red/green bar reader and red/green glasses are used along with age-appropriate reading material. The patient, wearing red/green glasses, is instructed to view age-appropriate reading material with about 20/30-size print. The bar reader is placed on top of the reading material. Start with +0.50/−0.50 lenses and empirically determine the lenses that the patient can just clear with minimal effort. This will be the starting point. It is common for some patients to have more difficulty with either plus or minus at this stage, depending on their underlying problem. Flip lenses are held before the patient's eyes and he or she is instructed to clear the print. The patient reads one line of print and the flip lenses are flipped to the other side, presenting a new accommodative stimulus. The patient is again asked to clear the print and read one line through the flip lenses. The therapist emphasizes

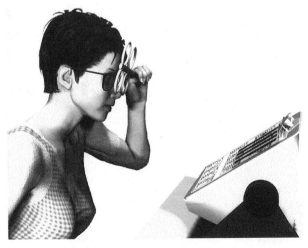

FIG. 6.4. Binocular accommodative facility using a bar reader.

that the reading material should always be visible through the four stripes of the red/green material.

After repeating this several times, the patient is asked to describe the differences he or she experiences through the minus and plus lenses. The questions should be open-ended at first. If the patient is unable to describe any differences, ask the following questions:

With which lens is the print larger or smaller?
With which lens do you feel more strain or effort?
Does this lens make you look close or far?
With which lens is it easiest to see all four lines?

The objective is for the patient to realize that he or she can either stimulate or relax the accommodative system and to learn to voluntarily do this. Any other questions that will lead the patient to this objective would be appropriate.

Once the patient can consistently describe that the print becomes smaller with the minus lenses and appears either closer or farther away, the second objective is to help the patient develop a kinesthetic awareness of accommodation. We want the patient to be able to appreciate the difference in feeling between relaxing and stimulating accommodation. Often it is necessary to use questions and statements such as:

Does it feel like you are working harder or straining your eyes now? That is the feeling of focusing. If you cannot see clearly through this lens, try to get the feeling of straining, looking close, or focusing your eyes. (Conversely, with plus lenses you would ask the patient to get the feeling of looking far away, relaxing the eyes—the sensation of drifting off to sleep.)

The same procedure can be performed using Polaroid glasses and a Polaroid bar reader.

Procedure 2

BAF therapy can also be performed using any fusional vergence therapy target. Procedures such as Vectograms, Tranaglyphs, the Aperture Rule, and Eccentric Circles are all very valuable techniques for BAF (Fig. 6.5). These techniques are described in Chapter 5.

Important factors to be considered along with methods of increasing and decreasing the level of difficulty of the task are listed in Tables 6.1 and 6.2.

Endpoint

Discontinue this therapy technique when the patient is able to successfully clear +2.50 and −2.50, 20 cpm without suppression.

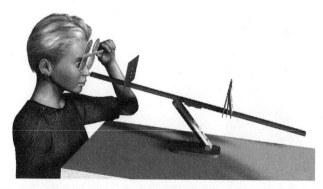

FIG. 6.5. Aperture Rule used for binocular accommodative facility.

ACCOMMODATIVE PROCEDURES (PAPER, PENCIL, AND MISCELLANEOUS TASKS)

Hart Chart Distance to Near Accommodative Rock (Monocular)

Objective

The objectives of Hart chart rock are to restore normal accommodative amplitude and facility. Both the range over which the patient can accommodate and the speed of the accommodative response are considered important in this technique.

Equipment Needed

1. Large Hart chart suitable for distance viewing[a,b]
2. Small Hart chart suitable for near viewing[a,b]
3. Eye patch

Description and Setup

The setup for this procedure is illustrated in Fig. 6.6.

1. Level One Have the patient cover his or her left eye with the eye patch. Ask the patient to hold the small chart at 40 cm, focus on the top line, and read the line aloud when it is clear. After reading the top line on the near chart, ask him or her to look at the second line of the far Hart chart and read it aloud when it is clear. The patient continues to alternate from the near to the far Hart chart for several minutes. Repeat the entire sequence with the right eye covered and the left eye open.

2. Level Two Ask the patient to hold the small chart at arm's length and to call off the letters on the top line as he or she slowly moves the chart closer. When the patient can no longer keep it clear, have him or her shift to the second line of the larger chart, which is placed at about 10 ft. Have the patient repeat the procedure with the third line of the small chart, moving it closer as he or she calls off the letters. Repeat the procedure with the patch moved to the right eye.

3. Level Three To increase the level of difficulty, ask the patient to hold the near chart 1 to 2 in. farther away than the point at which he or she reports blurred vision and switch fixation

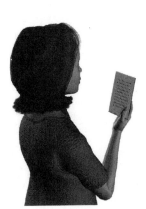

FIG. 6.6. Hart chart for accommodative rock.

from the larger distance chart to the smaller near chart. Each time the patient switches fixation, he or she reads a line.

Important factors to consider and methods of increasing and decreasing the level of difficulty of the task are listed in Tables 6.1 and 6.2.

ENDPOINT

For patients younger than 20 years old, discontinue this therapy technique when the patient is able to successfully clear the near chart when it is held 3 in. from his or her eyes and then change fixation and clear the far Hart chart held at 10 ft. For patients older than 20 years, the endpoint will depend on the amplitude of accommodation. Discontinue this procedure when the patient can successfully clear the near chart, which is held at a distance equal to half of his amplitude.

STUDY QUESTIONS

1. How can you increase the level of difficulty with red–red rock?
2. Would you expect a patient to have more difficulty sorting five lenses with 0.5 D increments or 1 D increments? Explain your reasoning.
3. Describe two methods of decreasing the level of difficulty of the lens-sorting task.
4. Describe two techniques you could use to help a patient who is experiencing difficulty with the BAF procedure.
5. How can you increase the level of difficulty of the Hart chart procedure?

SOURCES OF EQUIPMENT

a. Bernell Corporation: 4016 North Home Street, Mishawaka, IN 46545; 800-348-2225.
b. GTVT: 29425 144th Avenue SE, Kent, WA 98042; 800-848-8897.
c. Keystone View Company: 2200 Dickerson Road, Reno, NV 89503; 800-806-6569.

7
Ocular Motility Procedures

PROCEDURES
Lenses, Prisms, and Mirrors

Loose prism jumps

Paper, Pencil, and Miscellaneous Tasks

Hart chart saccadic therapy
Letter tracking
Symbol tracking
Visual tracing
Rotating pegboard
Flashlight tag
Computer software for saccades and pursuits

Afterimage Techniques

Afterimages used for saccades and pursuits

OCULAR MOTILITY PROCEDURES (LENSES, PRISMS, AND MIRRORS)
Loose Prism Jumps
Objective

The objectives of loose prism jumps are to improve the accuracy and speed of saccadic eye movements. The procedure is always performed monocularly.

Equipment Needed

1. Loose prisms in the following powers: 12, 10, 8, 6, 5, 4, 3, 2, 1, and 0.5 Δ[a,b]
2. A variety of fixation targets to be used at distance and near, ranging in size from 20/60 to 20/20

Description and Setup

While the patient views a target monocularly, a prism is placed before the fixating eye. Because the prism will displace the image of the fixation object off the fovea, a saccade will be necessary to regain foveal fixation. The objectives are for the patient to be able to quickly and accurately regain fixation. In addition, an important goal is for the patient to be sensitive to very small amounts of prism. As we discussed earlier in this chapter, a goal of therapy with saccades is to move from large gross saccadic movements to small fine movements. The procedure should, therefore, begin with large magnitude prism, with a gradual reduction in the magnitude of the prism until the patient can successfully work with 0.5 Δ. Another important variable is the size of the fixation object. Begin with larger targets (20/60) and decrease the target size until the patient can work with 20/20-size print with 0.5 Δ.

When the therapist works with the patient, the placement of the base of the prism should be varied each time (base-up, base-down, right, left, and any combination). Thus, the required direction of the saccadic eye movement will not be known in advance.

Endpoint

Discontinue this therapy technique when the patient is able to make an accurate rapid saccade using 0.5 Δ and a 20/20 target at both a distance and near working distance.

OCULAR MOTILITY PROCEDURES (PAPER, PENCIL, AND MISCELLANEOUS TASKS)

Hart Chart—Saccadic Therapy

Objective

The objectives of the Hart chart for saccadic therapy are to increase the speed and accuracy of saccadic fixation.

Equipment Needed

1. Large Hart chart for distance viewing
2. Eye patch

Description and Setup

Place the Hart chart about 5 to 10 ft from the patient. Occlude the patient's left eye with an eye patch and instruct the patient to call out the first letter in column 1 and then the first letter in column 10, the second letter from the top in column 1 and the second letter from the top in column 10, the third letter from the top in column 1 and the third letter from the top in column 10, and so forth. Continue until the patient has called out all letters from columns 1 and 10. As the patient calls out the letters, write down his or her responses and, when the task is completed, have the patient check his or her accuracy. Requiring the patient to check for errors is, in itself, another saccadic therapy technique. Now the patient will have to make saccades from far to near to check for errors.

Once this task can be completed in about 15 seconds without any errors, you can increase the level of difficulty several ways. Ask the patient to continue calling out letters in the other columns. Specifically, after completing columns 1 and 10, have the patient call out columns 2 and 9, 3 and 8, 4 and 7, and 5 and 6. The inner columns are more difficult because they are surrounded by other targets.

An even greater level of difficulty can be achieved by requiring saccades from the top of one column to the bottom of another. Instead of a left to right and right to left saccade, the patient will have to make an oblique saccade. For example, ask the patient to call out the top letter in column 1 and then the bottom letter in column 10, the second letter from the top in column 1 and the second letter from the bottom in column 10. Continue this pattern through the entire chart.

Many other variations to increase the level of difficulty are possible, including the use of multiple Hart charts, split Hart charts, incorporating the click of a metronome, and requiring the patient to maintain balance on a balance board while engaged in the task.

Letter and Symbol Tracking

Objective

The objectives of letter and symbol tracking are to increase the speed and accuracy of saccadic fixation. These procedures are generally used with children.

Equipment Needed

1. Letter and symbol tracking workbooks[a]
2. Plastic sheet, 8.5 × 11 in.
3. Paper clip
4. Pen used for overhead transparencies (washable type)
5. Eye patch

Description and Setup

Figures 7.1 and 7.2 illustrate the two workbooks. Both are designed to improve saccadic accuracy and speed. To permit the repeated use of the workbooks, we suggest that you cover the page being used with a plastic sheet and secure the plastic with a paper clip. We use overhead transparency sheets for this purpose.

As you can see in Fig. 7.1, each page of letter tracking has two or more paragraphs of what appear to be random letters. Occlude one of the patient's eyes and tell the patient to begin at the upper right and scan from left to right to find the first letter "a," and to make a line through the letter "a." Ask the patient to then find the very first "b," cross it out, and continue through the entire paragraph, finding the letters of the alphabet in order. The goal is to complete this task as quickly as possible. The therapist should time the therapy procedure. The patient's accuracy can also be evaluated. If the patient is scanning for the very first letter "d," for instance, and

A B C D E F G H I J K L M N O P Q R S T U V W X Y Z
a b c d e f g h i j k l m n o p q r s t u v w x y z   19

Iln chako evi nomd zeby thipg nare.

Zuth pirm nuroc dif stok. Nileg myt

lolf. Tixs nom raus zab tuin lugah.

Marb sewt rotsir puje. Yonak nesud

voz alee. Xart chod bugm turh sref

trea gen foru. Vab reps tique kowj.

Dagh meulb fwer ilg sida. Ubc they

bouf yed neoph vaik. Wolen kig peab

nad tenc xerb. Rait rebey fal zibt

_____ Min. _____ Sec.

FIG. 7.1. Letter tracking workbook.

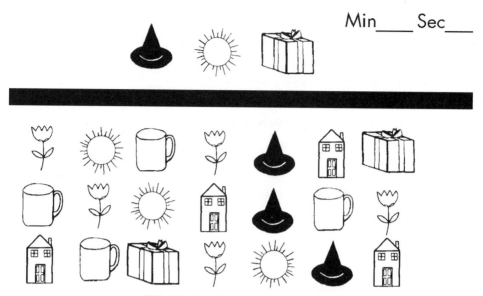

Min___ Sec___

FIG. 7.2. Symbol tracking workbook.

inadvertently misses it and finds a "d" later in the paragraph, he or she will be unable to find the entire alphabet sequence in the paragraph. The workbook has five different sizes of letters, creating another level of difficulty.

We suggest that after the child finds and marks a specific letter, the pen be lifted off the page so that the patient will have to use saccades to find the next letter.

If the child experiences difficulty with this task, symbol tracking (Fig. 7.2) can be used. Children in the first grade will sometimes have difficulty because of a lack of familiarity with the alphabet. This can cause great frustration and make the therapy technique very unpleasant for the child. In such cases, use symbol tracking, which utilizes large pictures, symbols, numbers, and fewer letters. The task is, therefore, considerably easier and is very useful with younger children or those with very severe ocular motility disorders.

Endpoint

Discontinue this technique when the performance in each eye is approximately equal and when the patient can successfully complete the paragraphs in about 1 minute.

Visual Tracing

Objective

The objectives of this technique are to improve the accuracy and speed of pursuit eye movements.

Equipment Needed

1. Visual tracing workbooks[a]
2. Plastic sheet, 8.5 × 11 in.
3. Paper clip

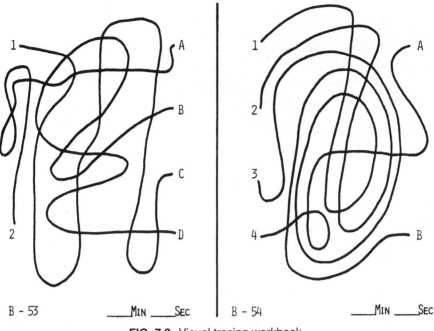

B - 53   ___MIN ___SEC | B - 54   ___MIN ___SEC

FIG. 7.3. Visual tracing workbook.

4. Pen used for overhead transparencies (washable type)
5. Eye patch

Description and Setup

Figure 7.3 provides an illustration of the visual tracing workbooks. The workbook contains tracing tasks that gradually increase in level of difficulty from the beginning to the end of the book. There are two therapy methods that can be used.

The easiest procedure is to occlude one of the patient's eyes and to ask the patient to place the pen on the letter "A" and to trace along the line, until the end of the line. The objective is for the patient to determine the number at the end of the line, beginning with the letter "A." Instruct the patient to then continue until he or she has found the answer for each line.

As the patient's accuracy and speed improve, the next level of difficulty can be added. In this technique, the patient must perform the same task just using his or her eyes. The patient must make a pursuit eye movement without the support of following the line with the pencil.

Endpoint

There are no specific clinical guidelines for this procedure. We continue this technique until the patient can perform with a reasonable degree of accuracy and speed.

Rotator-type Instruments

Objective

The objectives of this technique are to improve the accuracy and speed of pursuit eye movements.

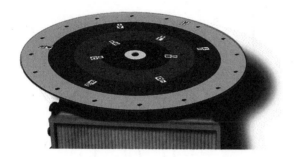

FIG. 7.4. Rotating pegboard (concentric circles are different colors: red, yellow, and blue).

Equipment Needed

1. Rotating pegboard[a]
2. Automatic rotating device[a]
3. Golf tees
4. Eye patch

Description and Setup

Figures 7.4 and 7.5 illustrate two automatic rotating devices that can be used to treat pursuit eye movement disorders. The instrument in Fig. 7.4 is called a rotating pegboard. Many different procedures can be performed with this instrument. After occluding one of the patient's eyes, instruct the patient to place a golf tee into a hole in the pegboard. Stress that you want the patient to first find the specific hole he or she will be using and then, in one motion, place the peg in the hole. Once the patient can accomplish this, turn on the rotating pegboard. Now

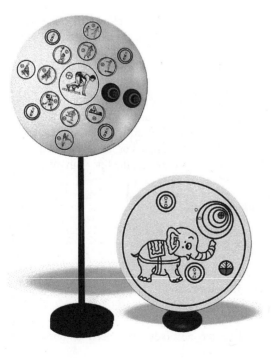

FIG. 7.5. Automatic rotator.

Comitancy

An important feature of divergence insufficiency is the comitant nature of the deviation (3,4,29,59). This means that versions are normal in all positions of gaze, and there is no difference in the magnitude of the phoria or strabismus when measured in different positions of gaze or with either eye fixating. Comitancy is a key finding that distinguishes divergence insufficiency from more serious conditions, such as sixth nerve palsy.

Symptoms

The most frequent symptom associated with divergence insufficiency is intermittent diplopia (3,4,29,59,60). The diplopia is most evident at distance. An important characteristic of this symptom is that the onset is not sudden. The patient usually reports that the diplopia has been a problem for a long time and has not changed in nature. The diplopia has been reported to decrease or disappear entirely after rest. Other reported symptoms include: headaches, ocular fatigue, nausea, dizziness, train and car sickness, panoramic headaches, blurred vision, difficulty focusing from far to near, and sensitivity to light (8).

Differential Diagnosis

Divergence insufficiency is considered to be a benign condition with no serious consequences other than the visual symptoms listed in Table 8.11. However, it resembles several other conditions and a careful differential diagnosis is important. These include convergence excess, basic esophoria, divergence paralysis, and sixth nerve palsy, all of which can present with an esodeviation at distance. The underlying cause of the last two conditions can often be life threatening. One must, therefore, be cognizant of the differential diagnosis of divergence insufficiency and first rule out the more serious disorders, such as divergence paralysis and sixth nerve palsy, which can mimic divergence insufficiency. Table 8.12 lists the various conditions that must be considered in the differential diagnosis of divergence insufficiency.

Convergence Excess and Basic Esophoria

Of the four conditions that must be ruled out, convergence excess and basic esodeviations are easily excluded because neither presents with greater eso at distance than at near or frequency of eso worse at distance than at near. Convergence excess is a condition in which there is greater eso at near than at distance and basic eso presents with approximately equal deviations at distance and near.

Sixth Nerve Palsy

Both unilateral and bilateral sixth nerve palsy more closely resemble divergence insufficiency, except that, in these conditions, a noncomitant deviation is present. A variety of clinical techniques, such as measurement of the deviation in the cardinal positions of gaze, the red glass test, and the Hess-Lancaster screen, can be used to determine comitancy.

TABLE 8.12. *Differential diagnosis of divergence insufficiency*

Functional disorders to rule out	Serious underlying disease to rule out
Convergence excess	Sixth nerve palsy
Basic esophoria	Divergence paralysis

TABLE 8.13. *Signs and symptoms of divergence paralysis*

Signs	Symptoms
Esophoria greater at distance than at near	Recent onset of intermittent diplopia at distance
Frequency of esodeviation worse at distance than at near	Recent onset of headaches
Low AC/A ratio (calculated method)	Recent onset of eyestrain
Decreased negative fusional vergence at distance	
No significant refractive error	
Comitant deviation	
Papilledema may be present	
"A" pattern esodeviation may be present	

Divergence Paralysis

The most difficult task for the clinician will be differentiating divergence insufficiency from divergence paralysis.

Signs and Symptoms

Table 8.13 lists the signs and symptoms of divergence paralysis. The most important characteristic is the *sudden* development of diplopia with marked esotropia at distance. The amount of diplopia at distance and the magnitude of the deviation decreases as the object of regard is brought toward the patient, until, at a certain distance, there is binocular vision. Duane (29) also reported that divergence paralysis, like divergence insufficiency, is a comitant deviation. Another symptom occasionally associated with divergence paralysis is headaches. The key difference between the headaches in divergence insufficiency and divergence paralysis is the sudden onset of the symptom in the latter condition.

Occasionally, but not always in patients with divergence paralysis, ophthalmoscopy reveals papilledema. An "A" pattern may be present with greater esodeviation in up-gaze and a decrease in down-gaze.

Is Divergence Paralysis a Distinct Entity?

Considerable controversy exists concerning the nature of divergence paralysis, and some authors question the validity of divergence paralysis as a diagnostic entity. Most authors (61–64) have described divergence paralysis as a condition consisting of the characteristics described above. However, Jampolsky (65) stated that the clinical signs and symptoms of so-called divergence paralysis are consistent with the diagnosis of a mild or moderate degree of sixth nerve paresis. It is quite possible that a mild bilateral sixth nerve palsy could resemble a divergence paralysis. Careful evaluation of comitancy should be part of the differential diagnosis of divergence paralysis. In addition, one should look carefully for endpoint nystagmus, which would tend to support a diagnosis of bilateral sixth nerve palsy.

Etiology of Divergence Paralysis

Divergence paralysis has been observed in a variety of conditions affecting the central nervous system. It has been seen in chorea, encephalitis, lues, multiple sclerosis, head trauma, cerebral hemorrhage, increased intracranial pressure, brain tumor, and vascular lesions of the brain stem.

Differential Diagnosis: Summary

Divergence insufficiency must be differentiated from divergence paralysis, as well as from sixth nerve paresis, convergence excess, and basic esophoria (Table 8.12). This differential diagnosis depends very much on the nature of the patient's symptoms. Typically, divergence insufficiency presents with a long history of intermittent diplopia that is most noticeable during distance viewing. In divergence paralysis and sixth nerve palsy, the diplopia is also worse for distance, but is sudden in onset. Although in both divergence insufficiency and divergence paralysis, the diplopia is essentially the same in all positions of gaze; in sixth nerve palsy, the deviation is noncomitant. In bilateral or unilateral sixth nerve palsy, endpoint nystagmus may be present. Divergence insufficiency, of course, can be distinguished from convergence excess in which the esodeviation is larger at near than at distance and symptoms are also more significant at near. Divergence insufficiency can also be differentiated from basic esophoria, in which the magnitude of the deviation is equal at distance and near. Other distinguishing features include:

- Divergence insufficiency worsens with fatigue, but divergence paralysis or sixth nerve palsy are stable in their manifestations. Thus, in divergence insufficiency, the diplopia becomes worse when the patient is tired.
- The diplopia noted by patients with divergence insufficiency is generally less than that in divergence paralysis or sixth nerve palsy.
- The range of single vision, as measured with a penlight, is large in divergence insufficiency and small in divergence paralysis.
- Papilledema is sometimes associated with divergence paralysis and sixth nerve palsy.
- In divergence paralysis or sixth nerve palsy, the patient may have other associated signs or symptoms, such as dizziness, lethargy, vomiting, irritability, gait disturbance, and distal paresthesia.
- In sixth nerve palsy, the deviation is noncomitant and endpoint nystagmus may be present.

The differential diagnosis is critical because, as stated previously, the causes of the various conditions under consideration vary from insignificant to life threatening. Divergence insufficiency is a benign isolated phenomenon, whereas divergence paralysis and sixth nerve palsy may be associated with brainstem pathology and vascular disorders. Acute neurologic oculomotor palsies suggest a serious condition. About one third of such patients do not survive 5 years (66). All patients suspected of having either divergence paralysis or sixth nerve palsy require immediate and careful neurological study.

Treatment

We recommend the management sequence outlined in Table 8.3.

Lenses

In all cases of binocular and accommodative dysfunction, the first management consideration is correction of any significant refractive error. In the case of divergence insufficiency, however, correction of refractive error generally has little beneficial effect on reduction of the angle of deviation. As stated previously, the prevalence of hyperopia in divergence insufficiency does not appear to be any greater than in the general population. In addition, divergence insufficiency is usually accompanied by a low calculated AC/A ratio. Both of these factors significantly decrease the likelihood of lenses being effective in the treatment of the condition. If hyperopia is present, however, one should certainly prescribe maximum plus to decrease the deviation as much as possible.

Prism

If a vertical deviation is present, vertical prism should be prescribed. For divergence insufficiency, horizontal prism is generally the most important treatment option. In the vast majority of cases, the use of horizontal relieving prism is necessary and represents the first and most effective treatment approach for divergence insufficiency.

Determination of the magnitude can be accomplished by several methods. One can use techniques that assess binocular status under dissociated conditions, such as the von Graefe phoria and vergence analysis using Sheard's criterion. A more desirable alternative is the use of fixation disparity analysis. Most authorities now consider fixation disparity analysis to be the method of choice because it evaluates binocularity under associated, and presumably more natural, conditions (41,67). In general, the minimum prism needed to eliminate the patient's symptoms should be prescribed. The prism prescription indicated by fixation disparity has generally been shown to be less than that revealed by other methods.

The associated phoria, as measured by the Mallett unit and the American Optical vectographic slide, tend to overestimate the amount of prism necessary (68) and is, therefore, not the preferred method for determination of horizontal prism. Rather, the Wesson card may be used to generate a forced vergence fixation disparity curve. This approach permits actual measurement of the fixation, disparity (along with the associated phoria), curve type, and slope of the curve. Of these four findings, it is the slope of the curve that provides the main information for prescribing prism (61). Guidelines for generating such curves and procedures for prescribing prism based on this information are described in detail in Chapter 14. However, the Wesson card is designed only for near testing. The B-VAT is a commercially available instrument that can be used for evaluating fixation disparity at distance. This instrument can be used to generate a forced vergence fixation disparity curve at distance as well as to measure the associated phoria. The American Optical vectographic slide can be used to measure the associated phoria.

Because divergence insufficiency usually produces symptoms only at a distance, a correction can be prescribed for distance-related tasks only or for full-time wear. Often divergence insufficiency patients can tolerate this additional base-out at near because PFV is usually adequate. If a patient is unable to tolerate the base-out prism for near work, vision therapy to expand PFV can be prescribed.

Vision Therapy

If the prescription of prism is not successful in eliminating the patient's symptoms, vision therapy is indicated. Although there are no specific data available on the effectiveness of vision therapy in cases of divergence insufficiency, there is sufficient information with other types of esodeviations to indicate that vision therapy should be effective in the management of the esodeviation (9,10).

Generally the following guidelines are appropriate:

- Begin vision therapy at near where the patient can succeed and gradually move toward greater distances.
- At any particular distance, begin with peripheral fusion targets and proceed to the use of central targets.
- Begin therapy with third-degree stimuli and proceed to second- and then first-degree stimuli.

The overall goals are to increase the NFV amplitude at distance and to improve vergence facility, permitting the patient to make rapid changes in vergence and accommodation with comfort and without diplopia.

TABLE 8.14. *Vision therapy for divergence insufficiency*

Phase 1
Objectives
- Develop a working relationship with the patient
- Develop an awareness of the various feedback mechanisms that will be used throughout therapy
- Develop feeling of diverging
- Normalize negative fusional vergence (NFV) amplitudes at near (smooth or tonic vergence demand)
- Normalize accommodative amplitude and ability to stimulate and relax accommodation

Phase 2
Objectives
- Normalize positive fusional vergence (PFV) amplitudes (smooth or tonic vergence demand)
- Normalize NFV facility at near (jump or phasic vergence demand)
- Normalize PFV facility (jump or phasic vergence demand)

Phase 3
Objectives
- Normalize NFV amplitudes at intermediate and far distances
- Normalize NFV facility at intermediate and far distances

Specific Vision Therapy Program

Phase 1

This first phase of therapy is designed to accomplish the objectives listed in Table 8.14 under Phase 1.

The first goals are to teach the concept and feeling of diverging and begin working with NFV at near. Although the ultimate goal with divergence insufficiency is to improve NFV at distance, it is much easier to begin therapy at near. Procedures that can be used to accomplish these first objectives are the Brock string, bug on string, variable Tranaglyphs, and Vectograms.

Endpoint

Phase 1 of therapy ends when the patient can:

- fuse to about 15 base-in at near with a Tranaglyph or other comparable technique.
- complete 12 cpm of accommodative facility with +2.00/−2.00 lenses using a 20/30 target.

A sample vision therapy program for Phase 1 is summarized in Table 8.15.

Phase 2

This second phase of therapy is designed to accomplish the objectives listed in Table 8.14 under Phase 2.

Once smooth NFV is normalized at near, phasic or jump vergence demand should be emphasized. Variable Tranaglyphs and Vectograms can still be used. However, the specific modifications to create a step vergence demand (described in Chapter 5) must be implemented.

Other valuable techniques at this stage are nonvariable Tranaglyphs, the Aperture Rule, Eccentric Circles, Free Space Fusion Cards, Lifesaver Cards, and Computer Orthoptics Jump Vergence Program.

In contrast to Phase 1—in which speed was not a factor—during this second phase of therapy, the emphasis should be on the qualitative aspects of fusion rather than magnitude. It is important to increase the speed of the fusional vergence response and quality of the recovery of fusion. A second objective of this phase of therapy is to begin working with PFV amplitudes and facility.

TABLE 8.15. *Sample vision therapy program for divergence insufficiency*

Phase 1
Sessions 1 and 2
In-Office
- Discuss nature of vision problem, goals of vision therapy, various feedback cues, importance of practice
- Brock string
- Tranaglyph or Vectograms: base-in
  1. Begin with a peripheral target like Tranaglyph 515 or the Quoit Vectogram
- Computer Orthoptics Random Dot Program: base-in
Home Therapy
- Brock string

Sessions 3 and 4
In-Office
- Bug off string
- Tranaglyph or Vectograms: base-in
- Use targets with more central demand (Clown, Bunny Tranaglyphs; Clown, Topper Vectograms)
- Computer Orthoptics Random Dot Program: base-in

Sessions 5 through 8
In-Office
- Bug on string
- Tranaglyph or Vectograms: base-in
  1. Use even-more detailed targets such as Tranaglyphs Sports Slide and Faces targets and the Spirangle Vectogram)
- Computer Orthoptics Random Dot Program: base-in
Home Therapy
- Tranaglyph: base-in

Phase 2
Sessions 9 and 10
In-Office
- Tranaglyph or Vectograms with modifications to create jump vergence demand: base-in
- Nonvariable Tranaglyphs
- Tranaglyph 515 or the Quoit Vectogram: base-out
- Binocular accommodative therapy techniques: use any of the binocular techniques listed above with ± lenses
Home Therapy
- Non variable Tranaglyph

Sessions 11 and 12
In-Office
- Tranaglyph or Vectograms with modifications to create jump vergence demand: base-in
- Aperture Rule: base-in
- More central Tranaglyphs or the Vectograms: base-out
- Binocular accommodative therapy techniques: use any of the binocular techniques listed above with ± lenses
Home Therapy
- Nonvariable Tranaglyph with loose prism jumps

Sessions 13 through 16
In-Office
- Aperture Rule: base-in
- Eccentric Circles or Free Space Fusion Cards: base-in
- Computer Orthoptics Random Dot Vergence Program: both base-in and base-out
- Aperture Rule: base-out
- Tranaglyph or Vectograms with modifications to create jump vergence demand: base-out
- Binocular accommodative therapy techniques: use any of the binocular techniques listed above with ± lenses
Home Therapy
- Eccentric Circles: base-in

Phase 3
Sessions 17 through 20
In-Office
- Tranaglyph or Vectograms at 1 m

TABLE 8.15. *Continued.*

- Eccentric Circles or Free Space Fusion Cards: base-in at 1 m
- Computer Orthoptics Random Dot Vergence Program: step–jump vergence at 1 m
Home Therapy
- Large Eccentric Circles at 1 m
Sessions 20 through 24
In-Office
- Tranaglyph or Vectograms projected with overhead projector
- Large Eccentric Circles at distance
Home Therapy
- Large Eccentric Circles at distance

Endpoint

The endpoint of Phase 2 is reached when the patient can:

- fuse card 12 using convergence and card 6 using divergence with the Aperture Rule.
- fuse the Eccentric Circles or Free Space Fusion Cards using convergence (12 cm separation) and divergence (6 cm separation).

A sample vision therapy program for Phase 2 is summarized in Table 8.15.

Phase 3

After achieving the objectives of Phases 1 and 2, the goal is to begin moving the training distance from near to far. This can be accomplished in several steps. For example, after working with techniques like the Tranaglyphs, Vectograms, and Eccentric Circles at 40 cm, the same procedures can be repeated at 1 m. Once success is achieved at this distance, other targets must be used as the distance is increased. The Tranaglyphs and Vectograms can also be projected on an overhead projector or large Eccentric Circles printed on 8.5 × 11 in. paper can be used. Another technique that can be used for training NFV at distance is the use of loose prism with appropriate targets containing suppression controls. Samples of such targets are illustrated in Chapter 5 (Figs. 5.30 and 5.31).

Vision therapy may also be necessary when base-out prism is prescribed for divergence insufficiency. Occasionally this prism is successful in relieving the patient's symptoms at distance, but creates discomfort at near when the prism is worn for full-time wear. One option is to prescribe two pairs of glasses, using prism only in the distance glasses. Another option is vision therapy to expand PFV at near to allow the patient to function comfortably with the additional convergence demand. A vision therapy program similar to that described earlier in this chapter for convergence insufficiency would be appropriate.

A reevaluation should be performed about halfway through the therapy program and again at the end of therapy. Refer back to the original complaints and determine if the patient is now comfortable. All tests of binocular and accommodative function should be repeated and compared to the initial findings as well as the expected findings.

When all vision therapy objectives have been reached and the vision therapy program is completed, we recommend the home vision therapy maintenance program outlined in Table 8.10.

Summary of Vision Therapy for Divergence Insufficiency

In contrast to convergence insufficiency, which is the easiest heterophoric binocular vision disorder to treat with vision therapy, divergence insufficiency is the most difficult. If the use of lenses and base-out prism is not totally effective in eliminating the patient's symptoms, the therapy program outlined above should be attempted.

Surgery

Optometric treatment of divergence insufficiency involves the judicious application of lenses, prism, and vision therapy. Fortunately, only in very extreme cases, is a surgical consultation necessary. Prangen and Koch (2) stated that divergence insufficiency patients appear to be poor surgical risks. Dunnington (68) recommended surgery only for the more resistant types of this condition. Burian (4) believed that bilateral lateral rectus resection is the procedure of choice, but only after prism therapy has been attempted.

Case Studies

Case 8.9

History

Suzanne, a 16-year-old girl in the eleventh grade, presented with a complaint of occasional double vision. The double vision was particularly bothersome when she had to take notes off the board in school and when driving. Her last eye examination was about 2 years ago and no problem was found. Her mother remembers, however, that about 4 years ago, Suzanne was also complaining of double vision. At that time, the doctor suggested that there was a vision problem, but it was not serious enough to treat.

Suzanne was in good health and was not taking any medication. She was doing well in school, had a normal appetite, and her sleep patterns were normal.

Examination Results

VA (distance, uncorrected):	OD: 20/20
	OS: 20/20
VA (near, uncorrected):	OD: 20/20
	OS: 20/20
Near point of convergence:	
Accommodative target:	6 cm
Penlight:	6 cm
Cover test (distance):	12 esophoria
Cover test (near):	2 exophoria
Subjective:	OD: +1.00, 20/20
	OS: +1.00, 20/20
Distance lateral phoria:	12 esophoria
Base-in vergence (distance):	X/2/−4
Base-out vergence (distance):	12/28/18
Vertical associated phoria (distance):	no vertical deviation
Near lateral phoria:	orthophoria
−1.00 gradient:	2 esophoria
Gradient AC/A ratio:	2:1
Calculated AC/A ratio:	1.2:1
Base-in vergence (near):	X/16/12

Base-out vergence (near):	12/26/12
Vertical associated phoria (near):	no vertical deviation
NBA:	+2.50
PRA:	−2.50
Accommodative amplitude (push-up):	OD: 12 D, OS: 12 D
MAF:	OD: 9 cpm, OS: 9 cpm
BAF:	8 cpm
MEM retinoscopy:	+0.50 OD and OS

Pupils were normal, all external and internal health tests were negative, the deviation was comitant, and color vision testing revealed normal function.

Case Analysis

All of the near point data are normal in this case. However, there is a significant degree of esophoria at distance, and the NFV at distance is reduced. The most likely diagnosis is divergence insufficiency. However, in such cases, it is important to think about the differential diagnosis listed in Table 8.12. The history suggests that this is not an acute problem. Suzanne complained of diplopia at least 4 years ago. It is likely that she is bothered more now because of the need to take more notes off the board at school and the fact that she is beginning to drive. The health history is negative and she is eating and sleeping well. Her school performance has not shown any signs of deterioration. Thus, Suzanne is a teenager who appears to be thriving and doing well in all areas, except for the occasional complaint of diplopia. This history suggests divergence insufficiency and the comitant nature of the deviation precludes a sixth nerve paresis. Thus, a diagnosis of divergence insufficiency is most likely.

Management

Because the lenses reduced the deviation slightly, they were prescribed to correct the hyperopia, even though the AC/A ratio is low. In addition, base-out prism was incorporated into her glasses. The amount of prism was determined, based on the associated phoria measured at distance using the American Optical Fixation Disparity target. The associated phoria with this device was 6 base-out. The final prescription was:

OD: +1.00 with 3 base-out
OS: +1.00 with 3 base-out

Suzanne was asked to wear these glasses for school and driving for 4 weeks and scheduled for a reevaluation. At the reevaluation, she reported elimination of her symptoms with the new glasses. The cover test with her glasses was 3 esophoria at distance and 6 exophoria at near. Base-in vergence at distance was X/7/3.

Suzanne was told to continue to wear the glasses in the same manner and to return in 1 year or sooner if she experienced any additional problems. This is a very typical case of divergence insufficiency. Glasses with low plus and base-out prism were effective without the need for vision therapy.

Case 8.10

History

Greg, a 22-year-old accountant, presented with a complaint of intermittent double vision and eyestrain. The double vision only bothered him when driving or when engaged in other tasks at a distance, like movies. At the end of the day, he often experienced eyestrain that he described as a general feeling of pulling around his eyes. He had complained for years about these problems and had been given glasses in the past. The glasses relieved, but did not entirely eliminate, the problems. In fact, the most recent glasses he received a year ago made it a little less comfortable when he read. He sometimes experienced eyestrain, even when reading with the newer glasses. His medical history was negative and he was not taking any medication.

Examination Results

Current prescription	OD: plano with 5 base-out	
	OS: plano with 5 base-out	
VA (distance, uncorrected):	OD: 20/20, corrected:	OD: 20/20
	OS: 20/20,	OS: 20/20
VA (near, uncorrected):	OD: 20/20, corrected	OD: 20/20
	OS: 20/20,	OS: 20/20
Near point of convergence:		
Accommodative target:	5 cm	
Penlight:	5 cm	
Cover test (distance, uncorrected):	15 esophoria	
Cover test (near, uncorrected):	orthophoria	
Cover test (near, corrected):	10 exophoria	
Subjective:	OD: plano, 20/20	
	OS: plano, 20/20	
Distance lateral phoria:	15 esophoria	
Base-in vergence (distance):	X/2/−4	
Base-out vergence (distance):	10/14/8	
Vertical associated phoria (distance):	no vertical deviation	
Near lateral phoria:	orthophoria	
−1.00 Gradient:	2 esophoria	
Gradient AC/A ratio:	2:1	
Base-in vergence (near):	12/18/9	
Base-out vergence (near):	10/14/10	
Vertical associated phoria (near):	no vertical deviation	
NRA:	+2.25	
PRA:	−2.50	
Accommodative amplitude (push-up):	OD: 10 D, OS: 10 D	
MAF:	OD: 9 cpm, OS: 9 cpm	
BAF:	7 cpm	
MEM retinoscopy:	+0.50 OD and OS	

Pupils were normal, all external and internal health tests were negative, the deviation was comitant, and color vision testing revealed normal function.

Case Analysis

The long-standing history of diplopia and asthenopia, along with the high esophoria at distance with a low AC/A ratio, clearly establishes a diagnosis of divergence insufficiency. This patient had already been treated with prism in the past and, while these glasses had helped, they had not totally eliminated his symptoms. The challenge in this case is the management rather than the diagnosis.

Management

There are two problems that had to be addressed in this case. The first problem is that, even with his current prescription (10 base-out prism), the patient reported that he still had some diplopia and discomfort. The second issue is that, with his glasses on, the patient had an additional problem of asthenopia when reading. Analysis of his near data, with his prescription, reveals the reason for this problem. The cover test at near through his prescription was 10 exophoria. The PFV at near without the glasses was 10/14/10. With the 10 base-out prism, the PFV measurement would be reduced about 10 Δ. Thus, with glasses on, he had a high degree of exophoria with reduced PFV ranges at near.

The use of additional prism was not indicated in this case. The associated phoria determined with fixation disparity testing confirmed that 8 to 10 base-out was an appropriate amount of prism. Vision therapy was prescribed to solve both problems described above. The first goal was to improve PFV at near and the second was to improve NFV at distance. This vision therapy program lasted about 3 months with 14 in-office visits. We followed the vision therapy sequence outlined in Table 8.15.

After vision therapy, the patient was able to wear the prism glasses more comfortably during reading tasks and he no longer had complaints about distance-related tasks. The cover test through his prescription was 4 esophoria at distance and 10 exophoria at near. The PFV at near with the glasses was 18/28/24 and the NFV at distance was X/7/5.

Summary and Conclusions

Divergence insufficiency represents a disorder of considerable clinical significance, even though it is the least prevalent binocular vision problem. Patients with greater esodeviation at distance than at near, a comitant deviation, and diplopia present a challenging diagnostic puzzle for the clinician. Divergence insufficiency, a benign condition, must be differentiated from divergence paralysis and sixth nerve palsy, which often have underlying etiologies of a serious nature. Knowledge of the characteristic signs and symptoms of these disorders is, therefore, important.

A diagnosis of either divergence paralysis or sixth nerve palsy would necessitate a referral for a neurological examination. Once a tentative diagnosis of divergence insufficiency is reached, the condition is generally managed by a combination of prism, lenses, and vision therapy.

STUDY QUESTIONS

1. Why are added lenses not a very effective treatment approach for low AC/A conditions?
2. Why is prism considered to be a more important treatment tool for divergence insufficiency than for convergence insufficiency?
3. Describe two modifications to the traditional near point of convergence test that can be used to detect more subtle cases of convergence insufficiency.
4. What are the key findings that would differentiate classical convergence insufficiency from convergence insufficiency associated with accommodative excess and pseudoconvergence insufficiency?
5. Outline a 3-phase vision therapy program for convergence insufficiency and indicate the key objectives for each phase of therapy.

6. Describe the recommendations you would make after a patient completes vision therapy for convergence insufficiency. What would the clinical care be like for the next 3 to 12 months?

SOURCES OF EQUIPMENT

a. RC Instruments: 21444 Hague Road, Noblesville, IN 46060; 800-348-2225.
b. Available from Bruce Wick, O.D., PhD., University of Houston, College of Optometry, 4901 Calhoun, Houston, TX 77204.

REFERENCES

1. London RF, Wick B. The effect of correction of vertical fixation disparity on the horizontal forced vergence fixation disparity curve. *Am J Optom Physiol Opt* 1987;64:653–656.
2. Prangen A, Koch FL. Divergence insufficiency: a clinical study. *Am J Ophthalmol* 1938;21:510–518.
3. Oaks LW. Divergence insufficiency as a practical problem. *Arch Ophthalmol* 1949;41:562–569.
4. Burian HM. Anomalies of convergence and divergence functions and their treatment. *Symposium on strabismus*, 3rd ed. St. Louis: Mosby, 1971:223–232.
5. Hermann JS. Surgical therapy for convergence insufficiency. *J Pediatr Ophthalmol Strabismus* 1981;18:28–31.
6. von Noorden GK. Resection of both medial rectus muscles in organic convergence insufficiency. *Am J Ophthalmol* 1976;81:223–230.
7. Haldi BA. Surgical management of convergence insufficiency. *Am J Ophthalmol* 1978;28:106–109.
8. Scheiman M. Divergence insufficiency: characteristics, diagnosis, and treatment. *Am J Optom Physiol Opt* 1986;63(6):425–431.
9. The efficacy of optometric vision therapy. The 1986/1987 AOA Future of Visual Development/Performance Task Force. *J Am Optom Assoc* 1988;59:95–105.
10. Suchoff IB, Petito GT. The efficacy of visual therapy. *J Am Optom Assoc* 1986;57:119–125.
11. Grisham JD. Visual therapy results for convergence insufficiency: a literature review. *Am J Optom Physiol Opt* 1988;65:448–454.
12. Hoffman L, Cohen A, Feuer G. Effectiveness of non-strabismic optometric vision training in a private practice. *Am J Optom & Arch Am Acad Opt* 1973;50:813–816.
13. Daum K. The course and effect of visual training on the vergence system. *Am J Optom Physiol Opt* 1982;59:223–227.
14. Daum K. Convergence insufficiency. *Am J Optom Physiol Opt* 1984;61:16–22.
15. Daum K. Double blind placebo-controlled examination of timing effects in the training of positive vergences. *Am J Optom Physiol Opt* 1986;63:807–812.
16. Vaegan JL. Convergence and divergence show longer and sustained improvement after short isometric exercise. *Am J Optom Physiol Opt* 1979;56:23–33.
17. Cooper J, Selenow A, Ciuffreda KJ, et al. Reduction of asthenopia in patients with convergence insufficiency after fusional vergence training. *Am J Optom Physiol Opt* 1983;60:982–989.
18. Daum K. A comparison of results of tonic and phasic training on the vergence system. *Am J Optom Physiol Opt* 1983;60:769–775.
19. Wick B. Vision therapy for presbyopic nonstrabismic patients. *Am J Optom Physiol Opt* 1977;54:244–247.
20. Cohen AH, Soden R. Effectiveness of visual therapy for convergence insufficiencies for an adult population. *J Am Optom Assoc* 1984;55:491–494.
21. Birnbaum MH, Soden R, Cohen AH. Efficacy of vision therapy for convergence insufficiency in an adult male population. *J Am Optom Assoc* 1999;70:225–232.
22. Duke-Elder S. *System of ophthalmology: ocular motility and strabismus*, vol. 7. London: Henry Kimpton, 1973:570–571.
23. Hugonnier R, Hugonnier SC. *Strabismus, heterophoria, and ocular motor paralysis*. St. Louis: Mosby, 1969:427–429.
24. von Noorden GK, Burian HM. *Binocular vision and ocular motility: theory and management of strabismus*, 5th ed. St. Louis: Mosby-Year Book, 1996:470–471.
25. Lyle TK, Wybar KC. *Practical orthoptics in the treatment of squint*, 5th ed. London: NK Lewis, 1967:427–429.
26. Griffin JR, Grisham JD. *Binocular anomalies: procedures for vision therapy*, 3rd ed. Boston: Butterworth-Heineman, 1995:431–435.
27. Pickwell LD. *Binocular vision anomalies: investigation and treatment*, 2nd ed. London: Butterworth-Heineman, 1989.
28. Press LJ. *Applied concepts in vision therapy*. Boston: Mosby, 1997.
29. Duane A. A new classification of the motor anomalies of the eye based upon physiological principles. *Ann Ophthalmol Otolaryngol* 1886:247–260.
30. Norn MS. Convergence insufficiency: incidence in ophthalmic practice—results of orthoptics treatment. *Acta Ophthalmol* 1966;44:132–138.

31. Kent PR, Steeve JH. Convergence insufficiency: incidence among military personnel and relief by orthoptics methods. *Milit Surg* 1953;112:202–205.
32. Scheiman M, Gallaway M, Coulter R, et al. Prevalence of vision and ocular disease conditions in a clinical pediatric population. *J Am Optom Assoc* 1996;67:193–202.
33. Rouse MW, Hyman L, Hussein M, et al. Frequency of convergence insufficiency in optometry clinic settings. *Optom Vis Sci* 1998;75:88–96.
34. Rouse MW, Borsting E, Hyman L, et al. Frequency of convergence insufficiency among fifth and sixth graders. *Optom Vis Sci* 1999;76:643–649.
35. Porcar E, Nartinez-Palomera A. Prevalence of general dysfunctions in a population of university students. *Optom Vis Sci* 1997;74:111–113.
36. Cooper J, Duckman R. Convergence insufficiency: incidence, diagnosis, and treatment. *J Am Optom Assoc* 1978;49:673–680.
37. Borsting E, Rouse MW, De Land PN, et al. Prospective comparison of convergence insufficiency and normal binocular vision on CIRS symptom surveys. *Optom Vis Sci* 1999;76:221–228.
38. Rouse MW, Hyman L, Hussein M, et al. *J Optom Vis Devel* 1997;28:91–97.
39. Hayes GJ, Cohen BE, Rouse MW, et al. Normative values for the near point of convergence of elementary schoolchildren. *Optom Vis Sci* 1998;75:506–512.
40. Scheiman M, Gallaway M, Frantz KA, et al. Near point of convergence: test procedure, target selection, and expected findings. *Optom Vis Sci* 2001 *(in press)*.
41. Wick BC. Horizontal deviations. In: Amos J, ed. *Diagnosis and management in vision care*. Boston: Butterworth-Heineman, 1987:473.
42. Mohindra I, Molinari J. Convergence insufficiency: its diagnosis and management—Part 1. *Optom Monthly* 1980;71(3):38–43.
43. Davis CE. Orthoptics treatment in convergence insufficiency. *J Can Med Assoc* 1956;55:47–49.
44. Capobianco M. The subjective measurement of the near point of convergence and its significance in the diagnosis of convergence insufficiency. *Am Orthoptic J* 1952;2:40–42.
45. Rosner J. *Pediatric optometry*. Boston: Butterworth-Heineman, 1982:258.
46. von Noorden GK, Brown DJ, Parks M. Associated convergence and accommodative insufficiency. *Doc Ophthalmol* 1973;34:393–403.
47. Pickwell LD, Dorth, Stephens LC. Inadequate convergence. *Brit J Physiol Opt* 1975;30:34–37.
48. Pickwell LD, Hampshire R. The significance of inadequate convergence. *Ophthalmic Physiol Opt* 1981;1:13–18.
49. Richman JE, Cron MT. *Guide to vision therapy*. South Bend, IN: Bernell Corporation, 1989.
50. Burde RM, Savino PJ, Trobe JD. Clinical decisions in neuro-ophthalmology. 2nd ed. St. Louis: Mosby-Year Book, 1992:284–285.
51. Scheiman M, Cooper J, Mitchell GL, et al. A survey of treatment modalities for convergence insufficiency. *Optom Vis Sci* 2001;79:151–157.
52. Duke-Elder S, Wybar K. Ocular motility and strabismus. In: Duke-Elder S. *System of ophthalmology* St. Louis: Mosby, 1973;6:547–551.
53. Gallaway M, Scheiman M, Malhotra K. The effectiveness of pencil pushups treatment for convergence insufficiency. *Optom Vis Sci* 2001 *(in press)*.
54. Cooper J, Feldman J. Operant conditioning of fusional convergence ranges using random dot stereograms. *Am J Optom Physiol Opt* 1980;57:205–213.
55. Cooper J, Citron M. Microcomputer produced anaglyphs for evaluation and therapy of binocular anomalies. *J Am Optom Assoc* 1983;54:785–788.
56. Cooper J, Selenow A, Ciuffreda KJ, et al. Reduction of asthenopia in patients with convergence insufficiency after fusional vergence training. *Am J Optom Physiol Opt* 1983;60:982–989.
57. Cooper J. Review of computerized orthoptics with specific regard to convergence insufficiency. *Am J Optom Physiol Opt* 1988;65:455–463.
58. Swartout JB. *Manual of procedures and forms for in-office and out-of-office optometric vision training programs*. Santa Ana, CA: Vision Extension, 1991.
59. Moore S, Harbison JW, Stockbridge L. Divergence insufficiency. *Am Orthop J* 1971;21:59–63.
60. Lyle DJ. Divergence insufficiency. *Arch Ophthalmol* 1954;52:858–864.
61. Chamlin M, Davidoff LM. Divergence paralysis with increased intracranial pressure. *J Neurosurg* 1950;7:539–543.
62. Bruce GM. Ocular divergence: its physiology and pathology. *Arch Ophthalmol* 1935;13:639–660.
63. Bielchowsky A. Lectures on anomalies of the eyes. III. Paralysis of conjugate movements of the eyes. *Arch Ophthalmol* 1935;13:569–583.
64. Bender MB, Savitsky N. Paralysis of divergence. *Arch Ophthalmol* 1940;23:1046–1051.
65. Jampolsky A. Ocular divergence mechanisms. *Trans Am Ophthalmol Soc* 1971;68:730–822.
66. Higgins JD. Oculomotor system. In: Barresi BJ, ed. *Ocular assessment: the manual of diagnosis for office practice*. Boston: Butterworth-Heineman, 1984:201.
67. London R. Fixation disparity. In: Barresi BJ, ed. *Ocular assessment: the manual of diagnosis for office practice*. Boston: Butterworth-Heineman, 1984:148.
68. Dunnington JH. Paralysis of divergence with report of three cases due to epidemic encephalitis. *Arch Ophthalmol* 1923;52:39–49.

9

High AC/A Conditions: Convergence Excess and Divergence Excess

In this chapter, we discuss the characteristics, diagnosis, and management of nonstrabismic binocular disorders associated with a high AC/A ratio. As we described previously, the AC/A ratio is the major factor that determines the sequence of management decisions in patients with heterophoria (Chapter 3). Consequently, certain general treatment strategies are shared by all binocular conditions associated with a high AC/A ratio. However, there are also important differences among patients with high AC/A ratios who have convergence excess and those who have divergence excess. After a review of the general principles that apply to all high AC/A disorders, each condition will be described separately to highlight the differences in characteristics, diagnosis, and management.

The specific conditions that will be discussed in this chapter are the various forms of convergence excess and divergence excess.

OVERVIEW OF GENERAL MANAGEMENT PRINCIPLES FOR HETEROPHORIA ASSOCIATED WITH HIGH AC/A RATIO

For binocular vision disorders associated with a high AC/A ratio, the specific management sequences are listed in Tables 9.1 and 9.2. The major difference that distinguishes high AC/A problems from conditions associated with low and normal AC/A ratios is the relative effectiveness of added lenses in effecting a change in the size of the heterophoria. An example of this is the patient with convergence excess described in Case 9.1.

Case Studies

Case 9.1

A 10-year-old boy presented with a complaint of eyestrain, blurred vision, and inability to concentrate when reading after 10 minutes. These problems had been bothering him since the beginning of the school year. The refraction was +1.00 D OD and OS, the distance phoria was 4 esophoria, and the near phoria was 20 esophoria (IPD = 58 mm). The calculated AC/A ratio in this case is 8:1. Near point testing through the subjective revealed the following:

Negative relative accommodation (NRA):	+2.50
Positive relative accommodation (PRA):	−1.00
Near lateral phoria (NLP):	3 esophoria
Base-in near (N):	4/10/4
Base-out near (N):	16/26/16
Vergence facility:	0 cpm, diplopia with base-in
Monocular estimation method (MEM):	+1.25 OD and OS

TABLE 9.1. *Sequential considerations in the management of convergence excess*

Optical correction of ametropia	Vision therapy for amblyopia
Added lens power	Vision therapy for suppression
Vertical prism	Vision therapy for sensory motor function
Horizontal prism	Surgery
Occlusion for amblyopia	

Binocular accommodative facility (BAF):	diplopia with −2.00, 0 cpm
Monocular accommodative facility (MAF):	12 cpm

Since the AC/A ratio is high, it is important to prescribe for the ametropia in this case. Prescribing +1.00 will reduce the near phoria to about 2 esophoria. Analysis of the near point data indicates that all of the direct and indirect measures of negative fusional vergence (NFV) are low. The use of added plus lenses in this case is indicated and will eliminate the remaining esophoria, balance the NRA/PRA relationship, and normalize the MEM and base-in findings. The near point analysis in this case suggests that a +0.75 to a +1.00 add is appropriate.

Case 9.2

A 4-year-old girl was brought for an examination because her parents had noticed that her right eye was drifting out toward the end of the day and when she was tired. They had noticed it for the last year and felt that the proportion of time that the eye turned was increasing. The refraction was +0.25 OD and OS. The cover test at distance was an intermittent 25 Δ, right exotropia (deviates 10% of the time). At near, the cover test was 5 exophoria. The calculated AC/A ratio is 13:1.

The ametropia is insignificant in this case but the use of added lenses can be helpful in the treatment of this patient. Because of the high AC/A ratio, glasses can be prescribed to help control the deviation. The use of −1.50 OU would significantly reduce the angle at distance. Since it could also lead to a high degree of esophoria at near, investigation of the use of a bifocal is also appropriate. In this case, the use of −1.50 with a +1.00 add OU is a valuable optical management technique because of the high AC/A ratio. If this child were older, vision therapy would probably be adequate to treat the divergence excess. In preschool children who may be difficult to treat using vision therapy, added lenses are an important temporary treatment option.

Another example of the effectiveness of added lenses in high AC/A cases is illustrated in Case 9.2.

TABLE 9.2. *Sequential considerations in the management of divergence excess*

Optical correction of ametropia	Vision therapy for suppression
Vertical prism	Vision therapy for sensory motor function
Added minus lens power	Horizontal prism
Occlusion for amblyopia	Surgery
Vision therapy for amblyopia	

Optical correction of ametropia still remains the first issue that should be considered. However, as evidenced by the preceding case report, the consideration of added lenses is close to the top of the list in Table 9.1. In high AC/A cases, correction of the refractive error may be helpful for two reasons. The first is that the presence of an uncorrected refractive error may create an imbalance between the two eyes, leading to sensory fusion disturbances, or it may create decreased fusional ability due to blurred retinal images. The second reason is that, because of the high AC/A, correction of the ametropia may have a beneficial effect on the magnitude of the deviation.

When considering the final prescription for these patients, it is important to first determine if a vertical deviation is present. As discussed in previous chapters, correction of even small amounts of vertical deviations can have a positive effect on the horizontal deviation. We suggest prescribing for vertical deviations as small as 0.5 Δ (Chapter 13).

A key difference between the sequential management of convergence excess and divergence excess is that esophores are more likely to benefit from horizontal prism than exophores. The use of base-out prism is an early management consideration in convergence excess, but the use of base-in is near the bottom of the list for divergence excess (see Tables 9.1 and 9.2). Because of the effectiveness of added lenses, prism is rarely necessary for convergence excess associated with normal tonic vergence (orthophoria at distance). An example of the value of base-out prism in the treatment of convergence excess, however, is the case illustrated below.

Case 9.3

A 21-year-old woman presented with a chief complaint of intermittent diplopia when driving and when reading. The diplopia was worse when reading and she also complained of eyestrain when reading for more that 15 minutes. Although she had always had these problems, they seemed worse since she started a new job in which she worked at a desk 8 hours a day doing paperwork. The cycloplegic refraction revealed plano OD and OS. The cover test was 8 esophoria at distance and 16 esophoria at near. The calculated AC/A ration is 9.4:1 (IPD = 62 mm).

This is a case of convergence excess with high tonic vergence or a moderate degree of esophoria at distance. Since there is no refractive error, the use of lenses in a distance prescription is not an option. The patient does have a high AC/A ratio, and the near deviation can be decreased easily using added lenses. However, a prescription, such as plano with a +1.50 add, would only eliminate the patient's near complaints. She would still experience diplopia when driving. The use of base-out prism is an important option in this type of case. The magnitude of the prism should be determined based on fixation disparity assessment (Chapter 14). A final prescription in this case might be:

OD: plano, 2 base-out
OS: plano, 2 base-out
+1.00 add

Thus, in cases of convergence excess associated with high tonic vergence, horizontal prism is an important consideration. When convergence excess is associated with a normal or low tonic vergence, prism is generally not necessary.

Although amblyopia is uncommon in nonstrabismic binocular vision anomalies, it can occur if the phoria is associated with a significant degree of anisometropia. Although anisometropic amblyopia is typically shallow (about 20/60 to 20/80), one of the early considerations should be treatment of amblyopia using occlusion and vision therapy. The use of occlusion and specific vision therapy procedures for the treatment of the amblyopia, and any associated suppression, always needs to be considered immediately after prescribing for the anisometropia and considering prism to compensate for a vertical phoria. In cases of convergence excess or divergence excess associated with anisometropia, we recommend part-time occlusion. Several (2 to 4) hours of occlusion using an opaque patch along with active amblyopia therapy is usually sufficient to resolve the amblyopia. Details about the evaluation and management of anisometropic amblyopia are described in Chapter 16. In almost all cases, however, amblyopia will not be present in either convergence or divergence excess. Thus, after consideration of ametropia, added lenses, and prism, vision therapy is the next treatment issue.

In many cases of convergence excess, the use of added lenses and prism will be sufficient to successfully treat the patient. If NFV is severely reduced, the magnitude of the esophoria is very large, or the patient remains uncomfortable even after wearing the glasses, vision therapy should be recommended. In contrast, vision therapy is the primary treatment option for divergence excess. In general, vision therapy is more effective for divergence excess, while base-out prism and added plus lenses tend to be more effective for convergence excess.

The final sequential management consideration listed in Tables 9.1 and 9.2 is surgery. Convergence excess can almost always be successfully managed with a combination of nonsurgical methods. Divergence excess may at times present with a very large magnitude exotropia at distance. When the size of the deviation is greater than 30 to 35 Δ, surgery will sometimes be necessary to supplement other nonsurgical approaches.

Prognosis for Binocular Vision Disorders Associated with High AC/A Ratios

The prognosis for successful treatment of convergence excess is excellent. In many cases the use of lenses, added lenses, and prism will be sufficient. If the patient is still symptomatic after these other interventions, vision therapy can be used and will generally lead to success. It would be rare, therefore, to be unable to successfully treat a patient with convergence excess. Failures with these patients are almost always associated with refusal to wear glasses or poor compliance with vision therapy.

The treatment of convergence excess with vision therapy has received some recent attention in the literature. In a record review of 12 patients with convergence excess who underwent vision therapy, Shorter and Hatch (1) found that 8 of 12 (66%) patients reported improved symptoms, and 5 of the 8 patients with complete data (62.5%) showed increased NFV. The changes were not statistically significant, however. Grisham et al. (2) and Wick (3) each reported a case of convergence excess that showed increased NFV and reduced symptoms after vision therapy. Ficarra et al. (4) performed a retrospective review of 31 patients (mean age 15.9 years) with convergence excess. The mean number of vision therapy visits was 19.4. There was a significant reduction in symptoms and significant improvement in NFV and PRA. The authors found that the most important factor in determining success was the magnitude of the pre-vision therapy near phoria. Gallaway and Scheiman (5) also performed a retrospective analysis of 83 consecutive patients treated with vision therapy for convergence excess. In contrast to the study by Ficarra et al. (4), which took place at an optometry school clinic, this study consisted of private practice patients. Thus, the testing was standardized within a practice and two clinicians performed all measurements. Statistically significant changes were found in direct and indirect measures of NFV, and 84% of patients reported total elimination of symptoms. Vision therapy does appear to be a viable alternative for patients with convergence excess.

In contrast to the success of added lenses with convergence excess, divergence excess responds best to vision therapy. Many studies have evaluated the efficacy of vision therapy for divergence excess. Goldrich (6) reported on the success of vision therapy in a sample of

28 divergence excess patients. He developed excellent, good, fair, and poor criteria for cure. To be placed in the excellent category a patient had to be free from asthenopia, have a phoria at all times, and have normal binocular findings. Placement in the good category meant that the patient was also free from asthenopia and had a phoria at all times, but could have deficiencies on some binocular testing. A fair result meant that an intermittent strabismus was occasionally observed on cover testing, and a poor result suggested that little improvement had occurred.

Twenty (71.4%) patients achieved an excellent rating and three (10.7%) patients had a good rating. Thus, in 82.1% of the patients, vision therapy was successful in eliminating the intermittent strabismus and asthenopia. For the subjects in the excellent category, the mean number of therapy visits was 20.2 sessions and for the good category, 28.3 sessions. Only one patient was rated poor after treatment.

Pickwell (7) reported on the results of vision therapy on 14 divergence excess patients. Ten patients achieved a satisfactory level, two patients showed measurable improvement, and two others discontinued therapy before completion. Daum (8) did a retrospective study of 18 divergence excess patients. The duration of treatment was unusually short, only 5.2 weeks, which raises questions about the meaning of his treatment results. However, he did suggest several interesting points relative to prognosis. He found that success was significantly better in subjects who had lower angles of deviation and no vertical deviation.

Other authors who have studied the effectiveness of vision therapy for intermittent exotropia did not differentiate divergence excess from other types of intermittent exotropia. Although this makes the results more difficult to analyze, the results still have relevance for understanding the effectiveness of vision therapy for divergence excess. Divergence excess is the most common type of intermittent exotropia for which surgery is likely to be recommended. As a result, it is reasonable to suggest that many of the patients reported in the following studies had divergence excess strabismus.

In a study of 37 exotropes, Sanfilippo and Clahane (9) found an excellent result in 64.5%, a good result in 9.7%, and a fair result in 22.6%. Only one patient (or 3.2%) had a poor result. The authors considered 64.5% to be "cured," and 32.3% to have immediate improvement in status. They also provided useful data about various factors that influence the effectiveness of treatment. Amblyopia, a constant deviation, noncomitancy, and a vertical component were negative factors.

Cooper and Leyman (10) reported on a retrospective study of 182 intermittent exotropes treated with orthoptics alone. They found a good result in 58.7% and a fair result in 38.4%. Only 5.6% of their sample failed to make significant progress with orthoptics.

Coffey et al. (11) reviewed 59 studies of intermittent exotropia treatment and they compiled pooled success rates. They calculated the following pooled success rates: 28% for over minus therapy, 28% for prism therapy, 37% for occlusion, 46% for surgery, and 59% for vision therapy. Cooper et al. (12) also reviewed the literature and concluded that divergence excess under the age of 6 years should be treated cautiously, so as to reduce or eliminate the possibility of developing amblyopia or permanent loss of stereopsis. They suggested various nonsurgical intervention approaches such as patching, minus lens therapy, and home-based antisuppression treatment initially. Only if the deviation persists or increases, should surgical intervention be considered. They suggested that in children over 6 years of age, vision therapy is the treatment of choice unless the deviation is large ($>35 \Delta$).

Thus, the literature supports the effectiveness of vision therapy in the treatment of divergence excess and, when compared to the cure rates for surgery described later in this chapter, suggests that vision therapy should be the first treatment option. It is important to keep in mind some of the negative prognostic factors suggested by the studies described above. Negative factors include a large angle of deviation ($>35 \Delta$), a large vertical component, and a noncomitancy.

Summary of Key Points in Treating Phoria Patients Associated with High AC/A

The primary determinant of the management sequence of high AC/A binocular vision problems is the effectiveness of added lenses. Because of the high AC/A ratio, added lenses have a significant effect on the angle of deviation and are, therefore, an important early treatment consideration. When esophoria is present at distance and correction of hyperopia is not sufficient to decrease the phoria to a manageable level, base-out prism is sometimes useful. At times, the use of lenses, added lenses, and prism will not be enough to restore comfort and vision therapy is necessary.

CONVERGENCE EXCESS

Convergence excess is a condition in which there is an esophoria at near, orthophoria or low to moderate esophoria at distance, reduced NFV, and a high AC/A ratio. Of the various nonstrabismic binocular vision problems seen in clinical practice, convergence excess is one of the most common. Hokoda (13) found a prevalence rate of 5.9% in a population of symptomatic individuals seeking vision care. In contrast, 4.2% were found to have convergence insufficiency. Scheiman et al. (14) also found a higher prevalence of convergence excess than convergence insufficiency. They performed a prospective study on 1,650 children between the ages of 6 and 18 years and found prevalence of 8.2%. In a university population, Porcar and Nartinez-Palomera (15) found a 1.5% prevalence of convergence excess.

Characteristics

Symptoms

Most symptoms are associated with reading or other close work. Common complaints include eyestrain and headaches after short periods of reading, blurred vision, diplopia, sleepiness, difficulty concentrating, and loss of comprehension over time (Table 9.3). Some patients with convergence excess are asymptomatic. This may be due to suppression, avoidance of near visual tasks, high pain threshold, or occlusion of one eye when reading. Clinicians should always inquire about avoidance of reading or other near tasks if a patient with convergence excess reports an absence of other symptoms.

Avoidance is often as important a reason for recommending therapy as any of the other symptoms associated with convergence excess.

TABLE 9.3. *Signs and symptoms of convergence excess*

Signs	Indirect Tests of Negative Fusional Vergence
Esophoria greater at near than at distance	Low positive relative accommodation
Frequency of esodeviation worse at near than at distance	Fails −2.00 on binocular accommodative facility testing
High AC/A ratio (calculated method)	High MEM retinoscopy finding
Moderate degree of hyperopia	**Symptoms**
Comitant deviation	Eyestrain associated with reading
Direct Tests of Negative Fusional Vergence	Headaches associated with reading
	Inability to attend and concentrate when reading
Reduced smooth negative fusional vergence (NFV) at near	Problems with reading comprehension
Reduced jump NFV at near	Occasional double vision
	Blurred vision

Signs

Signs of convergence excess are shown in Table 9.3.

Refractive Error

Convergence excess may be associated with hyperopia. This is a desirable characteristic. Because of the high AC/A ratio, correction of the hyperopia will lead to a decrease in the magnitude of the esophoria at near and at distance. As we stated earlier, one of the primary reasons for a lack of success in the treatment of convergence excess is the patient's refusal to wear glasses. Although this is very rare, there is another treatment alternative that can be considered in such cases.

When all efforts to have the patient wear eyeglasses or contact lenses fail, pharmacologic treatment is a last resort that can be attempted. Because of the side effects and complications associated with these drugs, this approach should only be used when the patient is either very symptomatic or the deviation is intermittent and the proportion of time the eye deviates is significant and is increasing. Pharmacologic treatment involves the use of echothiophate iodide (Phospholine Iodine) drops or diisopropyl flurophosphate (DFP) ointment. Both are anticholinesterase agents that cause miosis and ciliary spasm. This reduces or eliminates the need for accommodative effort and thereby leads to less accommodative convergence and reduced esophoria.

Echothiophate iodide solution comes in concentrations of 0.03, 0.06, 0.125, and 0.25%. We recommend using 0.03% echothiophate iodide solution once a day (at night) for 1 week. The use of Tylenol for the first week helps reduce the headaches associated with the ciliary spasm, which occur initially. After the first week, increase the concentration to 0.06% and reevaluate the patient's status in 2 weeks. Side effects and complications associated with the use of echothiophate iodide include headaches, reversible iris cysts, cataracts, and a greater risk of retinal detachment. The use of 2.5% phenylephrine has been shown to minimize the formation of iris cysts.

DEP ointment is also an anticholinesterase that can be used to treat convergence excess. A 0.25 in. strip of 0.025% ointment is applied every night. Tylenol should be used the first week or two to reduce the headaches associated with ciliary spasm. Side effects are similar to those described for echothiophate iodide.

When either drug is used, monthly reevaluations should be scheduled to monitor the patient for any side effects or complications and to assess the effect of the treatment. If symptoms have decreased or the proportion of time the deviation occurs is significantly reduced, the treatment can be continued with monthly reevaluation.

Characteristics of the Deviation

Patients with convergence excess generally have greater esophoria at near, a high AC/A ratio, and decreased NFV.

Some authors have suggested that a 10 Δ difference from one distance to another is a useful guideline. Rather than depend on this guideline, we find it more useful to think about the difference one would expect based on the presence of a high AC/A ratio. Since an AC/A ratio of greater than 7:1 is considered high, as little as a 3 Δ difference between distance and near would be sufficient to fit the diagnosis of convergence excess.

Clinicians should use their judgment and generally rely on the other characteristics, in addition to the magnitude of the angle at distance and near, to reach a diagnosis. For instance, the near deviation may be an intermittent or constant strabismus versus a phoria at distance. This finding would also suggest a diagnosis of convergence excess. Thus, a comparison of the proportion of time the deviation is present, as well as the magnitude at distance and near, is an important part of the diagnostic process.

AC/A Ratio

A high AC/A ratio ($\geq 7:1$) is always present in convergence excess. This is well accepted, based on the calculated AC/A and is an important factor when treatment is considered.

Analysis of Binocular and Accommodative Data

All direct tests of NFV tend to be low in convergence excess (Table 9.3). This includes step, smooth, and jump vergences. In addition, all tests that indirectly assess NFV (Table 9.3) will also be low. Tests performed binocularly with minus lenses evaluate the patient's ability to stimulate accommodation and control binocular alignment using NFV. Two examples are PRA and BAF testing with minus lenses. A characteristic finding in convergence excess is a report of diplopia, rather than blur as the endpoint, on PRA and BAF testing. In fact, it is important to specifically ask about diplopia when performing these tests on a patient suspected of having convergence excess.

A low finding on either PRA or BAF testing may be due to an inability to stimulate accommodation or reduced NFV. The differential diagnosis is based on assessment of accommodation under monocular conditions. An easy and helpful technique is to simply cover one eye after the patient reports blur on the PRA test. If the blur continues, the problem is usually accommodative (accommodative insufficiency or ill-sustained accommodation). If the patient's vision clears, the problem is associated with binocular vision (NFV). Normal monocular accommodative ability on other tests suggests reduced NFV.

Another important indirect test of NFV is MEM retinoscopy. It is not unusual to find an abnormal result on this test in convergence excess. An MEM finding of greater plus than expected suggests that the patient is using as little accommodation as possible to decrease the use of accommodative convergence. This reduces the amount of esophoria and the demand on NFV.

In some instances of convergence excess, a low to moderate degree of esophoria is present at distance as well. This is due to a moderate to high degree of tonic vergence. In such cases, in addition to the low NFV at near, the distance findings will be low as well.

Differential Diagnosis

It is important to rule out serious underlying etiology in all cases of convergence excess. Differential diagnosis (Table 9.4) depends very much on the nature of the patient's symptoms.

TABLE 9.4. *Differential diagnosis of convergence excess*

Functional disorders to rule out
1. Basic esophoria
2. Divergence insufficiency
3. Accommodative disorders

Serious underlying disease to rule out
1. Spasm of accommodation/convergence due to local inflammation such as scleritis, iritis, uveitis
2. Spasm of accommodation/convergence due to sympathetic paralysis, syphilis
3. Spasm of accommodation/convergence due to drugs including:
   eserine
   pilocarpine
   excessive doses of vitamin B_1
   sulfonamides

Typically, convergence excess presents with long-standing chronic complaints. The health history is negative and the patient is not taking any medication known to affect accommodation. Convergence excess associated with serious underlying disease has an acute onset, and medical problems or neurological symptoms are usually present. The primary functional disorders that must be differentiated from true convergence excess are basic esophoria, divergence insufficiency, and esophoria at near secondary to accommodative anomalies.

Convergence excess is considered to be a benign condition, with no serious consequences other than the visual symptoms listed in Table 9.4. It is relatively easy to differentiate from other binocular vision disorders associated with esophoria, such as basic esophoria (equal deviation at distance and at near) and divergence insufficiency (greater esophoria at distance). Convergence excess must also be differentiated from esophoria at near, secondary to an accommodative anomaly. To do so requires a careful analysis of all accommodative and binocular vision data. Cases 1 to 4 in Chapter 2 are examples of the analytical process the clinician must follow.

Convergence excess or esophoria at near can also be associated with more serious underlying conditions. A condition called spasm of accommodation or convergence can occur, and one resulting clinical finding may be esophoria at near. Accommodative spasm can be functional, but it may also be caused by more serious underlying disease. Some of the more common causes include local inflammation and central nervous system lesions. Ocular inflammation such as scleritis, iritis, and uveitis can cause uniocular accommodative spasm and esophoria. This suggests that slit lamp evaluation is an important test in the differential diagnosis of convergence excess.

Central nervous system disorders, such as sympathetic paralysis and syphilis, may also lead to accommodative spasm and esophoria. In addition, a variety of drugs may produce bilateral accommodative spasm and esophoria. Some of the more common drugs that can produce these effects include eserine, pilocarpine, excessive doses of vitamin B_1, and sulfonamides.

When managing a case of convergence excess that is thought to have a functional basis, if improvement in symptoms and findings does not occur as expected, it is wise to reconsider the etiology of the condition.

Treatment

We recommend following the management sequence listed in Table 9.1.

Lenses

In all cases of binocular and accommodative dysfunction, the first management consideration is correction of any significant refractive error. With convergence excess, it is important to prescribe maximum plus if a significant degree of hyperopia is present (+0.50 or greater). When dealing with convergence excess associated with high tonic vergence, a cycloplegic examination should be performed before determining the prescription.

Added Lenses

Because of the high AC/A ratio, the use of added plus lenses at near is highly effective in cases of convergence excess. In Chapter 3, we discussed the important clinical data that are used to determine whether additional plus should be prescribed. Although the AC/A ratio is the key finding, it is important to consider all of the data listed in Table 9.5.

TABLE 9.5. *Consideration for prescribing added plus lenses*

Test	Consider the use of added plus	Added plus not indicated
AC/A ratio	High	Low
Refractive error	Hyperopia	Myopia
Near phoria	Esophoria	Exophoria
Negative relative accommodation (NRA)/ positive relative accommodation (PRA)	Low PRA	Low NRA
Base-out at near	Normal to high	Low
Monocular estimation method retinoscopy	High	Low
Amplitude of accommodation	Low	Normal
Accommodative facility testing	Fails −	Fails +

How Much Additional Plus Should Be Prescribed?

When prescribing added plus lenses, the objective is to determine the lowest amount of plus that will eliminate the patient's symptoms and normalize optometric data. A variety of methods have been suggested for calculating the amount of additional plus to prescribe for patients with convergence excess. Some of the more popular methods are analysis of the NRA/PRA relationship, MEM retinoscopy or other near point retinoscopy, use of the AC/A ratio, and fixation disparity analysis. We advocate the use of a group of findings, rather than relying on any one test. As we discussed in Chapter 2, reliance on any one test may be misleading at times. The optometric data listed in Table 9.5 can be used to determine the amount of plus to prescribe.

An example of this is Case 9.1, described earlier in this chapter. After prescribing +1.00 to correct the hyperopia, this patient was still 3 esophoric at near, with a low PRA, reduced base-in at near, an MEM finding of +1.25, and diplopia with minus lenses during BAF testing.

Both the NRA/PRA (NRA, +2.50; PRA, −1.00) relationship and MEM retinoscopy suggest a prescription of an additional +0.75 to +1.00 for near. In addition, the AC/A ratio suggests that the near phoria should be about 3 exophoria with this prescription.

Prism

If a vertical deviation is present, we recommend that vertical prism be prescribed. The most effective method for determining the amount of vertical prism is the associated phoria, which can be measured with any fixation disparity device (Chapter 14).

Because of the high AC/A ratio, the use of lenses is so effective that horizontal prism is rarely necessary, except for convergence excess associated with high tonic vergence (moderate to high esophoria at distance). When a moderate to high degree of esophoria is present at distance, base-out prism should be considered. The decision to prescribe base-out prism should be based on the presence or absence of distance-related symptoms. If a prism prescription is being considered, fixation disparity testing is the most effective method for determining the amount of horizontal prism (Chapter 14).

Vision Therapy

If NFV is severely reduced, the magnitude of the esophoria is very large, or the patient remains uncomfortable even after wearing the glasses, vision therapy should be recommended. A vision therapy program for convergence excess generally requires 12 to 24 office visits. If refractive correction and added lenses are used, the number of sessions may be less. The total number of therapy sessions also depends on the age of the patient, motivation, and compliance.

Specific Vision Therapy Program

All of the vision therapy techniques recommended below are described in detail in Chapters 5 to 7.

Phase 1

This first phase of therapy is designed to accomplish the objectives listed in Table 9.6 under Phase 1.

As we discussed in Chapter 8, vision therapy requires communication and cooperation between the therapist and patient, and it is important to develop a working relationship with the patient during the first few sessions.

The first goal of the therapy is to teach the concept and feeling of diverging and the ability to accurately diverge. The patient should be able to voluntarily converge and diverge to any distance from 2 in. to 20 ft. Commonly used procedures to accomplish this first objective are the Brock string and bug on string.

Convergence excess patients generally have very limited base-in blur, break, and recovery findings. Therefore, another objective of the first phase of vision therapy is to normalize NFV amplitudes. The initial goal is to reestablish a normal vergence range for smooth- or tonic-type vergence demand. A smooth vergence demand is easier for the patient to accomplish in the early part of a vision therapy program. Such a demand allows the patient to begin the procedure with accommodation and convergence at the same plane. A divergence demand can then be slowly introduced, which requires the patient to hold accommodation at 40 cm and move the convergence plane further away.

Another advantage of beginning with smooth vergence procedures is that, in some cases, the introduction of any divergence is enough to cause suppression or diplopia. Smooth vergence

TABLE 9.6. *Vision therapy for convergence excess: general objectives*

Phase 1
Objectives
• Develop a working relationship with the patient
• Develop an awareness of the various feedback mechanisms that will be used throughout therapy
• Develop voluntary convergence/divergence
• Normalize negative fusional vergence (NFV) amplitudes (smooth or tonic vergence demand)
• Normalize accommodative amplitude and ability to stimulate and relax accommodation.

Phase 2
Objectives
• Normalize positive fusional vergence (PFV) amplitudes (smooth or tonic vergence demand)
• Normalize NFV facility (jump or phasic vergence demand)
• Normalize PFV facility (jump or phasic vergence demand)

Phase 3
Objectives
• Develop ability to change from a convergence to a divergence demand
• Integrate vergence procedures with changes in accommodative demand
• Integrate vergence procedures with versions

techniques provide a starting point for therapy with such patients. If the patient is unable to fuse any divergence demand, the procedure can begin with a convergence demand. For example, a variable Tranaglyph can be set at 10 base-out and then gradually reduced to zero. This approach at least allows the patient to get started and experience some success. The change from 10 base-out to zero can be viewed as divergence therapy relative to the starting point. Speed is of little importance initially. Rather, we simply want the patient to be able to maintain fusion as the divergence demand is slowly increased. Instrumentation that can be used to create a smooth gradual increase in divergence demand includes the variable Tranaglyphs, variable Vectograms, and the variable Prismatic Stereoscope.

In some cases of convergence excess in pre-presbyopes, an accommodative problem may also be present. If so, the final objective of the first phase of therapy is to normalize accommodative amplitude and the ability to stimulate and relax accommodation. If, however, accommodative function is normal, there is generally no need to spend much time working with the accommodative system. Accommodative techniques can be found in Chapter 6. Lens sorting, loose lens rock, and Hart chart procedures are commonly used in this first phase of therapy.

Endpoint

Phase 1 of therapy ends when the patient can:

- accurately diverge using the Brock string to 10 ft.
- fuse to about 15 base-in at 40 cm using a Tranaglyph or other divergence technique.
- complete 12 cpm of MAF with +2.00/−2.00 lenses using a 20/30 target.

A sample vision therapy program for Phase 1 is summarized in Table 9.7.

Phase 2

This second phase of therapy is designed to accomplish the objectives listed in Table 9.6 under Phase 2.

Once smooth NFV is normalized, phasic or jump vergence demand should be emphasized. Variable Tranaglyphs and Vectograms can still be used. However, the specific modifications to create a step vergence demand (described in Chapter 5) must be implemented. These include:

1. Change of fixation from the target to another point in space
2. Cover/uncover one eye
3. Loose prism or flip prism
4. Flip lenses to create a step change in accommodative demand, requiring a compensatory vergence change to maintain fusion
5. Two different Tranaglyphs set up in a Dual Polachrome Illuminated Trainer
6. Polaroid or red/green flippers

Other valuable techniques at this stage are the nonvariable Tranaglyphs, the Aperture Rule, Eccentric Circles, Free Space Fusion Cards, Lifesaver Cards, and the Computer Orthoptics Jump Vergence Program.

In contrast to Phase 1, in which speed was not a factor, during this second phase of therapy, the emphasis should be on the qualitative aspects of fusion rather than magnitude. It is important to increase the speed of the fusional vergence response and the quality of the recovery of fusion.

TABLE 9.7. *Sample vision therapy program for convergence excess*

Phase 1
Sessions 1 and 2
In-Office
- Discuss nature of vision problem, goals of vision therapy, various feedback cues, importance of practice.
- Brock string; concentrate on developing feeling of diverging
- Lens sorting
- Loose lens rock (begin with plus if accommodative excess, with minus if accommodative insufficiency)
- Tranaglyph or Vectograms: divergence
  1. Begin with a peripheral target like Tranaglyph 515 or the Quoit Vectogram
- Computer Orthoptics Random Dot Program: divergence
Home Therapy
- Brock string

Sessions 3 and 4
In-Office
- Bug on string, concentrate on feeling of diverging
- Loose lens rock
- Tranaglyph or Vectograms: divergence
  1. Use targets with more central demand (Clown, Bunny Tranaglyphs; Clown, Topper Vectrograms)
- Computer Orthoptics Random Dot Program: divergence
Home Therapy
- Add loose lens rock

Sessions 5 through 8
In-Office
- Loose lens rock
- Tranaglyph or Vectograms: divergence
  Use even more detailed targets such as Tranaglyphs Sports Slide and Faces targets and the Spirangle Vectogram)
- Computer Orthoptics Random Dot Program: divergence
Home Therapy
- Tranaglyph: divergence

Phase 2
Sessions 9 and 10
In-Office
- Tranaglyph or Vectograms with modifications to create jump vergence demand: divergence
- Nonvariable Tranaglyphs
- Tranaglyph 515 or the Quoit Vectogram: convergence
- Binocular accommodative therapy techniques: use any of the binocular techniques listed above with ± lenses
Home Therapy
- Nonvariable Tranaglyphs

Sessions 11 and 12
In-Office
- Tranaglyph or Vectograms with modifications to create jump vergence demand: divergence
- Aperture Rule: divergence
- More central Tranaglyphs with loose prism jumps
- Binocular accommodative therapy techniques: use any of the binocular techniques listed above with ± lenses
Home Therapy
- Nonvariable Tranaglyphs with loose prism jumps

Sessions 13 through 16
In-office
- Aperture Rule: divergence
- Eccentric Circles or Free Space Fusion Cards: divergence
- Computer Orthoptics Random Dot Vergence Program: both divergence and convergence
- Aperture Rule: convergence
- Tranaglyph or Vectograms with modifications to create jump vergence demand: convergence
- Binocular accommodative therapy techniques: use any of the binocular techniques listed above with ± lenses

TABLE 9.7. *Continued.*

Home Therapy
- Eccentric Circles or Free Space Fusion Cards: divergence

Phase 3
Sessions 17 through 20
In-office
- Tranaglyph or Vectograms with Polaroid or red/greed flippers
- Eccentric Circles or Free Space Fusion Cards
- Computer Orthoptics Random Dot Vergence Program: step–jump vergence
Home Therapy
- Eccentric Circles or Free Space Fusion Cards: divergence

Sessions 21 through 22
In-office
- Tranaglyph or Vectograms with Polaroid or red/green flippers
- Eccentric Circles or Free Space Fusion Cards
- Lifesaver Cards
- Computer Orthoptics Random Dot Vergence Program: jump–jump vergence
Home Therapy
- Eccentric Circles or Free Space Fusion Cards: convergence and divergence

Sessions 23 and 24
In-office
- Tranaglyph or Vectograms with Polaroid or red/green flippers
- Eccentric Circles or Free Space Fusion Cards with rotation and versions
- Lifesaver Cards with rotation and versions
- Computer Orthoptics Vergence Program with rotation
Home Therapy
- Eccentric Circles or Free Space Fusion Cards: divergence and convergence

A second objective of this phase of therapy is to begin working with positive fusional vergence (PFV) amplitudes. The same techniques used in Phase 1, to work with NFV, are repeated for PFV. Finally, during the end of this phase of therapy, begin to incorporate PFV facility-type techniques, using the same procedures listed above for jump vergence demand for NFV.

Endpoint

The endpoint of Phase 2 is reached when the patient can:

- fuse card 12 using convergence and card 6 using divergence with the Aperture Rule.
- fuse the Eccentric Circles or Free Space Fusion Cards using convergence (12 cm separation) and divergence (6 cm separation).

A sample vision therapy program for Phase 2 is summarized in Table 9.7.

Phase 3

This third phase of therapy is designed to accomplish the objectives listed in Table 9.6 under Phase 3.

Until this point, the patient has either worked in the convergence or divergence directions separately. Now the objective is to develop the patient's ability to change from a convergence to a divergence demand and to integrate vergence procedures with versions and saccades. Several excellent procedures are available to help accomplish these objectives. Vectograms with

Polaroid flippers or Tranaglyphs with red/green flippers can be used. Each time the flippers are changed, the demand switches from divergence to convergence. Transparent Keystone Eccentric Circles or transparent Bernell Free Space Fusion Cards are excellent inexpensive methods for achieving this objective. By this time, the patient has already learned to fuse these cards using divergence or convergence. Now the patient is taught to switch from divergence and then back to convergence. As this skill improves, speed or the number of cycles per minute is emphasized.

The final objective of therapy is to integrate vergence procedures with versions and saccades. Under normal seeing conditions, patients are constantly trying to maintain vergence while changing fixation from one location to another. We feel that it is, therefore, important to combine vergence therapy with versions and saccades. Techniques such as the Brock string with rotation, Eccentric Circles and Free Space Fusion Cards with rotation and/or lateral movements, and the Lifesaver Cards with rotation can be used to accomplish this goal. The Computer Orthoptics Program that combines horizontal vergence with rotation is also useful for this objective.

Endpoint

The endpoint for this phase of therapy is reached when the patient is able to maintain clear single binocular vision with the Eccentric Circle or Free Space Fusion Cards together, while slowly rotating the cards.

Since the objectives of vision therapy are to eliminate the patient's symptoms and normalize binocular and accommodative findings, a reevaluation should be performed about 6 weeks into the therapy program and again at the end of therapy. Refer back to the original complaints and determine if the patient is now comfortable. All tests of binocular and accommodative function should be repeated and compared to the initial findings as well the expected findings.

When all vision therapy objectives have been reached and the vision therapy program is completed, we recommend the home vision therapy maintenance program outlined in Table 8.10, and described in Chapter 8.

Summary of Vision Therapy for Convergence Excess

The phases and objectives outlined above and in Tables 9.6 and 9.7 represent one approach that will lead to successful elimination of a patient's symptoms and normalization of optometric data. The number of sessions is approximate and will vary from one patient to another. In our experience, adults generally can complete a vision therapy program in about half the time necessary for children. Another variable is the use of home therapy techniques to supplement the activities used for in-office therapy. Home therapy can be useful with a highly motivated adult patient. It may also be effective when the patient is a motivated compliant child with a parent that has the capability to function as the home therapist. In some cases, however, the parent may not interact well with the child in this role, and home therapy will not be helpful. Appendix A (at the end of the book) lists a variety of instructional sheets for vision therapy that can be used for home therapy. Using the approach suggested above should lead to the achievement of the very high success rates reported in the literature for convergence excess.

Surgery

The use of lenses, prism, and vision therapy in the treatment of convergence excess is so successful that surgery is seldom necessary.

Case Studies

Case 9.4

History

Jessica, a 10-year-old fifth grader, presented with complaints of eyestrain and blurry vision after 15 to 20 minutes of reading. She said that these problems began in fifth grade when the teachers began giving more homework. She never had an eye examination. Her medical history was negative and she was not taking any medication.

Examination Results

VA (distance, uncorrected):	OD: 20/20
	OS: 20/20
VA (near, uncorrected):	OD: 20/20
	OS: 20/20
Near point of convergence:	
Accommodative target:	5 cm
Penlight:	5 cm
Cover test (distance):	orthophoria
Cover test (near):	10 esophoria
Subjective:	OD: plano, 20/20
	OS: plano, 20/20
Distance lateral phoria:	orthophoria
Base-in vergence (distance):	X/7/4
Base-out vergence (distance):	12/24/15
Near lateral phoria:	10 esophoria
−1.00 gradient:	18 esophoria
Gradient AC/A ratio:	8:1
Calculated AC/A ratio:	10:1
Base-in vergence (near):	X/4/-4
Base-out vergence (near):	14/30/18
Vergence facility	0 cpm, diplopia with base in
NRA:	+2.50
PRA:	diplopia with −0.25
Accommodative amplitude (push-up):	OD: 15 D, OS: 15 D
MAF:	OD: 12 cpm, OS: 12 cpm
BAF:	diplopia with −2.00
MEM retinoscopy:	+1.50 OD and OS

Pupils were normal, all external and internal health tests were negative, the deviation was comitant, and color vision testing revealed normal function.

Case Analysis

Based on the large esophoria at near, the best way to approach this case is to analyze the NFV group data. For this patient, all of the direct and indirect findings that probe NFV are abnormal. The direct findings, NFV at near, and vergence facility are severely reduced. In addition, the indirect tests—PRA, BAF, and MEM retinoscopy—all suggest an esophoria/low NFV problem.

The distance phoria is ortho and the calculated and gradient AC/A ratios are both high. This set of findings clearly suggests a diagnosis of convergence excess with normal tonic vergence.

Management

Since there was no refractive error, our initial approach in this case was to prescribe added lenses just for near. To determine the amount of plus to prescribe, we analyzed several key findings including the AC/A ratio, NRA/PRA relationship, fusional vergence findings, and MEM retinoscopy. In this case, the NRA/PRA relationship suggested an add of about +1.25, as did MEM retinoscopy. The AC/A ratio showed that an add of +1.25 would reduce the near phoria to about ortho and increase the NFV ranges at near by about 10 Δ. We, therefore, prescribed +1.25 OD and OS for all near work.

A decision that clinicians must make when prescribing added plus lenses is whether to recommend single vision lenses or bifocals. We generally recommend a bifocal prescription for elementary schoolchildren so that they do not have to remove their glasses when looking at the teacher or the chalkboard. In our experience, young children wearing single vision glasses often lose, break, or scratch their glasses because of the continual need to remove the prescription.

As children become more mature and able to care properly for their glasses, a single vision prescription becomes a viable option. For older children (adolescent) and adults, we outline the advantages and disadvantages of single vision and bifocal lenses and allow the patient to help with the final decision. However, most patients find that a properly prescribed bifocal is the most satisfactory alternative.

Although a bifocal is our first recommendation for elementary schoolchildren, we do sometimes encounter resistance from parents about the idea of a bifocal for a child. When this occurs, it is best to review and demonstrate the benefits of a bifocal, and, if the parent is still uneasy, prescribe a single vision prescription. We ask the parent to carefully monitor the child's compliance with the wearing instructions and the child's ability to care for the glasses. The parent always has the option to switch, at a later date, to a bifocal and will often be more accepting of this suggestion after they personally experience the problems associated with a single vision prescription.

In this case, a follow-up visit after 6 weeks revealed that Jessica was doing well with the glasses, and she reported a complete relief of symptoms. We, therefore, did not have to recommend any additional treatment.

Case 9.5

History

Marilyn, a 16-year-old high school junior, complained of an inability to read comfortably for more than 10 minutes. When she read for longer periods of time, she felt a pulling sensation that would soon develop into a headache over her eyes. She experienced difficulty with comprehension and sometimes fell asleep when reading. Her last eye examination was about 1 year ago when she had complained of similar symptoms. The doctor prescribed reading glasses that did help. However, even with glasses, Marilyn continued to feel uncomfortable when reading. Her health history was negative.

Examination Results

VA (distance, uncorrected):   OD: 20/20
                                                OS: 20/20

VA (near, uncorrected):	OD: 20/20
	OS: 20/20
Near point of convergence:	
Accommodative target:	5 cm
Penlight:	5 cm
Cover test (distance):	Orthophoria
Cover test (near):	15 esophoria
Subjective:	OD: plano, -0.25×180, 20/20
	OS: plano, 20/20
Distance lateral phoria:	1 exophoria
Base-in vergence (distance):	X/8/5
Base-out vergence (distance):	X/20/10
Near lateral phoria:	16 esophoria
-1.00 gradient:	25 esophoria
Gradient AC/A ratio:	9:1
Calculated AC/A ratio:	12.5:1
Base-in vergence (near):	X/2/−2
Base-out vergence (near):	10/16/6
Vergence facility	0 cpm, diplopia with base in
NRA:	+2.50
PRA:	diplopia at plano
Accommodative amplitude (push-up):	OD: 13 D, OS: 13 D
MAF:	OD: 10 cpm, OS: 11 cpm
BAF:	diplopia with −2.00
MEM retinoscopy:	+1.50

Pupils were normal, all external and internal health tests were negative, the deviation was comitant, and color vision testing revealed normal function.

Her current near prescription was OD +1.75 and OS +1.75

Case Analysis

The analysis is very similar to Case 9.4. Because of the presence of the esophoria, analysis should begin with inspection of all NFV data. We reached a diagnosis of convergence excess with normal tonic vergence, based on the high AC/A and the low NFV findings on both direct and indirect measures. Both the MEM finding and the NRA/PRA relationship suggested a near prescription of about +1.25.

Management

The interesting thing about this case was that Marilyn was already wearing a near prescription of +1.75 OD and OS. This was essentially the prescription that we would have given, based on our analysis. She reported a decrease in symptoms with her glasses, but was still not happy with her reading comfort. We, therefore, recommended that she continue to wear her glasses and begin a program of vision therapy.

The vision therapy program lasted 20 visits, and we followed the sequence recommended in Table 9.7. She came in 2 times a week and was given home vision therapy techniques to practice about 10 minutes, 5 days a week. A reevaluation at the end of therapy revealed the following findings:

(All through plano)	
Near lateral phoria:	14 esophoria
Base-in (near):	12/16/12
Base-out (near):	22/32/24
Vergence facility:	9 cpm
NRA:	+2.50
PRA:	−1.25
MEM:	+1.00 OD and OS

Marilyn continued to wear her reading prescription and reported that she was able to read with comfort as long as she desired. We recommended the maintenance schedule outlined in Table 9.9.

Case 9.6

History

Paul, a 6-year-old first grader, was brought for an evaluation by his mother because she noticed that he often rubbed his eyes and occasionally covered one eye when he read.

These problems began after the first month of first grade. His mother had a history of surgery for crossed eyes when she was 3 years old. She said that, when Paul was younger, she occasionally noticed his eyes crossing, but it seemed to stop. Paul had never had an eye examination before. His health history was negative.

Examination Results

IPD:	54 mm
VA (distance, uncorrected):	OD: 20/20
	OS: 20/20
VA (near, uncorrected):	OD: 20/20
	OS: 20/20
Near point of convergence:	
Accommodative target:	5 cm
Penlight:	5 cm
Cover test (distance):	15 Δ esophoria
Cover test (near):	22 Δ, intermittent (deviates with prolonged cover), alternating esotropia
Cover test (near) (near with +2.00):	6 esophoria
Subjective:	OD: +1.00, 20/20
	OS: +1.00, 20/20
Cycloplegic	OD: +1.50, 20/20
	OS: +1.50, 20/20
Base-in vergence (distance):	X/2/0
Base-out vergence (distance):	X/14/10
Associated phoria measured with the	
AO vectographic target:	3 base-out
Gradient AC/A ratio:	8:1
Calculated AC/A ratio:	8.8:1

Treatment

We recommend the management sequence listed in Table 10.2.

Lenses

The symptoms commonly found in fusional vergence dysfunction may also be present in patients with uncorrected refractive error or latent hyperopia. It is, therefore, important to eliminate latent hyperopia as a cause, by performing a cycloplegic refraction, and to correct any significant refractive error.

Prism

If a vertical deviation is present, we recommend that vertical prism be prescribed before vision therapy begins. The most effective method for determining the amount of vertical prism is the associated phoria that can be measured with any fixation disparity device (Chapter 14).

The use of horizontal relieving base-in prism is not necessary in fusional vergence dysfunction because the phoria is normal at both distance and near.

Vision Therapy

A vision therapy program for fusional vergence dysfunction generally requires between 12 to 24 in-office visits, if vision therapy is office based. The total number of therapy sessions depends on the age of the patient, motivation, and compliance. Motivated adults can sometimes successfully complete vision therapy for fusional vergence dysfunction in 10 to 12 visits.

Specific Vision Therapy Program

All of the vision therapy techniques recommended below are described in detail in Chapters 5 to 7.

Phase 1

This first phase of therapy is designed to accomplish the objectives listed in Table 10.7 under Phase 1.

TABLE 10.7. *Vision therapy for fusional vergence dysfunction*

Phase 1
Objectives
- Develop a working relationship with the patient
- Develop an awareness of the various feedback mechanisms that will be used throughout therapy
- Develop voluntary convergence and divergence
- Normalize positive and negative fusional vergence amplitudes (smooth or tonic vergence demand)
- Normalize accommodative amplitude and ability to stimulate and relax accommodation

Phase 2
Objectives
- Normalize positive fusional vergence facility (jump or phasic vergence demand)
- Normalize negative fusional vergence facility (jump or phasic vergence demand)

Phase 3
Objectives
- Develop ability to change from a convergence to a divergence demand
- Integrate vergence procedures with changes in accommodative demand
- Integrate vergence procedures with versions and saccades

As we discussed in earlier chapters, it is important to develop a working relationship with the patient during the first few sessions and to make the patient aware of the various feedback mechanisms that will be used throughout therapy. The basic approach used for fusional vergence dysfunction is to work toward establishing both normal PFV and NFV ranges and facility. Since it is generally easier to work with PFV, we suggest starting the therapy using convergence techniques.

The first goal of the therapy, therefore, is to teach the concept and feeling of converging. The patient should be able to voluntarily converge and diverge to any distance from 2 in. to 20 ft. Once the patient can voluntarily initiate a controlled convergence movement, the other goals of the vision therapy program become much easier to accomplish. Three commonly used procedures to accomplish this first objective are the Brock string, bug on string and the red/green barrel card.

Simultaneously try to normalize PFV amplitudes. The initial goal is to reestablish a normal vergence range for smooth- or tonic-type vergence demand. A smooth vergence demand is easier for the patient to accomplish in the early part of a vision therapy program (Chapter 4). Instruments that can be used to accomplish this objective are the variable Tranaglyphs, variable Vectograms, and the variable Prismatic Stereoscope from Bernell. These three devices can be used to create a smooth gradual increase in convergence demand. As the patient begins to make progress with PFV, begin working with NFV as well, using the same techniques.

By definition, patients with a diagnosis of fusional vergence dysfunction do not have accommodative problems. Nevertheless, accommodative training techniques are often useful in the initial phase of therapy because they can aid in the process of establishing the feeling of looking close and far and of converging and diverging. Certainly, if the patient has an accommodative disorder in addition to the fusional vergence dysfunction, accommodative techniques are important. Accommodative techniques are described in Chapter 6. Lens sorting, loose lens rock, and Hart chart procedures are commonly used in this first phase of therapy.

Endpoint

Phase 1 of therapy ends when the patient can:

- demonstrate voluntary convergence.
- fuse to about 30 base-out and 15 base-in using a Tranaglyph or other comparable technique.
- complete 12 cpm of accommodative facility with +2.00/−2.00 lenses using a 20/30 target.

A sample vision therapy program for Phase 1 is summarized in Table 10.8. This program includes several techniques that can be used by the patient at home to supplement the in-office therapy.

Phase 2

This second phase of therapy is designed to accomplish the objectives listed in Table 10.7 under Phase 2.

Once smooth PFV and NFV are normalized, phasic or jump vergence demand should be emphasized. Variable Tranaglyphs and Vectograms can still be used. However, the specific modifications to create a step vergence demand (described in Chapter 5) must be implemented. These include:

1. Changing fixation from the target to another point in space
2. Cover/uncover one eye

TABLE 10.8. *Sample vision therapy program for fusional vergence dysfunction*

Phase 1
Sessions 1 and 2
In-office
- Discuss nature of vision problem, goals of vision therapy, various feedback cues, importance of practice
- Brock string
- Lens sorting
- Loose lens rock (begin with plus if accommodative excess, with minus if accommodative insufficiency)
- Tranaglyph or Vectograms: convergence
  1. Begin with a peripheral target like Tranaglyph 515 or the Quoit Vectogram
- Computer Orthoptics Random Dot Program: convergence
Home Therapy
- Brock string

Sessions 3 and 4
In-office
- Bug on string
- Loose lens rock
- Tranaglyph or Vectograms: convergence and divergence
  1. Use targets with more central demand (Clown, Bunny Tranaglyphs; Clown, Topper Vectograms)
- Computer Orthoptics Random Dot Program: convergence and divergence
Home Therapy
- Add loose lens rock

Sessions 5 through 8
In-office
- Barrel card
- Voluntary convergence
- Loose lens rock
- Tranaglyph or Vectograms: convergence and divergence
  1. Use even more detailed targets such as Tranaglyphs Sports Slide and Faces targets and the Spirangle Vectogram)
- Computer Orthoptics Random Dot Program: convergence and divergence
Home Therapy
- Tranaglyph: convergence and divergence

Phase 2
Sessions 9 and 10
In-office
- Tranaglyph or Vectograms with modifications to create jump vergence demand: convergence
- Nonvariable Tranaglyphs: convergence
- Binocular accommodative therapy techniques: use any of the binocular techniques listed above with ± lenses
Home Therapy
- Nonvariable Tranaglyphs: convergence

Sessions 11 and 12
In-office
- Tranaglyph or Vectograms with modifications to create jump vergence demand: convergence and divergence
- Aperture Rule: convergence and divergence
- Binocular accommodative therapy techniques: use any of the binocular techniques listed above with ± lenses
Home Therapy
- Non-variable Tranaglyphs with loose prism jumps: convergence and divergence

Sessions 13 through 16
In-office
- Aperture Rule: convergence and divergence
- Eccentric Circles or Free Space Fusion Cards: convergence and divergence
- Computer Orthoptics Random Dot Vergence Program: both divergence and convergence
- Binocular Accommodative therapy techniques: use any of the binocular techniques listed above with ± lenses

TABLE 10.8. *Continued.*

Home Therapy
• Eccentric Circles or Free Space Fusion Cards
Phase 3
Sessions 17 through 20
In-office
• Tranaglyph or Vectograms with Polaroid or red/green flippers.
• Eccentric Circles or Free Space Fusion Cards
• Computer Orthoptics Random Dot Vergence Program: step–jump vergence.
Home Therapy
• Eccentric Circles or Free Space Fusion Cards: convergence
Sessions 21 and 22
In-office
• Tranaglyph or Vectograms with Polaroid or red/green flippers.
• Eccentric Circles or Free Space Fusion Cards
• Lifesaver Cards
• Computer Orthoptics Random Dot Vergence Program: jump–jump vergence
Home Therapy
• Eccentric Circles or Free Space Fusion Cards: divergence
Sessions 23 and 24
In-office
• Tranaglyph or Vectograms with Polaroid or red/green flippers.
• Eccentric Circles or Free Space Fusion Cards with rotation and versions
• Lifesaver Cards with rotation and version
• Computer Orthoptics Vergence Program with rotation
Home Therapy
• Eccentric Circles or Free Space Fusion Cards: divergence/convergence

3. Loose prism or flip prism
4. Flip lenses to create a step vergence change in vergence demand
5. Two different Tranaglyphs set up in a Dual Polachrome Illuminated Trainer
6. Polaroid or red/green flippers

Other valuable techniques at this stage are: nonvariable Tranaglyphs, the Aperture Rule, Eccentric Circles, Free Space Fusion Cards, Lifesaver Cards, and Computer Orthoptics Jump Vergence activities.

In contrast with Phase 1, in which speed was not a factor, during this second phase of therapy, the emphasis should be on the qualitative aspects (speed, accuracy) of fusion rather than quantitative (magnitude) aspects. It is important to increase the speed of the fusional vergence response and quality of the recovery of fusion.

Endpoint

The endpoint of Phase 2 is reached when the patient can:

• fuse card 12 using convergence and card 6 using divergence with the Aperture Rule.
• fuse the Eccentric Circles or Free Space Fusion Cards using convergence (12 cm separation) and divergence (6 cm separation).

A sample vision therapy program for Phase 2 is summarized in Table 10.8. This program includes several techniques that can be used by the patient at home to supplement the in-office therapy.

Phase 3

This third phase of therapy is designed to accomplish the objectives listed in Table 10.7 under Phase 3.

Until this point, the patient has either worked separately with convergence techniques or divergence techniques. Now the objective is to develop the patient's ability to change from a convergence to a divergence demand and to integrate vergence procedures with versions. Several excellent procedures are available to help accomplish this objective. Vectograms with Polaroid flippers or Tranaglyphs with red/green flippers can be used. Each time the flippers are changed, the demand switches from divergence to convergence. The transparent Keystone Eccentric Circles or transparent Bernell Free Space Fusion Cards are excellent inexpensive methods for achieving this objective. The patient has already learned, by this time, to fuse these cards with a divergence or convergence demand separately. Now the patient is taught to switch from convergence and then back to divergence. As this skill improves, speed or the number of cycles per minute is emphasized.

The final objective of therapy is to integrate vergence procedures with versions and saccades. Under normal seeing conditions, patients are constantly trying to maintain accurate vergence while changing fixation from one location to another. It is, therefore, important to combine vergence therapy with versions and saccades. Techniques such as the Brock string with rotation and Eccentric Circles and Free Space Fusion Cards or Lifesaver Cards with rotation or lateral movements and saccades can be used to accomplish this goal. The Computer Orthoptics Program that combines horizontal vergence with rotation is also useful for this objective.

Endpoint

The endpoint for Phase 3 is reached when the patient can:

* maintain clear single binocular vision with the Eccentric Circles and Free Space Fusion Cards held together, while slowly rotating the cards and converging and diverging.

Since the objectives of vision therapy are to eliminate the patient's symptoms and normalize binocular and accommodative findings, a reevaluation should be performed about halfway through the therapy program and again at the end of therapy. A reference point for determining when to perform the first reevaluation is when the patient can begin working with jump vergence techniques, such as the Aperture Rule. During these evaluations, the clinician should refer back to the original complaints and determine if the patient is now comfortable. All tests of binocular and accommodative function should be repeated and compared to the initial findings as well as the expected findings.

When all vision therapy objectives have been reached and the vision therapy program is completed, we recommend the home vision therapy maintenance program outlined in Table 8.10.

Summary of Vision Therapy for Fusional Vergence Dysfunction

The sample vision therapy program described above and outlined in Table 10.8 represents one approach that will lead to successful elimination of a patient's symptoms and normalization of optometric data. The number of sessions is approximate and will vary from one patient to another. Remember that it is often not necessary to work with every procedure suggested in this chapter. The objective is to achieve a successful result as quickly as possible. If it becomes apparent that a recommended procedure is easy for the patient, go on to the next technique.

Surgery

Surgery is unnecessary in fusional vergence dysfunction.

Case Studies

Case 10.1

History

John, a 16-year-old junior in high school, presented with complaints of eyestrain and blurry vision after about 20 minutes of reading. He had these problems for several years, but, in his previous visits to eye doctors, no one has been able to help him. The last doctor who examined him about 1 year ago, gave him reading glasses. John did not feel that these helped and stopped wearing them after about 4 weeks. His medical history was negative and he was not taking any medication.

Examination Results

Previous prescription	+0.50
	+0.50
IPD:	62 mm
VA (distance, uncorrected):	OD: 20/20
	OS: 20/20
VA (near, uncorrected):	OD: 20/20
	OS: 20/20
Near point of convergence:	
Accommodative target:	5 cm
Penlight:	5 cm
Cover test (distance):	orthophoria
Cover test (near):	2 exophoria
Subjective:	OD: +0.25 − 0.25 × 180, 20/20
	OS: +0.25 − 0.25 × 180, 20/20
Cycloplegic:	OD: +0.75 − 0.25 × 180, 20/20
	OS: +0.75 − 0.25 × 180, 20/20
Distance lateral phoria:	Orthophoria
Base-in vergence (distance):	X/4/2
Base-out vergence (distance):	6/10/6
Near lateral phoria:	3 exophoria
−1.00 gradient:	1 esophoria
Gradient AC/A ratio:	4:1
Calculated AC/A ratio:	4.8:1
Base-in vergence (near):	4/8/6
Base-out vergence (near):	6/10/2
Vergence facility	3 cpm, difficulty with base-out and base-in
NRA:	+1.50
PRA:	−1.25
Accommodative amplitude (push-up):	OD: 11 D, OS: 11 D

MAF:	OD: 11 cpm, OS: 11 cpm
BAF:	2 cpm
Monocular estimation method (MEM) retinoscopy:	+0.25

Pupils were normal, all external and internal health tests were negative, the deviation was comitant, and color vision testing revealed normal function.

Case Analysis

Because the phoria was normal at both distance and near, the most likely cause for John's symptoms was an accommodative disorder. Analysis of the results of accommodative testing revealed a normal amplitude, facility, and accommodative response. The NRA and PRA were both low, but, given the normal accommodative function, these findings reflected a problem with fusional vergence. The next most likely hypothesis was fusional vergence dysfunction. Both PFV and NFV findings were reduced on direct measures and indirect tests of fusional vergence. The low NRA, PRA, and reduced BAF results suggested problems with fusional vergence. These findings led to a diagnosis of fusional vergence dysfunction.

Management

We advised John that the previous prescription would not be expected to relieve his problem. The ametropia was considered insignificant and, since there was no vertical deviation, glasses were not prescribed. We prescribed a program of vision therapy to normalize his fusional vergence findings and eliminate symptoms.

John was seen twice a week and was also given home vision therapy procedures to practice. We followed the sequence outlined in Table 10.8, and 16 visits of in-office vision therapy were necessary to achieve a successful result. At the end of therapy, John reported that he was able to read for as long as he wanted without any discomfort.

A reevaluation after 16 visits revealed the following findings:

Base-in vergence (distance):	X/8/6
Base-out vergence (distance):	X/20/16
Near lateral phoria:	2 exophoria
Base-in vergence (near):	14/26/22
Base-out vergence (near):	20/32/28
Vergence facility	14 cpm
NRA:	+2.50
PRA:	−2.50
BAF:	11 cpm

The maintenance program suggested in Table 8.10 was followed, and a reevaluation in 6 months revealed that John continued to feel comfortable and his findings remained normal.

BASIC ESOPHORIA

Background Information

Basic esophoria was first described by Duane (18). It is a condition in which tonic vergence is high and the AC/A ratio is normal. As a result, there is an equal amount of esophoria at distance and near with reduced NFV at both distances.

The prevalence of this condition has not been clearly established in our literature. Scheiman et al. (16) studied 1,650 children (ages 6 to 18 years) and found a prevalence of only 0.7%. Porcar and Nartinez-Palomera (17) studied a university population and found a prevalence of 1.5%.

Characteristics

Symptoms

Because esophoria is present at all distances, patients may present with symptoms associated with reading and other close work, as well as symptoms associated with distance activities. Common reading and near point complaints include eyestrain, headaches, blurred vision, diplopia, sleepiness, difficulty concentrating, and loss of comprehension over time (Table 10.9). Problems associated with distance include blurred vision and diplopia when driving and watching television and movies as well as in a classroom situation. Like other binocular vision disorders, it is possible for patients to have basic esophoria and yet be asymptomatic.

Signs

Signs of basic esodeviations are presented in Table 10.9.

Refractive Error

Basic esophoria is often associated with hyperopia. This is a desirable characteristic because, with a normal AC/A ratio, correction of the hyperopia will lead to a decrease in the magnitude of the esophoria at both near and at distance.

Characteristics of the Deviation

Patients with basic esophoria have an equal amount of esophoria at distance and at near, with decreased NFV at both distances. Generally, if the deviations are within 5 Δ of one another, they are considered equal. The deviation can be a phoria, an intermittent, or a constant strabismus. There is little information in our literature, however, about the prevalence of these various forms of basic esophoria. In our experience, most cases of basic esophoria are either heterophorias or intermittent strabismics.

TABLE 10.9. *Signs and symptoms of basic esodeviations*

Signs	Symptoms
Esophoria equal at distance and near	Long-standing
Normal AC/A ratio (calculated method)	Headaches
Hyperopia often present	Eyestrain
Direct tests of negative fusional vergence at both distance and near	Blurred vision
Low step vergence	
Low smooth vergence	
Low jump vergence	
Indirect tests of negative fusional vergence at near	
Low positive relative accommodation	
Low binocular accommodative facility testing with minus lenses	
High monocular estimation method retinoscopy	

AC/A Ratio

A normal AC/A ratio is always present in basic esophoria. This is well accepted, based on the calculated AC/A, and is an important factor when treatment is considered.

Analysis of Binocular and Accommodative Data

As illustrated in Chapter 2, Fig. 2.3, the entry point into the analysis of data for basic esophoria is the esodeviation at both distances. Direct tests of NFV, at both distance and near, will be low in basic esophoria (Table 10.9). This includes step-, smooth-, and jump-type vergences. In addition, all near point tests that indirectly assess NFV (Table 10.9) also will be low. Tests performed binocularly with minus lenses evaluate the patient's ability to stimulate accommodation and control binocular alignment using NFV. Two examples are the PRA and BAF testing with minus lenses. A characteristic finding in basic esophoria is a report of diplopia, rather than blur, on the PRA and BAF testing. In fact, it is important to specifically ask about diplopia when performing these tests on a patient suspected of having basic esophoria.

Another important indirect test of NFV is MEM retinoscopy. It is not unusual to find an abnormal result on this test in basic esophoria. An MEM finding of greater plus than expected suggests that the patient is using as little accommodation as possible to decrease the use of accommodative convergence. This reduces the demand on NFV.

Differential Diagnosis

The differential diagnosis of basic esodeviation is presented in Table 10.10.

Basic esophoria is considered to be a benign condition with no serious consequences other than the visual symptoms listed in Table 10.10. It is relatively easy to differentiate from other binocular vision disorders associated with esophoria, such as convergence excess (greater esophoria at near) and divergence insufficiency (greater esophoria at distance).

Basic esophoria or esophoria at near can also be associated with more serious underlying conditions. Of particular importance is the history. As we have stated previously, an acute onset of a binocular vision problem is suspicious. The sudden onset of esophoria warrants consideration of problems such as sixth nerve palsy and divergence paralysis.

Differential Diagnosis: Summary

A serious underlying etiology must be ruled out in all cases of basic esophoria. This differential diagnosis depends very much on the nature of the patient's symptoms. Typically, basic esophoria presents with long-standing chronic complaints. The health history is negative and the patient is not taking any medication known to affect accommodation. Basic esophoria associated with serious underlying disease has an acute onset and medical problems or neurological symptoms are usually present. The primary functional disorders that must be differentiated from true basic esophoria are convergence excess and divergence insufficiency.

When managing a case of basic esophoria that is thought to have a functional basis, if improvement in symptoms and findings does not occur as expected, it is wise to reconsider the etiology of the condition.

TABLE 10.10. *Differential diagnosis of basic esodeviation*

Functional disorders to rule out	Serious underlying disease to rule out
Divergence insufficiency	Sixth nerve palsy
Convergence excess	Divergence paralysis

Treatment

We recommend following the management sequence listed in Table 10.3.

Lenses

With basic esophoria, it is important to prescribe maximum plus if a significant degree of hyperopia is present. It is best to perform a cycloplegic examination before determining the prescription.

Added Lenses

Because of the normal AC/A ratio, the use of added plus lenses at near is moderately effective in cases of basic esophoria. In Chapter 3 we discussed the important clinical data that are used to determine whether additional plus should be prescribed. Although the AC/A ratio is the key finding, it is important to consider all of the data listed in Table 10.11.

How Much Additional Plus Should Be Prescribed

When prescribing added plus lenses, the objective is to determine the lowest amount of plus that will eliminate the patient's symptoms and normalize optometric data. A variety of methods have been suggested for calculating the amount of additional plus to prescribe for patients with basic esophoria. Some of the more popular methods are analysis of the NRA/PRA relationship, MEM retinoscopy or other near point retinoscopy, use of the AC/A ratio, and fixation disparity analysis. We advocate the use of a group of findings rather than relying on any one test. As we discussed in Chapter 3, reliance on any one test may be misleading at times. The optometric data listed in Table 10.11 can be used to determine the amount of plus to prescribe.

Prism

If a vertical deviation is present, we recommend that vertical prism be prescribed. The most effective method for determining the amount of vertical prism is the associated phoria that can be measured with any fixation disparity device (Chapter 14).

Because of the normal AC/A ratio, the use of lenses alone will not always be effective. This is particularly true when there is no significant degree of hyperopia. In such cases, horizontal relieving prism certainly should be considered. If a base-out prism prescription is being considered, fixation disparity testing is the most effective method for determining the amount of horizontal prism (Chapter 14).

TABLE 10.11. *Consideration for prescribing added plus lenses*

Test	Consider the use of added plus	Added plus not indicated
AC/A ratio	High	Low
Refractive error	Hyperopia	Myopia
Near phoria	Esophoria	Exophoria
Negative relative accommodation (NRA)/ positive relative accommodation (PRA)	Low PRA	Low NRA
Base-out at near	Normal to high	Low
Monocular estimation method retinoscopy	High	Low
Amplitude of accommodation	Low	Normal
Accommodative facility testing	Fails −	Fails +

Vision Therapy

If basic esophoria is not associated with hyperopia, vision therapy is generally necessary. Other important variables include the status of NFV and the magnitude of the esophoria. The larger the degree of esophoria at distance and near, the more likely that vision therapy will be necessary. A vision therapy program for basic esophoria generally requires from 12 to 24 in-office visits. The total number of therapy sessions depends on the age of the patient, motivation, and compliance.

The vision therapy program for basic esophoria is identical to that recommended for convergence excess in Chapter 9 except that, during Phases 2 and 3, therapy is performed at intermediate and far distances.

Specific Vision Therapy Program

All of the vision therapy techniques recommended below are described in detail in Chapters 5 to 7.

Phase 1

This first phase of therapy is designed to accomplish the objectives listed in Table 10.12 under Phase 1.

The first goal of the therapy itself is to teach the concept and feeling of diverging, and the ability to accurately diverge. The patient should be able to voluntarily converge and diverge to any distance from 2 in. to 20 ft. Commonly used procedures to accomplish this first objective are the Brock string and bug on string.

Basic esophoria patients generally have very limited base-in blur, break, and recovery findings. Therefore, another objective of the first phase of vision therapy is to normalize NFV amplitudes. The initial goal is to reestablish a normal vergence range for smooth- or tonic-type vergence demand.

TABLE 10.12. *Vision therapy for basic esodeviations*

Phase 1
Objectives
- Develop a working relationship with the patient
- Develop an awareness of the various feedback mechanisms that will be used throughout therapy
- Develop the feeling of diverging
- Normalize negative fusional vergence (NFV) amplitudes (smooth or tonic vergence demand)
- Normalize accommodative amplitude and ability to stimulate and relax accommodation

Phase 2
Objectives
- Normalize positive fusional vergence (PFV) amplitudes (smooth or tonic vergence demand)
- Normalize NFV facility (jump or phasic vergence demand)
- Normalize PFV facility (jump or phasic vergence demand)
- Normalize NFV at intermediate distances

Phase 3
Objectives
- Develop ability to change from a convergence to a divergence demand
- Integrate vergence procedures with changes in accommodative demand
- Integrate vergence procedures with versions
- Normalize NFV at distance

TABLE 10.13. *Sample vision therapy program for basic esodeviations*

Phase 1
Sessions 1 and 2
In-office
- Discuss nature of vision problem, goals of vision therapy, various feedback cues, importance of practice
- Brock string, concentrate on developing feeling of diverging
- Lens sorting
- Loose lens rock (begin with plus if accommodative excess, with minus if accommodative insufficiency)
- Tranaglyph or Vectograms: divergence
  1. Begin with a peripheral target like Tranaglyph 515 or the Quoit Vectogram
- Computer Orthoptics Random Dot Program: divergence
Home Therapy
- Brock string

Sessions 3 and 4
In-office
- Bug on string, concentrate on feeling of diverging
- Loose lens rock
- Tranaglyph or Vectograms: divergence
  1. Use targets with more central demand (Clown, Bunny Tranaglyphs; Clown, Topper Vectograms)
- Computer Orthoptics Random Dot Program: divergence
Home Therapy
- Add loose lens rock

Sessions 5 through 8
In-office
- Loose lens rock
- Tranaglyph or Vectograms: divergence
  1. Use even more detailed targets such as Tranaglyphs Sports Slide and Faces targets and the Spirangle Vectogram)
- Computer Orthoptics Random Dot Program: divergence
Home Therapy
- Tranaglyph: divergence

Phase 2
Sessions 9 and 10
In-office
- Tranaglyph or Vectograms with modifications to create jump vergence demand: divergence
- Nonvariable Tranaglyphs
- Tranaglyph 515 or the Quoit Vectogram: convergence
- Binocular accommodative therapy techniques: use any of the binocular techniques listed above with ± lenses
Home Therapy
- Nonvariable Tranaglyphs

Sessions 11 and 12
In-office
- Tranaglyph or Vectograms with modifications to create jump vergence demand: divergence
- Aperture Rule: divergence
- More central Tranaglyphs or the Vectograms: convergence
- Binocular accommodative therapy techniques: use any of the binocular techniques listed above with ± lenses
Home Therapy
- Nonvariable Tranaglyphs with loose prism jumps

Sessions 13 through 16
In-office
- Aperture Rule: divergence and convergence
- Eccentric Circles or Free Space Fusion Cards: divergence
- Computer Orthoptics Random Dot Vergence Program: both divergence and convergence
- Tranaglyph or Vectograms with modifications to create jump vergence demand: convergence
- Tranaglyph or Vectograms at one meter
Home Therapy
- Eccentric Circles or Free Space Fusion Cards: divergence

TABLE 10.13. *Continued.*

Phase 3
Sessions 17 through 20
In-office
- Tranaglyph or Vectograms with Polaroid or red/green flippers.
- Eccentric Circles or Free Space Fusion Cards
- Computer Orthoptics Random Dot Vergence Program: step–jump vergence
- Tranaglyph or Vectograms at 1 m
- Eccentric Circles or Free Space Fusion Cards: divergence at 1 m
- Computer Orthoptics Random Dot Vergence Program: step–jump vergence at 1 m
Home Therapy
- Eccentric Circles or Free Space Fusion Cards: divergence
Sessions 21 and 22
In-office
- Tranaglyph or Vectograms with Polaroid or red/green flippers.
- Eccentric Circles or Free Space Fusion Cards
- Lifesaver Cards
- Computer Orthoptics Random Dot Vergence Program: jump–jump vergence
- Tranaglyph or Vectograms projected with overhead projector
- Large Eccentric Circles at distance
Home Therapy
- Eccentric Circles or Free Space Fusion Cards: convergence and divergence
Sessions 23 and 24
In-Office
- Tranaglyph or Vectograms with Polaroid or red/green flippers.
- Eccentric Circles or Free Space Fusion Cards with rotation and versions
- Lifesaver Cards with rotation and versions
- Computer Orthoptics Vergence Program with rotation
- Tranaglyph or Vectograms projected with overhead projector
- Large Eccentric Circles at distance
Home Therapy
- Eccentric Circles or Free Space Fusion Cards: divergence and convergence

In some cases of basic esophoria in pre-presbyopes, an accommodative problem may also present. If so, the final objective of the first phase of therapy is to normalize accommodative amplitude and the ability to stimulate and relax accommodation. If, however, accommodative function is normal, there is generally no need to spend a lot of time working with the accommodative system. Lens sorting, loose lens rock, and Hart chart procedures are commonly used in this first phase of therapy.

Endpoint

Phase 1 of therapy ends when the patient can:

- accurately diverge using the Brock string to 10 ft.
- fuse to about 15 base-in with a Tranaglyph or other comparable technique.
- complete 12 cpm of accommodative facility with $+2.00/-2.00$ lenses using a 20/30 target.

A sample vision therapy program for Phase 1 is summarized in Table 10.13.

Phase 2

This second phase of therapy is designed to accomplish the objectives listed in Table 10.12 under Phase 2.

Once smooth NFV is normalized, phasic or jump vergence demand should be emphasized. Variable Tranaglyphs and Vectograms can still be used. However, the specific modifications to create a step vergence demand (described in Chapter 5) must be implemented. Valuable techniques at this stage are the nonvariable Tranaglyphs, the Aperture Rule, Eccentric Circles, Free Space Fusion Cards, Lifesaver Cards, and Computer Orthoptics Jump Vergence activities.

In contrast with Phase 1, in which speed was not a factor, during this second phase of therapy, the emphasis should be on the qualitative aspects of fusion rather than magnitude. It is important to increase the speed of the fusional vergence response and the quality of the recovery of fusion.

A second objective of this phase of therapy is to begin working with PFV amplitudes. The same techniques used in Phase 1 to work with NFV are repeated for PFV. During the end of this phase of therapy, begin to incorporate PFV facility-type techniques, using the same procedures as listed above for jump vergence demand for NFV.

Finally, an important objective of this phase of therapy is to begin performing the treatment at intermediate distances. Now that the patient can successfully work with the various instruments and procedures at near, it is usually very easy to repeat similar techniques at greater distances. A very effective procedure is to use Tranaglyphs projected on the wall or a screen by an overhead projector. This technique works well because the patient is very familiar with the task and simply has to try and apply the same skills learned during earlier sessions.

Another method of presenting stimuli at intermediate distances is through the use of stereo-scopes. The working distance can be conveniently changed on most Brewster-type stereoscopes and a very wide variety of targets are readily available.

Endpoint

The endpoint of Phase 2 is reached when the patient can:

- fuse card 12 using convergence and card 6 using divergence with the Aperture Rule.
- fuse the Eccentric Circles or Free Space Fusion Cards using convergence (12 cm separation) and divergence (6 cm separation).
- fuse up to 20 Δ base-out and 10 Δ base-in with Tranaglyph targets projected at 10 ft using the overhead projector.

A sample vision therapy program for Phase 2 is summarized in Table 10.13.

Phase 3

This third phase of therapy is designed to accomplish the objectives listed in Table 10.12 under Phase 3.

Until this point, the patient has worked in the convergence or divergence directions sepa-rately. Now the objective is to develop the patient's ability to change from a convergence to a divergence demand and to integrate vergence procedures with versions and saccades. Sev-eral excellent procedures are available to help accomplish these objectives. Vectograms with Polaroid flippers or Tranaglyphs with red/green flippers can be used. Each time the flippers are changed, the demand switches from divergence to convergence. The transparent Keystone Eccentric Circles or transparent Bernell Free Space Fusion Cards are excellent inexpensive methods for achieving this objective.

Another objective of therapy is to integrate vergence procedures with versions and saccades. Techniques such as the Brock string with rotation, Eccentric Circles and Free Space Fusion Cards with rotation and/or lateral movements, and the Lifesaver Cards with rotation can be used to accomplish this goal. The Computer Orthoptics Program that combines horizontal vergence with rotation is also useful for this objective.

The final objective of this final phase of therapy is to work with divergence at distances of from 10 to 20 ft. The same procedures used at 5 to 10 ft during Phase 2 can be repeated at even greater distances. In addition, the techniques recommended for training the divergence excess patient at distance can be used (Chapter 9).

Endpoint

The endpoint for Phase 3 is reached when the patient can:

- maintain clear single binocular vision with the Eccentric Circles and Free Space Fusion Cards held together, while slowly rotating the cards and performing convergence and divergence therapy.
- maintain clear single binocular vision with the large Eccentric Circles and other targets at distance.

When all vision therapy objectives have been reached, the vision therapy program is completed, and we recommend the home vision therapy maintenance program outlined in Table 8.10 and described in Chapter 8.

Summary of Vision Therapy for Basic Esophoria

The phases and objectives outlined above and in Tables 10.12 and 10.13 represent one approach that will lead to successful elimination of a patient's symptoms and normalization of optometric data. The number of sessions is approximate and will vary from one patient to another.

Surgery

The use of lenses, prism, and vision therapy in the treatment of basic esophoria is so successful that surgery is virtually never necessary.

Case Studies

Case 10.2

History

Susan, a 14-year-old ninth grader, presented with a complaint of intermittent double vision in school. The double vision was worse when she was looking up at the teacher or chalkboard. She had complained on and off about this problem for several years, but had not received any treatment. Her mother remembered that when Susan was about 2 or 3 years old she brought her to an eye doctor because her eyes looked crossed. The doctor said that Susan had a mild eye turn and she would outgrow it. Her health was normal and she was not taking any medication.

Examination Results

IPD:	58 mm
VA (distance, uncorrected):	OD: 20/20
	OS: 20/20
VA (near, uncorrected):	OD: 20/20
	OS: 20/20
Near point of convergence:	5 cm

Cover test (distance):	16 Δ esophoria
Cover test (near):	14 Δ esophoria
Subjective:	OD: +1.00, 20/20
	OS: +1.00, 20/20
Cycloplegic:	OD: +1.50
	OS: +1.50
Distance lateral phoria:	18 esophoria
Base-in vergence (distance):	diplopia; needs 8 base-out to fuse
Base-out vergence (distance):	diplopia; needs 8 base-out to fuse, breaks at 26 base-out, and recovers at 18 base-out
Near lateral phoria:	16 esophoria
−1.00 gradient:	22 esophoria
Gradient AC/A ratio:	6:1
Calculated AC/A ratio:	5:1
Base-in vergence (near):	X/2/−4
Base-out vergence (near):	X/28/20
Vergence facility	0 cpm, diplopia with base in
NRA:	+2.50
PRA:	−0.25
Accommodative amplitude (push-up):	OD: 12 D, OS: 12 D
MAF:	OD: 10 cpm, OS: 10 cpm
BAF:	diplopia with −2.00
MEM retinoscopy:	+1.50 OU

Fixation disparity testing with the American Optical (AO) vectographic slide at distance revealed an associated phoria of 4 base-out.

Pupils were normal, all external and internal health tests were negative, the deviation was comitant, and color vision testing revealed normal function.

Case Analysis

The entry point into analysis of the data in this case is the large magnitude esophoria at distance and near. NFV at both distance and near are very reduced with diplopia on base-in testing at distance. The equal magnitude esophoria at distance and near, reduced NFV, poor vergence facility, and normal AC/A ratio clearly suggest a diagnosis of basic esophoria.

Management

Following the management sequence in Table 10.3, we prescribed for the full amount of hyperopia, which reduced the angle of deviation to about 12 Δ at distance and 10 Δ at near. Based on the fixation disparity results, we also prescribed 4 base-out prism. The final prescription given was OD +1.00 and OS +1.00, with a +1.00 add and 2 base-out in each eye. Susan wore these glasses for 4 weeks and returned for reevaluation. She reported relief of symptoms, and no further treatment was necessary.

BASIC EXOPHORIA

Background Information

Basic exophoria was first described by Duane (18). It is a condition in which tonic vergence is low and the AC/A ratio is normal. As a result, there is an equal amount of exophoria at distance and at near with reduced PFV at both distances. In a recent study, Daum (1) reported on a population of 177 patients with exodeviations. Convergence insufficiency was the most common type of exodeviation, with a prevalence of 62.1%. Basic exophoria was the next most prevalent exodeviation, with a prevalence of 27.6%.

The prevalence of this condition has not been clearly established in our literature. Scheiman et al. (16) studied 1,650 children (ages 6 to 18 years) and found a prevalence of only 0.3%. Porcar and Nartinez-Palomera (17) studied a university population and found a prevalence of 3.1%.

Characteristics

Symptoms

Because exophoria is present at all distances, patients may present with symptoms associated with reading and other close work, as well as symptoms associated with distance activities. Common reading and near point complaints include eyestrain, headaches, blurred vision, diplopia, sleepiness, difficulty concentrating, and loss of comprehension over time (Table 10.14). Problems associated with distance include blurred vision and diplopia when driving and watching television and movies, as well as in a classroom situation. Like other binocular vision disorders, it is possible for patients to have basic exophoria and yet be asymptomatic.

Signs

Signs of basic exodeviations are presented in Table 10.14.

Refractive Error

Refractive error is not a significant etiological factor in basic exophoria (7). If myopia is present, correction of the refractive error will lead to a moderate decrease in the magnitude of the exophoria at both near and at distance.

Near Point of Convergence

Because the magnitude of the exodeviation tends to be large in basic exophoria, the near point of convergence is often receded.

TABLE 10.14. *Symptoms and signs of basic exodeviations*

Signs
Receded near point of convergence
Equal exophoria at near and at distance
Normal AC/A ratio
Direct tests of positive fusional vergence at both distance and near
Low step vergence
Low smooth vergence
Low jump vergence
Indirect tests of negative fusional vergence at near
Low negative relative accommodation
Low binocular accommodative facility testing with plus lenses
Low retinoscopy monocular estimation method
Symptoms
These symptoms are generally related to the use of the eyes for reading or other near tasks:

Eyestrain	Difficulty concentrating on reading material
Headaches	Loss of comprehension over time
Blurred vision distance and near	A pulling sensation around the eyes
Double vision at distance and near	Movement of the print
Sleepiness	

Characteristics of the Deviation

Patients with basic exophoria have an equal amount of exophoria at distance and at near, with decreased PFV at both distances. Generally, if the deviations are within 5 Δ of one another, they are considered equal. Daum (19) suggested that if the distant deviation is greater than 6 Δ, the near deviation can be within 9 Δ to be considered basic exophoria, and, if the distance deviation is 5 Δ or less, the near deviation has to be within 3 Δ. Another interesting finding from Daum's study is that basic exophoria had the largest percentage of constant strabismus of the three categories of exodeviations. Sixteen percent of the basic exodeviations in his sample were constant strabismics, 49% were intermittent, and 35% were latent. In contrast, only 2% of the convergence insufficiency patients and 1% of the divergence excess patients were constant. The mean angle of deviation was 15.5 Δ at both distance and near for basic exodeviations.

AC/A Ratio

A normal AC/A ratio is always present in basic exophoria. This is well accepted, based on the calculated AC/A and is an important factor when treatment is considered. Daum (1) found an AC/A ratio of 6.2:1 in his sample of 49 equal exodeviations.

Analysis of Binocular and Accommodative Data

The entry point into the analysis of data for basic exophoria is the exodeviation at both distances. Direct tests of PFV at both distance and near will tend to be low in basic exophoria (Table 10.14). This includes step-, smooth-, and jump-type vergences. In addition, all near point tests that indirectly assess PFV (Table 10.14) also will be low. Tests performed binocularly with plus lenses evaluate the patient's ability to relax accommodation and control binocular alignment using PFV. Two examples are the NRA and BAF testing with plus lenses. Another important, indirect test of PFV is MEM retinoscopy. It is not unusual to find an abnormal result on this test in basic exophoria. An MEM finding of less plus than expected suggests that the patient is using as much accommodation as possible to increase the use of accommodative convergence. This reduces the demand on PFV.

Differential Diagnosis

The differential diagnosis of basic exophorias is presented in Table 10.15.

Basic exophoria is considered to be a benign condition with no serious consequences other than the visual symptoms listed in Table 10.15. It is relatively easy to differentiate from

TABLE 10.15. *Differential diagnosis of basic exophorias*

Functional disorders to rule out	Medial rectus weakness due to:
• Convergence insufficiency	• Multiple sclerosis
• Divergence excess	• Myasthenia gravis
Serious underlying disease to rule out	• Previous strabismus surgery
Convergence paralysis secondary to:	
• Ischemic infarction	
• Demyelination	
• Flu or other viral infection	
• Parkinson's disease	
• Parinaud's syndrome	

other binocular vision disorders associated with exophoria, such as convergence insufficiency (greater exophoria at near) and divergence excess (greater exophoria at distance).

While it is unusual for basic exophoria to be associated with more serious underlying conditions, this possibility should always be considered. The key factor is the history of the deviation. Generally, functional exodeviations tend to be long-standing, with patients reporting a history of chronic symptoms and previous attempts to solve the problem. It is important to be suspicious about the etiology when the history suggests an acute onset of the deviation. Basic exophoria associated with serious underlying disease has an acute onset and medical problems or neurological symptoms are usually present.

Table 10.15 lists the conditions that should be considered in the differential diagnosis of basic exophoria. When managing a case of basic exophoria that is thought to have a functional basis, if improvement in symptoms and findings does not occur as expected, it is wise to reconsider the etiology of the condition.

Treatment

We recommend following the management sequence listed in Table 10.4.

Lenses

Significant refractive error is usually not present in basic exodeviations. If myopia is present, it is helpful to prescribe glasses. Because of the normal AC/A ratio, prescription of minus lenses will tend to moderately reduce the angle of deviation at both distance and near. In the presence of hyperopia, the decision about prescribing is more complex. With low to moderate degrees of hyperopia—up to about +1.50—we suggest waiting until the patient begins making progress in vision therapy. Prescribing before vision therapy will increase the magnitude of the exodeviation and may exacerbate the patient's symptoms. When the amount of hyperopia is greater than +1.50, it is generally wise to prescribe a partial prescription initially and make modifications as the patient progresses in vision therapy. As we have recommended previously, it is important to prescribe for significant degrees of astigmatism and anisometropia.

Added Lenses

Added lenses can be an effective tool in the treatment of basic exodeviations because of the normal AC/A ratio. With esodeviations, added lenses are often prescribed for full-time wear in a bifocal format. With exodeviations, added lenses are generally not worn full time. Rather, they are used as aids during vision therapy or to facilitate fusion in basic exodeviations. If the deviation is large, intermittent or constant, and the patient is experiencing difficulty in the early stages of vision therapy, added lenses may be helpful.

Prism

Daum (2) found that 51% of his sample had vertical deviations. If a vertical deviation is present under fused conditions, we recommend that vertical prism be prescribed. The most effective method for determining the amount of vertical prism is the associated phoria that can be measured with any fixation disparity device (Chapter 14).

Horizontal relieving prism should be a consideration in basic exodeviations. Because of the excellent prognosis with vision therapy, however, the use of base-in prism for this condition is generally not necessary. When the magnitude of the initial deviation is large (greater than

30 Δ), base-in prism may be helpful at the end of vision therapy if the patient is not totally comfortable.

Vision Therapy

A vision therapy program for basic exophoria generally requires from 12 to 24 in-office visits if the deviation is latent or intermittent. Treatment can sometimes take longer if a constant strabismus is present. The total number of therapy sessions depends on the age of the patient, motivation, and compliance.

The vision therapy program for basic exophoria is very similar to that recommended for convergence insufficiency in Chapter 8, except that, during Phases 2 and 3, therapy is performed at intermediate and far distances.

Specific Vision Therapy Program

All of the vision therapy techniques recommended below are described in detail in Chapters 5 to 7.

Phase 1

This first phase of therapy is designed to accomplish the objectives listed in Table 10.16 under Phase 1.

The first goal of the therapy itself is to teach the concept and feeling of converging. The patient should be able to voluntarily converge and diverge to any distance from 2 in. to 20 ft. Once the patient can voluntarily initiate a controlled convergence movement, the other goals of the vision therapy program become much easier to accomplish. Three commonly used procedures to accomplish this first objective are the Brock string, bug on string and the red/green barrel card.

Basic exophoria patients generally have very limited base-out blur, break, and recovery findings. Therefore, another objective of the first phase of vision therapy is to normalize PFV

TABLE 10.16. *Vision therapy for basic exophorias*

Phase 1
Objectives
- Develop a working relationship with the patient
- Develop an awareness of the various feedback mechanisms that will be used throughout therapy
- Develop voluntary convergence
- Normalize positive fusional vergence (PFV) amplitudes (smooth or tonic vergence demand)
- Normalize accommodative amplitude and ability to stimulate and relax accommodation

Phase 2
Objectives
- Normalize negative fusional vergence (NFV) amplitudes (smooth or tonic vergence demand)
- Normalize PFV facility (jump or phasic vergence demand)
- Normalize NFV facility (jump or phasic vergence demand)
- Normalize PFV at intermediate distances

Phase 3
Objectives
- Develop ability to change from a convergence to a divergence demand
- Integrate vergence procedures with changes in accommodative demand
- Integrate vergence procedures with versions and saccades
- Normalize PFV at distance

amplitudes. The initial goal is to reestablish a normal vergence range for smooth- or tonic-type vergence demand. It is important, however, to move to the next phase involving jump vergence as soon as possible. This tends to shorten the time course of therapy.

Instrumentation that can be used to accomplish these objectives includes variable Tranaglyphs, variable Vectograms, and the variable Prismatic Stereoscope from Bernell. These three devices can be used to create a smooth gradual increase in convergence demand.

If an accommodative problem is also present, the final objective of the first phase of therapy is to normalize accommodative amplitude and the ability to stimulate and relax accommodation. If accommodative function is normal, however, there is generally no need to spend a lot of time working with the accommodative system. Accommodative techniques are described in Chapter 6. Lens sorting, loose lens rock, and Hart chart procedures are commonly used in this first phase of therapy.

Endpoint

Phase 1 of therapy ends when the patient can:

- demonstrate voluntary convergence.
- fuse to about 30 base-out with a Tranaglyph or other comparable technique.
- complete 12 cpm of accommodative facility with +2.00/−2.00 lenses using a 20/30 target.

A sample vision therapy program for Phase 1 is summarized in Table 10.17. This program includes several techniques that can be used by the patient at home to supplement the in-office therapy.

Phase 2

This second phase of therapy is designed to accomplish the objectives listed in Table 10.16 under Phase 2.

Once smooth PFV is normalized, phasic or jump vergence demand should be emphasized. Variable Tranaglyphs and Vectograms can still be used. However, the specific modifications to create a step vergence demand (described in Chapter 5) must be implemented. Other valuable techniques at this stage are nonvariable Tranaglyphs, the Aperture Rule, Eccentric Circles, Free Space Fusion Cards, Lifesaver Cards, and Computer Orthoptics Jump Vergence activities.

In contrast to Phase 1, in which speed was not a factor, during this second phase of therapy, the emphasis should be on the qualitative aspects (speed, accuracy) of fusion rather than quantitative (magnitude) aspects. It is important to increase the speed of the fusional vergence response and quality of the recovery of fusion.

A second objective of this phase of therapy is to begin working with NFV amplitudes. Once the patient begins to demonstrate normal smooth PFV, it is important to also implement therapy with smooth negative vergence demand. The same techniques used in Phase 1 to work with PFV are repeated for NFV. Also incorporate NFV facility-type techniques, using the same procedures as listed above for jump vergence demand for PFV.

Finally, an important objective of this phase of therapy is to begin performing the treatment at intermediate distances. Now that the patient can successfully work with the various instruments and procedures at near, it is usually very easy to repeat similar techniques at greater distances. A very effective procedure is to use Tranaglyphs projected on the wall or a screen by an overhead projector. This technique works well because the patient is very familiar with the task and simply has to try and apply the same skills learned during earlier sessions. The targets, printed on 8.5 × 11 in. paper and discussed in Chapter 8 for divergence insufficiency, are helpful for basic exodeviations as well. Another method of presenting stimuli at

TABLE 10.17. *Sample vision therapy program for basic exophoria*

Phase 1
Sessions 1 and 2
In-office
- Discuss nature of vision problem, goals of vision therapy, various feedback cues, importance of practice
- Brock string
- Lens sorting
- Loose lens rock (begin with plus if accommodative excess, with minus if accommodative insufficiency)
- Tranaglyph or Vectograms: base-out
  1. Begin with a peripheral target like Tranaglyph 515 or the Quoit Vectogram
- Computer Orthoptics Random Dot Program: base-out
Home Therapy
- Brock string

Sessions 3 and 4
In-office
- Bug on string
- Loose lens rock
- Tranaglyph or Vectograms: base-out
  1. Use targets with more central demand (Clown, Bunny Tranaglyphs; Clown, Topper Vectograms)
- Computer Orthoptics Random Dot Program: base-out
Home Therapy
- Add loose lens rock

Sessions 5 through 8
In-office
- Barrel card
- Voluntary convergence
- Loose lens rock
- Tranaglyph or Vectograms: base-out
  1. Use even more detailed targets such as Tranaglyphs Sports Slide and Faces targets and the Spirangle Vectogram)
- Computer Orthoptics Random Dot Program: base-out
Home Therapy
- Tranaglyph: base-out

Phase 2
Sessions 9 and 10
In-office
- Tranaglyph or Vectograms with modifications to create jump vergence demand: base-out
- Nonvariable Tranaglyphs
- Tranaglyph 515 or the Quoit Vectogram: base-in
- Binocular accommodative therapy techniques: use any of the binocular techniques listed above with ± lenses
Home Therapy
- Nonvariable Tranaglyphs

Sessions 11 and 12
In-office
- Tranaglyph or Vectograms with modifications to create jump vergence demand: base-out
- Aperture Rule: base-out
- More central Tranaglyphs or the Vectograms: base-in
- Binocular Accommodative therapy techniques: use any of the binocular techniques listed above with ± lenses
Home Therapy
- Nonvariable Tranaglyphs with loose prism jumps

Sessions 13 through 16
In-office
- Aperture Rule: convergence and divergence
- Eccentric Circles or Free Space Fusion Cards
- Computer Orthoptics Random Dot Vergence Program: both base-in and base-out
- Tranaglyph or Vectograms with modifications to create jump vergence demand: base-in

TABLE 10.17. *Continued.*

- Binocular accommodative therapy techniques: use any of the binocular techniques listed above with ± lenses
- Tranaglyph or Vectograms at 1 m
Home Therapy
- Eccentric Circles or Free Space Fusion Cards

Phase 3
Sessions 17 through 20
In-office
- Tranaglyph or Vectograms with Polaroid or red/green flippers
- Eccentric Circles or Free Space Fusion Cards
- Computer Orthoptics Random Dot Vergence Program: step-jump vergence
- Tranaglyph or Vectograms at distance
Home Therapy
- Eccentric Circles or Free Space Fusion Cards: base-out

Sessions 21 and 22
In-office
- Tranaglyph or Vectograms with Polaroid or red/green flippers
- Eccentric Circles or Free Space Fusion Cards
- Lifesaver Cards
- Computer Orthoptics Random Dot Vergence Program: jump–jump vergence
- Distance fusion targets at distance
Home Therapy
- Eccentric Circles or Free Space Fusion Cards: base-in

Sessions 23 and 24
In-office
- Tranaglyph or Vectograms with Polaroid or red/green flippers
- Eccentric Circles or Free Space Fusion Cards with rotation and versions
- Lifesaver Cards with rotation and versions
- Computer Orthoptics Vergence Program with rotation
Home Therapy
- Eccentric Circles or Free Space Fusion Cards: base-in/base-out

intermediate distances is through the use of stereoscopes. The working distance can be conveniently changed on most Brewster-type stereoscopes, and a very wide variety of targets are readily available.

Endpoint

The endpoint of Phase 2 is reached when the patient can:

- fuse card 12 using convergence and card 6 using divergence with the Aperture Rule.
- fuse the Eccentric Circles or Free Space Fusion Cards using convergence (12 cm separation) and divergence (6 cm separation).
- fuse up to 20 Δ using convergence and 10 Δ using divergence with Tranaglyph targets projected at 10 ft using an overhead projector.

A sample vision therapy program for Phase 2 is summarized in Table 10.17.

Phase 3

This third phase of therapy is designed to accomplish the objectives listed in Table 10.16 under Phase 3.

Until this point, the patient has either worked in the convergence or divergence directions separately. Now the objective is to develop the patient's ability to change from a convergence to a divergence demand and to integrate vergence procedures with versions and saccades. Several excellent procedures are available to help accomplish this objective. Vectograms with Polaroid flippers or Tranaglyphs with red/green flippers can be used. Each time the flippers are changed, the demand switches from divergence to convergence. The transparent Keystone Eccentric Circles or transparent Bernell Free Space Fusion Cards are excellent inexpensive methods for achieving this objective.

Another objective of therapy is to integrate vergence procedures with versions and saccades. Techniques such as the Brock string with rotation, Eccentric Circles and Free Space Fusion Cards with rotation and/or lateral movements, and the Lifesaver Cards with rotation can be used to accomplish this goal. The Computer Orthoptics Program that combines horizontal vergence with rotation is also useful for this objective.

The final objective of this final phase of therapy is to work with convergence at distances of from 10 to 20 ft. The same techniques used in Phase 2 at intermediate distances are repeated at even greater distances.

Endpoint

The endpoint for Phase 3 is reached when the patient can:

- maintain clear single binocular vision with the Eccentric Circles and Free Space Fusion Cards held together, while slowly rotating the cards and performing convergence and divergence therapy.
- maintain clear single binocular vision with the large Eccentric Circles and other targets at distance.

When all vision therapy objectives have been reached and the vision therapy program is completed, we recommend the home vision therapy maintenance program outlined in Table 8.10 and described in Chapter 8.

Summary of Vision Therapy for Basic Exophoria

The phases and objectives outlined above and in Tables 10.16 and 10.17 represent one approach that will lead to successful elimination of a patient's symptoms and normalization of optometric data. The number of sessions is approximate and will vary from one patient to another.

Surgery

The use of lenses, prism, and vision therapy in the treatment of basic exophoria is so successful that surgery is virtually never necessary. If the magnitude of the deviation is greater than 30 Δ, however, some patients may not achieve full relief of symptoms. In these instances, a surgical referral should be considered.

REFERENCES

1. Daum K. A comparison of results of tonic and phasic training on the vergence system. *Am J Optom Physiol Opt* 1983;60:769–775.
2. Daum KM. Equal exodeviations: characteristics and results of treatment with orthoptics. *Aust J Optom* 1984;67: 53–59.

3. The efficacy of optometric vision therapy. In: The 1986/1987 AOA Future of Visual Development/Performance Task Force. *J Am Optom Assoc* 1988;59:95–105.

4. Suchoff IB, Petito GT. The efficacy of visual therapy. *J Am Optom Assoc* 1986;57:119–125.

5. Daum K. Double blind placebo-controlled examination of timing effects in the training of positive vergences. *Am J Optom Physiol Opt* 1986;63:807–812.

6. Vaegan JL. Convergence and divergence show longer and sustained improvement after short isometric exercise. *Am J Optom Physiol Opt* 1979;56:23–33.

7. Cooper J, Selenow A, Ciuffreda KJ, et al. Reduction of asthenopia in patients with convergence insufficiency after fusional vergence training. *Am J Optom Physiol Opt* 1983;60:982–989.

8. Wick B. Vision therapy for presbyopic nonstrabismic patients. *Am J Optom Physiol Opt* 1977;54:244–247.

9. Cohen AH, Soden R. Effectiveness of visual therapy for convergence insufficiencies for an adult population. *J Am Optom Assoc* 1984;55:491–494.

10. Hoffman L, Cohen A, Feuer G. Effectiveness of nonstrabismic optometric vision training in a private practice. *Am J Optom Arch Am Acad Opt* 1973;50:813–816.

11. Grisham JD. The dynamics of fusional vergence eye movements in binocular dysfunction. *Am J Optom Physiol Opt* 1980;57:205–213.

12. Grisham JD. Vergence orthoptics: validity and persistence of the training effect. *Am J Optom Physiol Opt* 1991;68:441–451.

13. Schapero M. The characteristics of ten basic visual training problems. *Am J Optom Arch Am Acad Optom* 1955;32:333–342.

14. Richman JE, Cron MT. *Guide to vision therapy.* South Bend, IN: Bernell Corp., 1988.

15. Faibish BH. Enhancing sensory fusion response through short training program. *Rev Optom* 1978(Oct):25–27.

16. Scheiman M, Gallaway M, Coulter R, et al. Prevalence of vision and ocular disease conditions in a clinical pediatric population. *J Am Optom Assoc* 1996;67:193–202.

17. Porcar E, Nartinez-Palomera A. Prevalence of general dysfunctions in a population of university students. *Optom Vis Sci* 1997;74:111–113.

18. Duane A. A new classification of the motor anomalies of the eye based upon physiological principles. *Ann Ophthalmol Otolaryngol* 1886(Oct):247–260.

19. Daum KM. Characteristics of exodeviations. I. A comparison of three classes. *Am J Optom Physiol Opt* 1986;63:237–243.

11

Accommodative Dysfunction

Many authors have suggested that anomalies of accommodation are commonly encountered in optometric practice (1–7). Although there are few studies on the prevalence of accommodative disorders in the general or clinical populations, those that are available do tend to confirm this contention. Hokoda (7) studied a sample of 119 symptomatic patients and found that accommodative dysfunction was the most commonly encountered condition. Twenty-five of the 119 subjects had binocular or accommodative disorders and 80% of the 25 had accommodative problems. Hoffman et al. (8) reported on the effectiveness of vision therapy for nonstrabismic vision therapy, using a sample of 129 subjects. Of the 129 subjects studied, 62% had accommodative dysfunction. In a study of 1,650 children between the ages of 6 and 18 years, Scheiman et al. (9) found that 2.2% of the children had accommodative excess, 1.5% had accommodative infacility, and, 2.3%, accommodative insufficiency. The overall prevalence of accommodative problems was 6%. In a study of 65 university students, Porcar and Nartinez-Palomera (10) found that 10.8% of the subjects had accommodative excess and 6.2% had accommodative insufficiency, for an overall prevalence of 17%.

One of the early attempts at classifying accommodative anomalies was by Duane in 1915 (11). He reported on the results of 170 patients and developed a classification including insufficiency of accommodation, ill-sustained accommodation, inertia of accommodation, excessive accommodation, inequality of accommodation, and paralysis of accommodation. This classification has received wide acceptance. Many other authors, discussing the classification, diagnosis, and management of accommodative anomalies, have essentially used Duane's initial classification with minor modifications (1,2,12–16). The classification of accommodative anomalies that we use in this chapter is also based on Duane's system and it is summarized below.

Classification of Accommodative Anomalies

Accommodative insufficiency

- Ill-sustained accommodation
- Paralysis of accommodation
- Unequal accommodation

Accommodative excess
Accommodative infacility

GENERAL TREATMENT STRATEGIES FOR ACCOMMODATIVE DYSFUNCTION

Sequential Management Considerations in the Treatment of Accommodative Dysfunction

Correction of ametropia
Added lenses
Vision therapy

The concepts that we discussed for the sequential management considerations of binocular vision disorders also apply to accommodative problems. Accommodative fatigue can occur secondary to uncorrected refractive error, such as hyperopia and astigmatism (14). A 3 D hyperope must accommodate 2,50 D, for a working distance of 40 cm and an additional 3 D, to overcome the hyperopia. The muscular fatigue resulting from 5.50 D of accommodation will often lead to the symptoms associated with accommodative problems. Low degrees of astigmatism and anisometropia can also lead to accommodative fatigue, if the accommodative level oscillates back and forth in an attempt to obtain clarity. It is also not unusual for myopes to experience discomfort when reading with their eyeglasses. This may be due to accommodative fatigue and must be considered in any management plan. The first management consideration, therefore, is correction of refractive error. We recommend applying the same criteria for prescribing that we discussed in Chapter 3.

Added lenses also play an important role in the treatment of accommodative dysfunction. Of the various accommodative problems, accommodative insufficiency and ill-sustained accommodation respond best to added plus lenses. The important concept is that any accommodative disorder in which the patient is experiencing problems stimulating accommodation will benefit from added plus lenses. Accommodative problems, in which the difficulty is with relaxation of accommodation or facility, do not respond as well to added lenses. Thus, accommodative excess and accommodative infacility generally require treatment other than added lenses.

Prism, which is so important in cases of binocular vision disorders, is not used for accommodative dysfunction unless there is an associated binocular problem. For purposes of this chapter, we will assume that the accommodative dysfunction is present in isolation. Therefore, prism is not listed as part of the sequential management for accommodative dysfunction.

The final treatment consideration is the use of vision therapy to restore normal accommodative function. Vision therapy is generally necessary in the management of accommodative excess and accommodative infacility. In many cases, it is also critical in the treatment of accommodative insufficiency and ill-sustained accommodation.

Surgery, which was a consideration for binocular vision problems, has no role relative to accommodative dysfunction.

Prognosis for Treating Accommodative Disorders

There have been many studies documenting the efficacy of vision therapy for improving accommodative function, along with several excellent reviews of the literature (17–19). In the most recent review, Rouse (19) reached the following conclusions:

- The literature provides a solid base of research supporting vision therapy as an effective treatment mode for accommodative deficiencies.
- Vision therapy procedures have been shown to improve accommodative function effectively and to eliminate or reduce associated symptoms.
- The actual physiological accommodative response variables modified by therapy have been identified, eliminating the possibility of Hawthorne or placebo effects accounting for treatment success.
- The improved accommodative function appears to be fairly durable after treatment.

The support in the literature comes from two sources, basic scientific investigation and clinical research. Basic scientists have shown that subjects can learn to voluntarily change accommodative response (20,21). These studies demonstrate that voluntary control of accommodation can be trained and transferred to a variety of stimulus conditions. Other researchers have tried to determine the underlying physiological basis for improved accommodative function. Liu et al. (3) and Bobier and Sivak (22) designed studies to identify which aspects of accommodation are affected by vision therapy. The importance of these two studies is that they used objective procedures to monitor accommodative function. These two investigations clearly demonstrated objective improvement in the dynamics of the accommodative response. The velocity of the accommodative response increased and the latency of the response decreased in both studies. In addition, both studies were able to show that the clinical testing of accommodative facility correlated well with the objective laboratory techniques. This result underscores the importance of the clinical use of accommodative facility testing.

Clinical studies of the efficacy of vision therapy for accommodative dysfunction have consistently demonstrated excellent success rates. The following retrospective studies included almost 300 patients. Hoffman et al. (8) reported on a sample of 80 patients with accommodative dysfunction and found an 87.5% success rate for normalizing accommodative ability. About 25 visits, on average, were required. Wold et al. (23) studied the effect of vision therapy on 100 consecutive patients. They found statistically significant changes in both accommodative amplitude and facility. Patients were seen 3 times per week, an average of about 35 visits. In a retrospective study of 114 patients with accommodative dysfunction, Daum (16) found that 96% achieved either total or partial success, with an average of about 4 weeks of therapy.

Several prospective studies have also been done to control for placebo or Hawthorne effects. In addition to the work done by Liu et al. (3) and Bobier and Sivak (22) discussed above, Cooper et al. (24) used a matched-subjects crossover design to control for placebo effects. They studied five subjects with accommodative disorders and asthenopia. The subjects were divided into control and experimental groups. The experimental group received twelve 30-minute sessions of accommodative therapy, while the control group received the same number of sessions of therapy using plano lenses. After the first phase of therapy, the experimental group received an additional 6 weeks of training, identical to that of the control group, and the control group received training identical to that of the experimental group. Four of the five subjects showed increased accommodative amplitude or facility and improvement in symptoms after therapy. These changes occurred only during the experimental phase of the training.

Two other controlled studies (25,26) not only showed improvements in accommodative function and elimination of symptoms, but also were able to demonstrate a transfer effect on performance. Weisz (25) showed that performance on a paper and pencil task improved after accommodative therapy and Hoffman (26) demonstrated improved perceptual performance after treatment.

Another important treatment option for accommodative dysfunction is the use of plus lenses. As we discuss later in this chapter, added plus lenses are indicated in accommodative insufficiency and ill-sustained accommodation. Daum (27) evaluated the effectiveness of plus lenses for the treatment of accommodative insufficiency. Of the 17 subjects in his study, 53% reported total relief of symptoms and 35% experienced partial alleviation of their difficulties. A greater percentage of patients received no relief at all with plus lenses compared to vision therapy (12% versus 4%). This suggests that even for the category of accommodative insufficiency, there are some situations in which vision therapy is the only effective treatment alternative. Daum concluded that

"For most patients, it would appear that the relative ease with which the training may be completed (and in view of the optical limitations and inconvenience of a near plus lens addition) makes orthoptic therapy the treatment method of choice."

ACCOMMODATIVE INSUFFICIENCY (ILL-SUSTAINED ACCOMMODATION, PARALYSIS OF ACCOMMODATION, UNEQUAL ACCOMMODATION)

Background Information

Accommodative insufficiency is a condition in which the patient has difficulty stimulating accommodation. The characteristic finding is an accommodative amplitude below the lower limit of the expected value for the patient's age. To determine the lower limit for a patient, we suggest using Hofstetter's formula, which states that the lower limit is equal to $15 - 0.25$ (age of patient) (26). If the amplitude is 2 D or more below this value, it is considered abnormal. In addition to the low amplitude of accommodation, which is the hallmark of accommodative insufficiency, there are other important characteristics that will be discussed in the next section.

It is important to realize that presbyopia, by definition, is a different entity than accommodative insufficiency. Presbyopia is a condition in which the amplitude of accommodation has diminished to the point where clear or comfortable vision at the near point is not achievable. This usually occurs between the ages of 40 and 45. The symptoms of presbyopia are identical to those of accommodative insufficiency. However, in presbyopia, the amplitude of accommodation is not abnormal relative to the patient's age. Rather, the amplitude is appropriate for the patient's age, although it is too low to permit clear comfortable vision at near. When we talk about accommodative insufficiency, therefore, we are generally referring to a condition that affects pre-presbyopes.

Ill-sustained accommodation or accommodative fatigue has been categorized by most authors as a subclassification of accommodative insufficiency. Both Duane (11) and Duke-Elder and Abrams (2) described ill-sustained accommodation as an early stage of accommodative insufficiency. It is a condition in which the amplitude of accommodation is normal under typical test conditions, but deteriorates over time. If ill-sustained accommodation is suspected, it is important, therefore, to repeat the amplitude of accommodation measurement several times (Chapter 1).

Another condition that can be categorized under accommodative insufficiency is accommodative paralysis. It is a very rare condition that is associated with a variety of organic causes, such as infections, glaucoma, trauma, lead poisoning, and diabetes. It can also occur as a temporary or permanent consequence of head trauma. Paralysis of accommodation can be unilateral or bilateral, sudden or insidious. If it is unilateral, it leads to the other category of accommodative dysfunction called unequal accommodation. Another possible cause of unequal accommodation is functional amblyopia.

Some authors have found that, of the various accommodative problems, accommodative insufficiency is the most common. In a study of the prevalence of accommodative and binocular vision disorders, Hokoda (7) found that 55% of the patients with accommodative anomalies had accommodative insufficiency. Daum (16) studied 114 patients who had been diagnosed as having accommodative dysfunction and found that 84% had accommodative insufficiency. However, Scheiman et al. (9) found about an equal mix of the three primary accommodative problems in their study (accommodative excess 2.2%, accommodative infacility 1.5%, and accommodative insufficiency 2.3%). Porcar and Nartinez-Palomera (10) found that 10.8% of the subjects had accommodative excess and 6.2% has accommodative insufficiency.

Characteristics

Symptoms

The symptoms of accommodative insufficiency are presented in Table 11.1.

TABLE 11.1. *Symptoms and signs of accommodative insufficiency*

Symptoms

These symptoms are generally related to the use of the eyes for reading or other near tasks:

Long-standing	Fatigue and sleepiness
Blurred vision	Loss of comprehension over time
Headaches	A pulling sensation around the eyes
Eyestrain	Movement of the print
Reading problems	Avoidance of reading and other close work

Signs

Direct measures of accommodative stimulation
Reduced amplitude of accommodation
Difficulty clearing −2.00 with monocular accommodative facility
High monocular estimation method finding
High fused cross-cylinder finding
Indirect measures of accommodative stimulation
Reduced positive relative accommodation
Difficulty clearing −2.00 with binocular accommodative facility
Low base-out to blur finding at near

The most common complaints include blur, headaches, eyestrain, double vision, reading problems, fatigue, difficulty changing focus from one distance to another, and sensitivity to light (16). Patients may also complain of an inability to concentrate, a loss of comprehension over time, and words moving on the page. All of these symptoms are associated with reading or other close work. Some patients with accommodative insufficiency are asymptomatic. For example, Daum (16) found 2% of the patients in his sample had no symptoms, although they clearly had accommodative insufficiency. In such cases, the most likely explanation is avoidance of reading and other close work. Since clinicians generally base their treatment decisions on the presence and severity of the patient's symptoms, it is important to remember that avoidance should be regarded as a symptom and is as important a reason for recommending therapy as any of the other symptoms associated with accommodative insufficiency.

Signs

The signs of accommodative insufficiency are presented in Table 11.1.

Accommodative insufficiency is a disorder in which the patient experiences difficulty with any optometric testing that requires stimulation of accommodation. Any test that involves the use of minus lenses will generally yield a reduced finding. The most characteristic sign is the reduced amplitude of accommodation. The patient with accommodative insufficiency will also have low findings on the positive relative accommodation (PRA), minus lenses with both monocular accommodative facility (MAF) and binocular accommodative facility (BAF) testing, and more plus than expected with MEM (monocular estimation method) retinoscopy and the fused-cross cylinder test.

Accommodative insufficiency may also be associated with a binocular vision problem. It is not unusual to find a small degree of esophoria in cases of accommodative insufficiency. A likely explanation is that the patient uses additional innervation to try and overcome the accommodative problem, which stimulates accommodative convergence, causing an esophoria. A condition called pseudoconvergence insufficiency has also been related to accommodative insufficiency (29). In such cases, the patient has difficulty accommodating and, therefore, underaccommodates relative to the stimulus. As a result, less accommodative convergence is available, the measured exophoria is larger, and a greater demand is placed on positive fusional convergence. Typically, such patients will also have a receded near point of convergence because of the reduced amplitude of accommodation and the lack of accommodative convergence. We presented a case of pseudoconvergence insufficiency in Chapter 8.

Analysis of Binocular and Accommodative Data

The entry point into the analysis of accommodative and binocular vision data is the phoria at distance and near. In cases of accommodative dysfunction, it is not unusual for the phoria to fall outside expected values. As we discussed above, accommodative insufficiency can be associated with exophoria or esophoria. It is important in such cases to carefully analyze the appropriate group data. For example, the patient in Case 11.1 presented with symptoms of blurred vision and eyestrain after reading for 15 minutes. The cover test at distance is ortho and, at near, 2 esophoria. After eliminating refractive error and organic causes, the best initial approach is to be concerned about an esophoria and a low negative fusional vergence (NFV)-type problem at near. We would, therefore, analyze the NFV group data, which includes base-in vergence at near, the PRA, BAF testing with minus lenses, MEM retinoscopy, and the fused cross-cylinder test. Case 11.1 illustrates that the indirect measures of NFV are abnormal. The patient has a low PRA and BAF finding, and MEM retinoscopy shows more plus than expected. This data can be a reflection of either an accommodative problem in which the patient has difficulty stimulating accommodation or convergence excess. The key to differentiating these two hypotheses is the direct measures of NFV. In this case, both the smooth and step vergence findings are essentially normal. This eliminates the possibility of a binocular problem. Once a binocular vision problem is eliminated, we recommend analysis of the accommodative system (ACC) group data. This data reveals a low amplitude of accommodation, inability to clear −2.00 with MAF along with the reduced PRA, high MEM finding, and inability to clear −2.00 lenses binocularly. These findings, analyzed as a group, suggest that the patient has difficulty with all tests requiring stimulation of accommodation, confirming a diagnosis of accommodative insufficiency.

Differential Diagnosis

The differential diagnosis of accommodative insufficiency is presented in Table 11.2.

Accommodative insufficiency is considered to be a benign condition, with no serious consequences other than the visual symptoms listed in Table 11.1. It is relatively easy to differentiate from other accommodative disorders. Accommodative insufficiency is the only condition associated with a reduced amplitude of accommodation. In addition, while the accommodative insufficiency patient has difficulty with all tests requiring stimulation of accommodation, the accommodative excess patient has difficulty with all tests requiring relaxation of accommodation. The accommodative facility patient has difficulty with both stimulation and relaxation of accommodation. Accommodative paralysis is a condition in which the amplitude of accommodation is dramatically reduced and there is usually some local or systemic disease or medication that can explain the problem.

While accommodative insufficiency generally has a functional etiology, it may occur in association with primary ocular disease, generalized systemic and neurologic disorders, as well as with lesions that produce focal interruption of the parasympathetic innervation of the ciliary body (10). A variety of ocular and systemic drugs can also lead to accommodative insufficiency. There are several comprehensive sources that describe these nonfunctional etiologies in detail (12,13). Table 11.2, compiled by London (13), is a list of the nonfunctional causes of

TABLE 11.2. *Differential diagnosis of accommodative insufficiency*

Functional disorders to rule out
Pseudoconvergence insufficiency
Basic exophoria
Divergence excess
Accommodative excess
Accommodative infacility

Nonfunctional causes of accommodative insufficiency

Bilateral[a]	Unilateral
Drugs	**Local eye disease**
Alcohol	Iridocyclitis
Artane	Glaucoma
Lystrone	Choroidal metastasis
Ganglion blockers	Tear in iris sphincter
Phenothiazides	Blunt trauma
Antihistamines	Ciliary body aplasia
Cycloplegics	Scleritis
CNS stimulants	Adie's syndrome
Marijuana	
General disease: adults	**General disease: adults**
Anemia	Sinusitis
Encephalitis	Dental caries
Diabetes mellitus	Posterior communicating artery
Multiple sclerosis	Aneurysm
Myotonic dystrophy	Parkinsonism
Malaria	Wilson's disease
Typhoid	Midbrain lesions
Toxemia	
Botulism	
General disease: children	
Anemia	Whooping cough
Mumps	Tonsillitis
Measles	Diphtheria
Scarlet fever	Lead and arsenic poisoning
Neuroophthalmic	**Neuroophthalmic**
Lesions in Edinger-Westphal syndrome	Fascicular nerve III lesion
Trauma to craniocervical region (whiplash)	Herpes zoster
Pineal tumor	Horner's syndrome
Parinaud's syndrome	
Polyneuropathy	
Anterior poliomyelitis	

[a] Bilateral problem may start unilaterally.
Source: From London R. Accommodation. In: Barresi BJ (ed), *Ocular assessment: The manual of diagnosis for office practice.* Boston: Butterworth-Heinemann, 1984:123–130, with permission.

accommodative problems. It is always important to rule out these nonfunctional causes before deciding on any treatment plan for accommodative insufficiency. This differential diagnosis depends very much on the case history. Patients presenting with accommodative insufficiency, secondary to any of the diseases listed in Table 11.2, will have a history of being ill in the past or at the present time. A history of diseases such as diabetes, encephalitis, multiple sclerosis, malaria, and typhoid, for example, would certainly be easy to elicit from a patient with any of these problems. The same is true of the various medications listed in Table 11.2. Accommodative insufficiency, secondary to functional causes, will present with long-standing chronic complaints and a negative health and medication history.

In most cases, therefore, the differential diagnosis is not difficult. However, if improvement in symptoms and findings does not occur as expected when managing a case of accommodative insufficiency that is thought to have a functional basis, it is prudent to reconsider the etiology of the condition.

Treatment

We recommend the management sequence listed on page 334.

Lenses

Because uncorrected refractive error can be a cause of accommodative fatigue, we recommend that correction of ametropia be the first management consideration. When dealing with patients with accommodative insufficiency, even small degrees of refractive error may be significant. Prescribing for small degrees of hyperopia, astigmatism, and small differences in refractive error between the two eyes, may provide some immediate relief of symptoms for the patient.

Added Lenses

Analysis of the near point findings in accommodative insufficiency clearly shows that these patients benefit from the use of added plus lenses. The low PRA, difficulty clearing minus during accommodative facility testing, the low amplitude of accommodation, and high MEM retinoscopy are all examples of data suggesting the need for plus lenses for near. The amount of added plus can easily be determined by analyzing this data. Referring to Case 11.1, the NRA was +2.50 and the PRA, −1.00. This suggests an add of +0.75. This patient could not clear −2.00 lenses during accommodative facility testing, and MEM retinoscopy was +1.00. Since the normal finding is +0.50, this suggests an add of +0.50.

Occasionally, myopic patients will experience difficulty with accommodation after they receive their first prescription or a large change in prescription. Esophoria at near is also a common finding in such cases. If the findings reveal accommodative insufficiency, a bifocal should be prescribed.

When there is an organic cause of the accommodative insufficiency or even paralysis of accommodation, added lenses are an important treatment consideration. In some cases, the accommodative paralysis is temporary. Added plus lenses are useful as a temporary solution, while treatment of the underlying condition occurs. If the underlying cause of the paralysis of accommodation cannot be eliminated and the condition is stable and nonprogressive, then added plus lenses may need to be permanent. A trial period of vision therapy can also be attempted, after medical concerns have been addressed.

Unequal accommodation, secondary to organic causes, also responds well to added plus lenses. In such cases, it is frequently necessary to consider prescribing unequal adds.

Vision Therapy

A vision therapy program for accommodative insufficiency generally requires from 12 to 24 in-office visits, if vision therapy is office-based. The total number of therapy sessions depends on the age of the patient, motivation, and compliance.

Specific Vision Therapy Program

All of the vision therapy techniques recommended below are described in detail in Chapters 5 to 7.

Phase 1

This first phase of therapy is designed to accomplish the objectives listed in Table 11.3 under Phase 1.

TABLE 11.3. *Vision therapy for accommodative insufficiency and ill-sustained accommodation*

Phase 1
Objectives
- Develop a working relationship with the patient
- Develop an awareness of the various feedback mechanisms that will be used throughout therapy
- Normalize accommodative amplitude and ability to stimulate accommodation
- Develop voluntary convergence
- Develop feeling of looking close and accommodating
- Normalize positive fusional vergence (PFV) amplitudes (smooth or tonic vergence demand)

Phase 2
Objectives
- Normalize ability to stimulate and relax accommodation
- Incorporate speed of response into accommodative techniques
- Normalize negative fusional vergence (NFV) amplitudes (smooth or tonic vergence demand)
- Normalize PFV facility (jump or phasic vergence demand)
- Normalize NFV facility (jump or phasic vergence demand)

Phase 3
Objectives
- Integrate accommodative facility therapy with binocular vision techniques
- Develop ability to change from a convergence to a divergence demand
- Integrate vergence procedures with versions and saccades

After establishing a working relationship with the patient and developing an awareness of the various feedback mechanisms that will be used throughout therapy, the first goal of the therapy itself is to improve the patient's ability to stimulate accommodation and normalize the amplitude of accommodation. The emphasis during this phase is on the magnitude rather than the speed of the accommodative response. Minus lenses are primarily used initially; however, toward the end of Phase 1, we begin to use plus and minus lenses. Useful procedures include lens sorting, the Hart chart, and loose lens rock.

Because of the interactions that occur between accommodation and vergence, it is also helpful to simultaneously work with convergence techniques. The objective is to help the patient appreciate the feeling and concept of looking close, converging, and accommodating. During Phase 1 it is, therefore, helpful to perform convergence procedures. Useful procedures include the Brock string, Tranaglyphs, and the Computer Orthoptics Random Dot program.

Endpoint

Phase 1 of therapy ends when the patient can:

- clear $+2.00/-6.00$ lenses monocularly with 20/30 size print.
- fuse up to 30 Δ using convergence with the Tranaglyphs or other convergence technique.
- fuse up to 45 Δ using convergence with the Computer Orthoptics Random Dot program.

A sample vision therapy program for Phase 1 is summarized in Table 11.4. This program includes several techniques that can be used by the patient at home to supplement in-office therapy.

Phase 2

This second phase of therapy is designed to accomplish the objectives listed in Table 11.3 under Phase 2.

In contrast to Phase 1, the speed of the accommodative response should now be emphasized. In addition, it is important to continue using plus as well as minus lenses. The objective is for the patient to be able to relax and stimulate accommodation as quickly as possible. The same techniques used during Phase 1 can be repeated using plus and minus lenses, with an emphasis on the speed of the accommodative response. We also begin working with BAF procedures, such as red–red rock and bar readers and binocular facility with targets such as Vectograms and Tranaglyphs.

We now incorporate divergence therapy, in addition to convergence therapy, and move toward binocular vision techniques that emphasize phasic vergence changes. By the end of this phase, the patient should be using the Aperture Rule and the Computer Orthoptics Random Dot Program for both convergence and divergence therapy.

Endpoint

The endpoint of Phase 2 is reached when the patient can:

- clear +2.00/−6.00 lenses monocularly with 20/30 size print, 20 cpm.
- clear +2.00/−2.00 lenses binocularly with 20/30 size print, 15 cpm.
- fuse card 12 using convergence and card 6 using divergence with the Aperture Rule.

A sample vision therapy program for Phase 2 is summarized in Table 11.4. This program includes several techniques that can be used by the patient at home to supplement the in-office therapy.

Phase 3

This third phase of therapy is designed to accomplish the objectives listed in Table 11.3 under Phase 3.

During Phase 3, the emphasis is on integration of accommodation and binocular therapy. Phasic binocular techniques, like the Aperture Rule, Eccentric Circles, Free Space Cards, and the step-jump vergence program of Computer Orthoptics are useful. BAF with flip lenses should be used with the phasic binocular techniques listed above. It is also important to integrate accommodative and binocular therapy with saccades and versions. Moving the Eccentric Circles or Free Space Fusion Cards into different positions of gaze or using several sets of cards in various positions, along with flip lenses, is an excellent procedure to accomplish this goal. Other techniques, such as the Brock string with rotation and Computer Orthoptics vergence with rotation, are useful.

Endpoint

The endpoint for this phase of therapy is reached when the patient is able to maintain clear single binocular vision with the Free Space Fusion Cards or the Eccentric Circle Cards together, while slowly rotating the cards and using +2.00/−2.00 flip lenses.

A reevaluation should be performed after about 3 to 4 weeks to determine if any progress has been made. If no improvement is evident, there may be an underlying organic basis to the low amplitude of accommodation and added plus lenses should be prescribed and vision therapy discontinued. If progress is adequate, reevaluate again at about halfway through the therapy program and again at the end of therapy. When all vision therapy objectives have been reached and the vision therapy program is completed, we recommend the home vision therapy maintenance program discussed in Chapter 8 (Table 8.10).

TABLE 11.4. *Sample vision therapy program for accommodative insufficiency*

Phase 1
Sessions 1 and 2
In-office
- Discuss nature of vision problem, goals of vision therapy, various feedback cues, importance of practice
- Lens sorting
- Loose lens rock (begin with minus lenses)
- Brock string
- Tranaglyph or Vectograms: base-out
  1. Begin with a peripheral target like Tranaglyph 515 or the Quoit Vectogram
- Computer Orthoptics Random Dot Program: base-out
Home Therapy
- Loose lens rock
- Brock string

Sessions 3 and 4
In-office
- Hart chart rock
- Loose lens rock; minus lenses
- Bug on string
- Tranaglyph or Vectograms: base-out
  1. Use targets with more central demand (Clown, Bunny Tranaglyphs; Clown, Topper Vectograms)
- Computer Orthoptics Random Dot Program: base-out
Home Therapy
- Loose lens rock
- Brock string

Sessions 5 through 8
In-office
- Hart chart rock
- Loose lens rock; add plus lenses
- Barrel card
- Voluntary convergence
- Tranaglyph or Vectograms: base-out
  1. Use even more detailed targets such as Tranaglyphs Sports Slide and Faces targets and the Spirangle Vectogram
- Computer Orthoptics Random Dot Program: base-out
Home Therapy
- Hart chart rock
- Tranaglyph: base-out

Phase 2
Sessions 9 and 10
In-office
- Loose lens rock; use both plus and minus lenses and incorporate speed as a factor
- Tranaglyph or Vectograms with modifications to create jump vergence demand: base-out
- Nonvariable Tranaglyphs
- Tranaglyph 515 or the Quoit Vectogram: base-in
- Binocular accommodative therapy techniques: use any of the binocular techniques listed above with ± lenses
Home Therapy
- Nonvariable Tranaglyphs
- Loose lens rock (emphasize speed)

Sessions 11 and 12
In-office
- Loose lens rock; use both plus and minus lenses and incorporate speed as a factor.
- Binocular accommodative therapy techniques: use any of the binocular techniques listed above with ± lenses
- Tranaglyph or Vectograms with modifications to create jump vergence demand: base-out
- Aperture Rule: base-out
- More central Tranaglyphs or the Vectograms: base-in

TABLE 11.4. *Continued.*

Home Therapy
• Nonvariable Tranaglyphs with ± flip lenses

Sessions 13 through 16
In-office
• Binocular accommodative therapy techniques: use any of the binocular techniques listed above with ± lenses
• Aperture Rule: base-out
• Eccentric Circles or Free Space Fusion Cards: base-out
• Computer Orthoptics Random Dot Vergence Program: both base-in and base-out
• Aperture Rule: base-in
• Tranaglyph or Vectograms with modifications to create jump vergence demand: base-in
Home Therapy
• Eccentric Circles or Free Space Fusion Cards: base-out

Phase 3
Sessions 17 through 20
In-office
• Binocular accommodative therapy with ± lenses and the Aperture Rule
• Tranaglyph or Vectograms with Polaroid or red/green flippers
• Eccentric Circles or Free Space Fusion Cards: base-out
• Computer Orthoptics Random Dot Vergence Program: step–jump vergence
Home Therapy
• Eccentric Circles or Free Space Fusion Cards: base-out

Sessions 21 and 22
In-office
• Binocular accommodative therapy with ± lenses and the Aperture Rule
• Tranaglyph or Vectograms with Polaroid or red/green flippers
• Eccentric Circles or Free Space Fusion Cards: base-in
• Computer Orthoptics Random Dot Vergence Program: jump–jump Vergence
Home Therapy
• Eccentric Circles or Free Space Fusion Cards: base-in

Sessions 23 and 24
In-office
• Binocular accommodative therapy with ± lenses and the Eccentric Circles
• Tranaglyph or Vectograms with Polaroid or red/green flippers
• Eccentric Circles or Free Space Fusion Cards with rotation and versions
• Lifesaver Cards with rotation and versions
• Computer Orthoptics Vergence Program with rotation
Home Therapy
• Eccentric Circles or Free Space Fusion Cards: base-in/base-out with ± flip lenses

Case Studies

The following case studies are representative of the types of accommodative insufficiency patients that clinicians will encounter in practice.

Case 11.1: Accommodative Insufficiency

History

Janet, a 17-year-old eleventh grader, presented with complaints of blurred vision and eyestrain after reading more than 15 minutes. Although she reported similar symptoms throughout high school, the problems were worse since the beginning of the school year. Her medical history was negative and she was not taking any medication. Janet had been examined about 2 years ago and the doctor said her eyes were fine.

Management

This is a typical presentation of ocular motor dysfunction. As we have emphasized throughout this chapter, there is often an associated accommodative or convergence disorder. In this case, we prescribed added plus lenses to manage the accommodative insufficiency. Both the MEM finding and the NRA/PRA relationship suggested an add of about +0.75. We prescribed OD = +0.25 and OS = plano with an add of +0.75 OU. We instructed Kevin to wear these glasses in school and for all near work. In addition, we prescribed a program of vision therapy to treat the ocular motor dysfunction and accommodative problems.

We followed the therapy sequence outlined in Table 12.6, and 18 therapy visits were required. A reevaluation after visit 18 revealed the following posttherapy results.

Cover test (distance):	orthophoria
Cover test (near):	2 exophoria
Subjective:	OD: +0.25
	OS: plano
Near lateral phoria:	3 base-in
Base-in vergence (near):	12/24/12
Base-out vergence (near):	20/30/22
NRA:	+2.50
PRA:	−2.25
Accommodative amplitude (push-up):	OD: 13 D, OS: 13 D
MAF:	OD: 10 cpm
	OS: 10 cpm
BAF:	8 cpm
MEM retinoscopy:	+0.75 OU
NSUCO saccades:	head movement 5, ability 5, accuracy 4
DEM:	ratio score: 45th percentile
	error score: 65th percentile
NSUCO Pursuits:	head movement 5, ability 4, accuracy 5

His parents and tutor reported a significant decrease in loss of place and skipping lines. In addition, his tutor found increased reading speed and comprehension and felt that she was now able to work with him more productively over the course of the 1-hour tutoring session. We discontinued therapy and instructed the patient to continue wearing his glasses for school and all reading.

This case demonstrates how ocular motor, accommodative, and convergence disorders can interfere with reading. These vision problems may cause inefficient slow reading with comprehension problems in children who have the basic reading abilities such as decoding and sight vocabulary skills. Treatment of these conditions can lead to increased reading speed and comprehension. Of course, children with such problems also may have other reading problems or lags and will generally require additional tutoring in reading to solve these problems.

Case 12.2

History

Bernadette, a 14-year-old ninth grader, was referred by another optometrist for vision therapy. The other optometrist had been treating Bernadette for about 1.5 years for increasing myopia. In addition, over the past 9 months, Bernadette had been complaining of difficulty reading music, with frequent loss of place. She also complained of eyestrain and discomfort associated with reading and other deskwork. The other optometrist prescribed bifocals about 3 months previously to try and relieve her symptoms. This approach was not successful, however.

Her current prescription was:

OD: $-1.75 - 0.75 \times 15$
OS: $-2.25 - 0.75 \times 165$
With a $+1.00$ add OU

Examination Results

VA (distance, corrected):	OD: 20/20 − 2
	OS: 20/20 − 2
VA (near, uncorrected):	OD: 20/25
	OS: 20/25
Near point of convergence:	
Accommodative target:	3 to 4 in.
Penlight:	3 to 5 in.
Cover test (distance):	orthophoria
Cover test (near):	2 esophoria, with a 2 Δ right hyperphoria

In down-gaze, the deviation was 10 esophoria. There was also a 2 Δ right hyperphoria in left gaze and a 2 Δ left hyperphoria in right gaze. Saccadic testing revealed great difficulty initiating saccades. The patient almost had to make a head movement to help initiate the saccade. The saccades were also inaccurate with significant undershoots.

Subjective:	OD: $-1.75 - 0.75 \times 15$
	OS: $-2.25 - 0.75 \times 165$
Distance lateral phoria:	orthophoria
Distance vertical phoria:	isophoria
Base-in vergence (distance):	x /6/2
Base-out vergence (distance):	8/17/12
Near lateral phoria:	3 esophoria
−1.00 gradient:	9 esophoria
Gradient AC/A ratio:	6:1
Calculated AC/A ratio:	7.2:1
Near vertical phoria:	1 base-down OD
Base-in vergence (near):	x /8/4
Base-out vergence (near):	x /12/6
NRA:	+1.75
PRA:	−1.75
Accommodative amplitude (push-up):	OD: 10 D, OS: 10 D
MAF:	OD: 3 cpm, OS: 3 cpm
BAF:	2 cpm
MEM retinoscopy:	+0.25 OU

Pupils were normal and all external and internal ealth tests were negative.

Case Analysis

Unless we look carefully at the cover test in different positions of gaze or eye movement testing, it is easy to see why the first optometrist referred this patient for vision therapy. Analysis of the accommodative and binocular data suggests problems with fusional vergence at near and accommodative infacility. Although the data do not suggest a specific diagnosis, there are certainly signs of fusional vergence dysfunction and accommodative infacility.

Of course, the results of saccadic testing and the vertical deviation and variation of the hyperphoria in different positions of gaze cannot be ignored. These are significant findings and suggest a possible serious underlying etiology. Based on these findings, we referred Bernadette for a neurological evaluation. As part of his evaluation, the neurologist referred her for magnetic resonance imaging (MRI). The results of this testing revealed the presence of an arachnoid cyst in the brainstem area. Based on this result, it was clear that the visual findings were secondary to the pressure on the brainstem due to the cyst. Neurosurgery was recommended.

Management

Two weeks later, Bernadette woke up at night vomiting and required neurosurgery to relieve the elevated intracranial pressure caused by the cyst. The surgical procedure was successful and a follow-up 4 weeks later revealed almost normal saccades. While the esophoria continued to be slightly larger in down-gaze, the hyperdeviation was no longer present.

This case underscores the importance of carefully evaluating eye movement skills and always being cognizant of the differential diagnosis of eye movement, as well as accommodative and binocular vision disorders.

SUMMARY

Assessing and treating ocular motility disorders has been a concern for clinicians because of the effect such problems may have on the functional capability of an individual. While saccadic and pursuit anomalies can be entirely functional in etiology, it is always important to first rule out the serious causes of ocular motor dysfunction in the differential diagnosis.

Once it is clear that a functional ocular motor dysfunction is present, following the sequential management sequence suggested in this chapter should lead to elimination of these problems, in most cases.

SOURCES OF EQUIPMENT

a. Instructional Communications Technology, Inc., 10 Stepar Place, Huntington Station, NY 11746.
b. Computer Aided Vision Therapy, Bernell Corporation, 750 Lincolnway East, P.O. Box 4637, Southbend, IN 46634; 800-348-2225.
c. RC Instruments, 1558 Eastport Court, P.O. Box 197, Cicero, IN 46034; 800-346-4925.

REFERENCES

1. Brookman KE. Ocular accommodation in human infants. *Am J Optom Physiol Opt* 1980;60:91–95.
2. Birch EE, Gwiazda J, Held R. Stereoacuity development for crossed and uncrossed disparities in human infants. *Vision Res* 1982;22:507–510.
3. Garzia RP, Richman JE, Nicholson SB, et al. A new visual-verbal saccade test: the Developmental Eye Movement test (DEM). *J Am Optom Assoc* 1990;61:124–135.

4. Grisham D, Simons H. Perspectives on reading disabilities. In: Rosenbloom AA, Morgan MW, eds. *Principles and practice of pediatric optometry.* Philadelphia: JB Lippincott, 1990:518–559.
5. Kulp MT, Schmidt PP. Effect of oculomotor and other visual skills on reading performance: a literature review. *Optom Vis Sci* 1996;73:283–292.
6. Solan HA. Eye movement problems in achieving readers: an update. *Am J Optom Physiol Opt* 1985;62:812–819.
7. Solan HA, Feldman J, Tujak L. Developing visual and reading efficiency in older adults. *Optom Vis Sci* 1995;72:139–145.
8. Rayner K. Eye movements in reading and information processing. *Psychol Bull* 1978;85:618–660.
9. Poynter HL, Schor C, Haynes HM, et al. Oculomotor functions in reading disability. *Am J Optom Physiol Optics* 1982;59:116–127.
10. Taylor EA. *Controlled reading.* Chicago: University of Chicago Press, 1937.
11. Gilbert LC. *Functional motor efficiency of the eye and its relation to reading.* University of California Press, Publications in Education, 1953;11:159–232.
12. Taylor EA. The spans, perception, apprehension and recognition. *Am J Ophthalmol* 1957;44:501–507.
13. Taylor SE. Eye movements in reading: facts and fallacies. *Am Educ Res J* 1965;2:4.
14. Zangwill OL, Blakemore C. Dyslexia: reversal of eye movements during reading. *Neuropsychologica* 1972;10:371–373.
15. Rubino CA, Minden H. An analysis of eye movements in children with a reading disability. *Cortex* 1973;9:217–220.
16. Griffin DC. Saccades as related to reading disorders. *J Learn Disabil* 1974;7:50–58.
17. Goldrich SG, Sedgwick H. An objective comparison of oculomotor functioning in reading disabled and normal children. *Am J Optom Physiol Opt* 1982;59:82P.
18. Raymond JE, Ogden NA, Fagan JE, et al. Fixational stability in dyslexic children. *Am J Optom Physiol Opt* 1982;65:174–179.
19. Jones A, Stark L. Abnormal patterns of normal eye movements in specific dyslexia. In: Rayner K, ed. *Eye movements in reading: perceptual and language processes.* New York: Academic Press, 1983:481–498.
20. Pavlidis GT. Eye movement differences between dyslexics, normal, and retarded readers while sequentially fixating digits. *Am J Optom Physiol Opt* 1985;62:820–832.
21. Pavlidis GT. Eye movements in dyslexia: diagnostic significance. *J Learn Disabil* 1985;18:42.
22. Flax N. Problems in relating visual function to reading disorder. *Am J Optom Arch Am Acad Optom* 1970;47:366–372.
23. Ludlam WM, Twarowski C, Ludlam DP. Optometric visual training for reading disability—a case report. *Am J Optom Arch Am Acad Optom* 1973;50:58–66.
24. Heath EJ, Cook P, O'Dell N. Eye exercises and reading efficiency. *Acad Therapy* 1976;11:435–445.
25. Pierce JR. Is there a relationship between vision therapy and academic achievement? *Rev Optom* 1977;114:48–63.
26. Getz D. Learning enhancement through vision therapy. *Acad Therapy* 1980;15(4):457–466.
27. Geiger G, Lettvin JY. Peripheral vision in persons with dyslexia. *N Engl J Med* 1987;316:1238–1243.
28. Adler-Grinberg D, Stark L. Eye movements, scanpaths, and dyslexia. *Am J Optom Physiol Opt* 1978;55:557–570.
29. Brown B, Haegerstrom-Portney G, Adams A, et al. Predictive eye movements do not discriminate between dyslexic and control children. *Neuropsychologica* 1983;21:121–128.
30. Olsen RK, Kliegl R, Davidson BJ. Dyslexic and normal readers eye movements. *J Exp Psychol (Hum Percept)* 1983;816–825.
31. Stanley G, Smith GA, Howell EA. Eye movements and sequential tracking in dyslexic and control children. *Br J Psychol* 1983;74:181–187.
32. Black JL, Collins DWK, De Roach JN, et al. Dyslexia: a detailed study of sequential eye movements for normal and poor reading children. *Percept Mot Skills* 1984;59:423–434.
33. Richman JE. Use of a sustained visual attention task to determine children at risk for learning problems. *J Am Optom Assoc* 1986;57:20–27.
34. Simon MJ. Use of a vigilance task to determine school readiness in preschool children. *Percept Mot Skills* 1982;54:1020–1022.
35. Richman JE. The influence of visual attention and automaticity on the diagnosis and treatment of clinical oculo-motor, accommodative, and vergence dysfunctions. *J Optom Vis Dev* 1999;30:132–141.
36. Coulter RA, Shallo-Hoffmann J. The presumed influence of attention on accuracy in the Developmental Eye Movement (DEM) test. *Optom Vis Sci* 2000;77:428–432.
37. Flax N. The relationship between vision and learning. In: Scheiman M, Rouse M, eds. *Optometric management of learning related vision problems.* St. Louis: CV Mosby, 1994.
38. Sherman A. Relating vision disorders to learning disability. *J Am Optom Assoc* 1973;44:140–141.
39. Hoffman LG. Incidence of vision difficulties in children with learning disabilities. *J Am Optom Assoc* 1980;51:447–451.
40. Lieberman S. The prevalence of visual disorders in a school for emotionally disturbed children. *J Am Optom Assoc* 1985;56:800–803.
41. Berthoz A, Melville Jones G. Preface: a review of an unanswered question? In: Berthoz A, Melville Jones G, eds. *Adaptive mechanisms in gaze control.* Amsterdam: Elsevier Science, 1985:1–3.

42. Optican LM. Adaptive properties of the saccadic system. In: Berthoz A, Melville Jones G, eds. *Adaptive mechanisms in gaze control.* Amsterdam: Elsevier Science, 1985:71–79.
43. (Deleted in proofs.)
44. Moidell BG, Bedell HE. Changes in oculocentric visual direction induced by the recalibration of saccades. *Vision Res* 1988;8:329–336.
45. McLaughlin SC. Parametric adjustment in saccadic eye movements. *Percept Psychophys* 1967;2:359–362.
46. Vissius G. Adaptive control of saccadic eye movements. *Bibl Ophthalmol* 1972;82:244–250.
47. Hallett PE, Lightstone AD. Saccadic eye movements towards stimuli triggered during prior saccades. *Vision Res* 1976;16:88–106.
48. Kommerell G, Olivier D, Theopold H. Adaptive programming of phasic and tonic components in saccadic eye movements: investigations in patients with abducens palsy. *Invest Ophthalmol Vis Sci* 1976;15:657–660.
49. Abel LA, Schmidt D, Dell'Osso LF, et al. Saccadic system plasticity in humans. *Ann Neurol* 1978;4:313–318.
50. Wold RM, Pierce JR, Keddington J. Effectiveness of optometric vision therapy. *J Am Optom Assoc* 1978;49:1047–1053.
51. Solan HA. The improvement of reading efficiency: a study of sixty-three achieving high school students. In: Solan HA, ed. *The psychology of learning and reading difficulties.* New York: Simon and Schuster, 1973:363–370.
52. Rounds BB, Manley CW, Norris RH. The effect of oculomotor training on reading efficiency. *J Am Optom Assoc* 1991;6:92–99.
53. Young BS, Pollard T, Paynter S, et al. Effect of eye exercises in improving control of eye movements during reading. *J Optom Vis Dev* 1982;13:4–7.
54. Fujimoto DH, Christensen EA, Griffin JR. An investigation in use of videocassette techniques for enhancement of saccadic movements. *J Am Optom Assoc* 1985;56:304–308.
55. Punnett AF, Steinhauer GD. Relationship between reinforcement and eye movements during ocular motor training with learning disabled children. *J Learn Disabil* 1984;17:16–19.
56. Goldrich SG. Emergent textual contours: a new technique for visual monitoring in nystagmus, oculomotor dysfunction, and accommodative disorders. *Am J Optom Physiol Opt* 1981;58:451–459.
57. Ciuffreda KJ, Goldrich SG, Neary C. Use of eye movement auditory feedback in the control of nystagmus. *Am J Optom Physiol Opt* 1982;59:396–409.
58. Abadi RV, Carden D, Simpson J. A new treatment for congenital nystagmus. *Br J Ophthalmol* 1980;64:2–4.
59. Flom MC, Kirschen DG, Bedell HE. Control of unsteady, eccentric fixation in amblyopic eyes by auditory feedback of eye position. *Invest Ophthalmol Vis Sci* 1980;19:1371–1381.
60. Fayos B, Ciuffreda KJ. Oculomotor auditory biofeedback training to improve reading efficiency. *J Behav Optom* 1998;9:143–152.
61. Sohrab-Jam G. Eye movement patterns and reading performance in poor readers: immediate effects of convex lenses indicated by book retinoscopy. *Am J Optom Physiol Optics* 1976;53:720–726.
62. Leigh RJ, Zee DS. *The neurology of eye movement,* 3rd ed. New York: Oxford University Press, 1999.
63. Lieberman S, Cohen AH, Rubin J. NYSOA K-D test. *J Am Optom Assoc* 1983;54:631–637.
64. Griffin JR. Pursuit fixations: an overview of training procedures. *Optom Monthly* 1976;67:35–38.
65. Groffman S. Visual tracing. *J Am Optom Assoc* 1966;37:139–141.
66. Burde RM, Savino PJ, Trobe JD. *Clinical decisions in neuro-ophthalmology,* 2nd ed. St. Louis: Mosby—Year Book, 1992:200–202.
67. Dejong JD, Melville Jones G. Akinesia, hypokinesia, and bradykinesia in the oculomotor system of patients with Parkinson's disease. *Exp Neurol* 1971;32:58–62.
68. Higgins JD. Oculomotor system. In: Barresi B, ed. *Ocular assessment.* Boston: Butterworth-Heinemann, 1984:201–208.
69. Griffin JR. Saccadic eye movements—recommended testing and training procedures. *Optom Monthly* 1981; 72(July):27–28.
70. Press LJ. *Computers and vision therapy programs.* Optometric Extension Program, Curriculum II, Series I. Santa Ana, CA: 1988;60.
71. Maino DM. Applications in pediatrics, binocular vision, and perception. In: Maino JH, Maino DM, Davidson DW, eds. *Computer applications in optometry.* Boston: Butterworth-Heinemann, 1989:99–113.
72. Vogel GL. Saccadic eye movements: theory. Testing and therapy. *J Behav Optom* 1995;6:3–12.

13

Cyclovertical Heterophoria

Uncorrected cyclovertical heterophorias frequently cause symptoms that prompt patients to seek visual care; yet, many practitioners are uncomfortable managing such deviations. Some reasons for the reluctance to prescribe treatment for cyclovertical heterophorias include a perception that these conditions are more difficult to understand, the occasional difficulty making an accurate assessment of the direction and magnitude using conventional measurement techniques, and a mistaken belief that therapy is not very successful. This chapter represents a review of the major clinical aspects of cyclovertical heterophoria. In it we include definitions, a brief historical review, a description of the expected frequency and diagnosis of cyclodeviations, and a discussion of applicable clinical management techniques.

CYCLOVERTICAL HETEROPHORIA: BACKGROUND

Definitions and Terminology

Vertical deviations, which are upward or downward misalignments of the visual axis of one eye from the object of regard (1), are typically measured in prism diopters (D) of vertical misalignment. Cyclodeviations are rotations or rotary displacements of the eye about an anteroposterior axis that are measured in degrees of rotation (1a). Both lateral and cyclovertical deviations are classified as:

Phorias are latent deviations from the relative positions necessary to maintain single binocular vision (1b). Latent deviations are held in check by fusional vergence (2).
Tropias are manifest deviations from the position of single binocular vision (1c).

Terminology for recording vertical deviations are hyper for upward deviations and hypo for downward deviations (3). Generally, vertical heterophorias are designated according to the eye that misaligns higher vertically. As a result of this convention, it is customary to speak of hyper, rather than hypo, phoria. In general, this convention should be followed unless there is a diagnosed pathology causing the vertical deviation. For example, in thyroid eye disease, a hypophoria often results from inferior rectus muscle involvement and it is more clinically correct to call this deviation a hypophoria of the eye with the involved muscle (as that is the actual deviation) than a hyperphoria of the other eye. In addition, when there is a strabismus, the strabismic eye is recorded and, thus, there are either hyper- or hypotropias. Current preferred terminology for torsional deviations is excyclophoria and encyclophoria. Excyclophoria is temporalward rotation (outturning) of the top of the vertical meridian of the cornea during dissociation, while encyclophoria is latent nasalward rotation (inturning) of the top of the vertical meridian of the cornea (1d).

Historical Perspective

The clinical importance of considering cyclovertical deviations when managing patients with binocular vision dysfunction has been recognized for many years. For example, the existence of latent hyperphoria has been debated since the early 1930s, and the role of prism adaptation in determining vertical prism corrections has been important in the clinical literature since the 1950s (4). Evaluation of cyclophorias has a similar history. In 1891, Savage reported "insufficiency of the oblique muscles" (5) and described detailed treatment for over 300 cases of cyclophoria. Jackson (6) agreed with Maddox (7) that "in nearly all cases, nonparalytic cyclophoria causes no symptoms and requires no treatment." Howe (8) implied that the small near excyclophoria that he found in about 25% of normal patients was probably not clinically significant. The contrasting opinions of Stevens (9) and Savage (5) (that cyclophoria plays a large role in binocular visual problems) and Maddox (7) (that cyclophoria is of no consequence) suggest that an intermediate view is probably correct.

Incidence

Hyperphoria

Estimates of the incidence of vertical deviations range from 7% (10) to 52% (11). Because of the wide range reported in the literature, it is difficult to be certain of the exact incidence, but, based on an average of the results reported in studies over the last 100 years (12), a reasonable estimate of the incidence of vertical deviations in a clinical population is approximately 20%. Probably about 10% of these have a type of latent vertical heterophoria that requires prolonged occlusion for diagnosis.

Cyclophoria

Measurement and analysis of cyclophoria includes differentiation between real and apparent torsion (rotation) of the eye(s) about the line of sight. In evaluation of cyclophoria, the important torsion is associated with fusional movements (cyclovergence). Average excyclophoria tested with horizontal Maddox rods at 20 ft is about 0.752 degrees ± 1.15 degrees (13). The excyclophoria that is usually present at distance increases as convergence increases, but it does not usually change for lateral version movements. Excyclophorias increase on up-gaze and decrease on down-gaze (14).

The significance of an increase in excyclophoria with convergence is a potential change in the astigmatic axis when fixation shifts from distance to near (14). Scobee (15) studied 247 patients and found that 77% had a shift in astigmatic axis of up to 10 degrees during near fixation (Table 13.1). Although a significant percentage of patients have a measurable change in near astigmatic axis, only a small portion will have the combination of sufficient astigmatism combined with a large enough change in axis to cause symptoms that justify treatment.

TABLE 13.1. *Near astigmatic axis shift*

	Patients tested (247)	
Near axis shift 189 (77%)		No shift 58 (23%)
	Patients with axis shift (189 of 247)	
	Monocular 104 (55%)	Binocular 85 (45%)
Right eye 75 (72%)	Left eye 29 (28%)	

Characteristics

Cause

Significant cyclovertical deviations can be caused by orbital, neuromuscular, or innervational factors. Little is known about the exact cause of either vertical phorias or cyclophorias, although a small amount of excyclophoria is physiologically normal. Increases in excyclophoria on convergence and up-gaze (16) are probably due to increased inferior oblique innervation through the third nerve nucleus associated with convergence (in the same way that accommodation, convergence, and pupil size are related). Cyclophoria also results from uncorrected oblique astigmatism. "Astigmatic" cyclophoria is due to perceived inclination of the images of vertical and horizontal lines that are inclined toward the corneal meridians of greatest curvature. Symptoms generally disappear after properly prescribed optical correction.

Motor and Sensory Fusion

Integration of similar ocular images into a single percept involves separate components of motor and sensory fusion (17). Since vertical heterophorias typically remain the same at distance and near (in the absence of a paretic muscle etiology), the average vertical motor fusion ranges of about 3 are also the same for distance and near (18). Cyclovergence ranges are greater for encyclovergence. For example, Sen et al. (19) found average encyclovergence in the primary position of 5.25 ± 2.73 degrees and average excyclovergence of 4.15 ± 1.86 degrees measured with vertical lines. However, cyclovertical vergence ranges are variable between subjects and for the same subject at different times, depending on the speed of disparity introduction (20), the targets used (21) and the attention of the subject (22).

Subjective measurements of fusion have sensory as well as motor components. The primary difference between cyclofusion and horizontal/vertical fusion is that the sensory component of cyclofusion is large, while it is small for horizontal/vertical fusion (23). For example, the motor component to cyclofusion is probably 50% to 60% of the total fusional response required (2.8 to 3.4 degrees, for a 5.75-degree torsional disparity) (24), depending on the size of the retinal area covered by the test used. Indeed, it is possible to produce solely sensory cyclofusion without motor cyclovergence (25).

Symptoms

As with other ocular conditions, eye related symptoms of cyclovertical heterophorias can be categorized as ocular, visual, and referred (26). Symptoms are variable, affected by the patient's mental and general physical state, and often similar to symptoms of other types of binocular dysfunction. Therefore, in addition to evaluating cyclovertical deviations, we suggest that a thorough examination of the lateral vergence and accommodative systems be carried out.

Symptoms of Cyclovertical Heterophorias
Lose place when reading
Eyes tire easily
Skips lines/reads same line
Slow reading
Burning sensations
"Eyestrain"
Headaches
Blurring of reading material

Ocular (asthenopic) symptoms are those directly associated with the use of the eyes. "Pulling" sensations, itching, "gritty" feelings, and burning are some of the ocular symptoms related to cyclovertical heterophoria. An asthenopic symptom particular to hyperphoria is carsickness. Visual symptoms—subjective observations such as blurred or double vision—may or may not be associated with ocular symptoms. Visual symptoms particular to cyclovertical heterophoria include loss of place while reading (hyperphoria), tilting or slanting of objects (cyclophoria), and problems when changing from distance to near fixation. Referred symptoms include headaches, nausea, dizziness, and nervousness.

In clinical practice, perhaps 15% to 20% of all patients have symptoms related to cyclovertical deviation. Patients with cyclovertical deviations may not be diagnosed early and may be anxious and apprehensive. This is not unusual, since a psychoneurotic factor has been found in 75% of ophthalmic patients, as compared to 50% in general medical practice (27).

Signs

An observable head tilt is a frequent sign exhibited by patients with cyclovertical deviations. Another sign that may be observed is a change in astigmatic axis from distance to near refraction, which can indicate cyclophoria associated with convergence. Corrective measures will be needed if excessive blur or near discomfort is noticed.

Another frequent manifestation of cyclovertical deviations is seen when patients appear to have normal muscle balance but have multiple pairs of eyewear, stating that none are "right." Careful diagnostic testing may reveal cyclovertical deviations or aniseikonia. When no binocular anomaly is found on conventional testing and symptoms are still present even after correction of refractive error, diagnostic monocular occlusion can be useful for determining a management strategy for the symptomatic patient who might otherwise be told "nothing is wrong with your eyes."

Differential Diagnosis

Dissociated Testing

The principle of dissociated testing is to measure the direction and magnitude of the cyclovertical phoria under conditions where fusion is prevented. When examining a patient with a cyclovertical deviation, it is important to assess the vertical component in the primary position, in all fields of gaze, and with the patient's head tilted to the right and left. This will often allow a determination of the muscle involved in causing the vertical phoria and assist in determining management options.

Three-step Test

When measures are made in all fields of gaze, the test is called the three-step test—named for the three diagnostic measures that are made. First, determine which eye is misaligned vertically (the "hyper" eye), then determine whether the hyper increases in right or left gaze, and finally assess whether the hyper increases on right or left head tilt. Table 13.2 indicates expected findings on the three-step test. For example, if there is right inferior rectus involvement, there will be a right hyper that increases on right gaze and on left head tilt (see bold area in table).

Three-step Test—Superior Oblique Palsies. Superior oblique palsies are relatively common, as it is moderately easy to injure the trochlear nerve (CNIV). The findings on the three-step test of superior oblique palsies are easy to remember, as they follow the marching cadence: RSO = right, left, right (**right** hyper, increases on **left** gaze and on **right** head tilt);

TABLE 13.2. *Three-step test*

Hyper	Increase on gaze	Increase on head tilt	Effected muscle
R	R	R	LIO
R	**R**	**L**	**RIR**
R	L	R	RSO
R	L	L	LSR
L	R	R	RSR
L	R	L	LSO
L	L	R	LIR
L	L	L	RIO

R, right; L, left; LIO, left inferior oblique; RIR, right inferior rectus; RSO, right superior oblique; LSR, left superior rectus; RSR, right superior rectus; LSO, left superior oblique; RIO, right inferior oblique; LIR, left inferior rectus.

LSO = left, right, left (**left** hyper, increases on **right** gaze, and **left** head tilt). The superior oblique palsy responses on the three-step test are common enough and easy enough to remember that all clinicians should easily be able to recall them.

The three commonly used techniques to assess the vertical deviation include the cover test, Maddox rods, and prism dissociation.

Cover Test

The cover test, which is used routinely in the diagnosis of lateral heterophorias and cyclovertical strabismus, is often of less value on diagnosis of small cyclovertical heterotropias. Because of the often very small nature of cyclovertical eye movements present in patients with heterophorias, even the most experienced observers may not always obtain a valid measure of cyclovertical heterophorias. As a result, Maddox rods are probably the most clinically used test for cyclovertical heterophorias.

Maddox Rod Evaluation for Vertical Phoria and Cyclophoria

Vertical Heterophoria—Single Maddox Rod

When testing for vertical phoria, a vertically aligned Maddox rod is placed before one eye and the amount of vertical misalignment between the horizontal line (seen by the eye behind the rod) and a light (seen by the fixing eye) is neutralized using a (Risley) prism. Figure 13.1 shows the technique needed to evaluate a hyperphoria. Because noncomitancy is frequent in cyclovertical deviations, assessment should be made in all fields of gaze (see three-step test results in Table 13.2).

Cyclophoria—Double Maddox Rod

When testing for cyclophoria, a Maddox rod is placed in front of each eye, prism is used to dissociate the rods, and the streaks are compared for parallelism. When cyclophoria is present, one image appears rotated. The corresponding Maddox rod can be rotated until the lines are parallel and the amount and kind of cyclophoria can be read directly from the indicators. For patients with unilateral superior oblique palsy, the excyclophoria is generally between 3 and 7 degrees, while, in bilateral superior oblique palsy, the excyclophoria is typically greater than 10 degrees. Care must be taken that the patient's gaze is in the primary position with no head tilt. Borish (22) suggests that the Maddox rod test for cyclophoria be incorporated into the examination between the "delayed subjective" and "ductions at far."

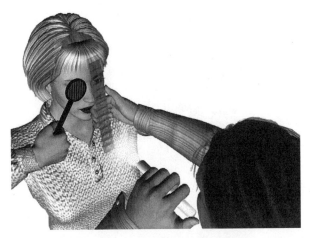

FIG. 13.1. Vertical eye alignment can be assessed with a single vertically oriented red Maddox rod and a penlight. With the patient observing the penlight with one eye and the horizontal red streak with the other, vertical prism power is slowly increased using base down prism over one eye, until the streak is reported to be aligned with the light. Changes in prism power should be at a slow steady rate.

Maddox Double Prism for Cyclophoria

Another useful clinical test for cyclophoria is the Maddox double prism, which is formed by placing two low-power (3 or 4 Δ) prisms base to base. Monocular diplopia results when an eye fixates with the horizontally oriented bases bisecting the pupillary axis. Thus, if a dot target is used, the eye with the double prism sees two dots, the other eye sees one, and three dots appear with both eyes open. The eye not behind the double prism is the eye being tested, so the subject's attention is directed to the center dot. Figure 13.2 shows the use of a trial frame for a patient with left excyclophoria. Provided the dots are not fused, the amount of cyclophoria can be quantified by rotating the prism until the dots are vertically aligned. Patient responses (especially children) are not extremely accurate on this test.

Prism Dissociation

Prism dissociation, an alternative to Maddox rods that is often used for clinical detection and quantification of vertical deviations, is used less often for cyclophorias. When using this technique for assessment of vertical heterophoria, nonfusable targets are dissociated (usually using horizontal prism) and the patient is required to respond when they are aligned vertically. Figure 13.3 shows the technique for prism dissociation evaluation of a patient with a left hyperphoria.

Fixation Disparity Tests

The principle of this testing is to measure the direction and magnitude of the cyclovertical phoria under conditions where fusion is present. Since the deviation is measured while the patient is fusing, fixation disparity tests probably correlate best with symptoms of cyclovertical heterophorias, just as they do for horizontal heterophoria (28,29). Both the horizontal and vertical associated phorias should be assessed. Additionally, the effects of small amounts of horizontal prism on the vertical associated phoria should be determined.

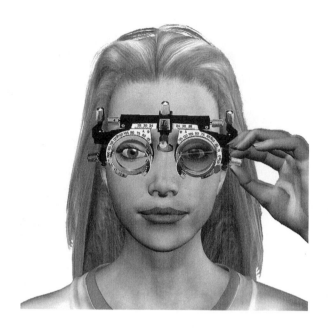

Measurement of cyclophoria

As the patient turns the knob on the trial frame, the appearance of the three dots
will change as shown below. The patient's goal is to adjust the orientation of the double
prism until the three dots appear to be vertically aligned (as if there were no cyclodeviation).

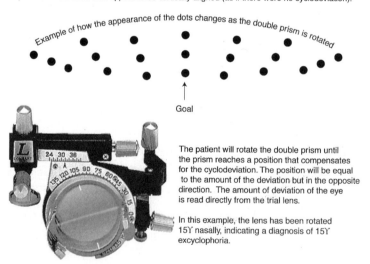

Example of how the appearance of the dots changes as the double prism is rotated

Goal

The patient will rotate the double prism until
the prism reaches a position that compensates
for the cyclodeviation. The position will be equal
to the amount of the deviation but in the opposite
direction. The amount of deviation of the eye
is read directly from the trial lens.

In this example, the lens has been rotated
15ϒ nasally, indicating a diagnosis of 15ϒ
excyclophoria.

FIG. 13.2. Top: Assessment of cyclophoria with the double 4△ prism test can be done using a
single dot as a target. **Middle:** When using the double 4△ prism, the patient will see three dots—
two seen by the eye observing through the double prism and one by the other eye. **Bottom:** The
double 4△ prism can be used to measure the amount of cyclophoria. With the prism mounted in
a trial frame, the patient rotates the prism until the dots are seen aligned; the amount of rotation
indicates the amount of cyclophoria.

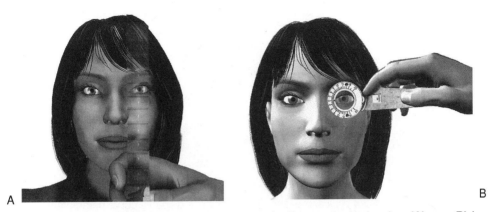

FIG. 13.3. Vertical eye alignment can be assessed with a vertical prism bar **(A)** or a Risley prism **(B).** The patient observes a short horizontal line or a diamond, and vertical diplopia is achieved using about 8△ of vertical prism. One eye is occluded and the target is briefly shown at intervals (flashed). The vertical prism power is slowly decreased until the two targets are reported to be in horizontal alignment. Changes in prism power should be at a slow steady rate. Small amounts of lateral prism (typically 6 to 10 △ base-in) may be needed to be sure that the targets are not fused, as the vertical prism power is reduced.

Horizontal Testing

It has been observed in some patients that small amounts of lateral prism can assist fusion to such an extent that a vertical associated phoria is reduced to zero (30); in these patients, no vertical prism is needed. The reason that these small lateral corrections affect the vertical deviation is not precisely known. However, it is prudent to evaluate this effect when there are small vertical associated phorias, generally less than 1.25 △. In general, patients with vertical deviations that respond to horizontal prism are candidates for horizontal fusional vergence therapy. They rarely require any prism after vision therapy programs are completed.

Vertical Testing

Vertical Associated Phoria

In general, the amount of prism to reduce the fixation disparity to zero can be prescribed with confidence that it will dramatically relieve the patient's symptoms. Since this measure is so easy to make, this form of fixation disparity testing has become the test of choice for vertical heterophoria and, when used properly, is also useful for diagnosis of patients with symptomatic cyclophoria. Associated phoria measures can be made using the American Optical (AO) Vectographic slide, Turville testing, and the Mallett near unit (Fig. 13.4).

A valuable addition to vertical associated phoria evaluation can be used to be certain that the endpoint has been reached. The principle is to align the eyes vertically so that there is no alteration in ocular alignment required when the patient blinks. This can be achieved by interposing vertical prism until the nonius lines seem to be stable through the prism. Then have the patient close both eyes for 1 to 2 seconds. When the eyes are first opened, the patient's task is to notice whether the nonius lines are exactly aligned or whether one line or the other had to move up or down to become aligned. Repeat the open–close eyes procedure and modify the prism prescription in 0.5 △ steps until the lines appear stable and aligned at all times. Frequently, small increases in vertical prism from that seen in standard eyes open associated phoria measure is required to reach the stable endpoint of alignment of the lines immediately

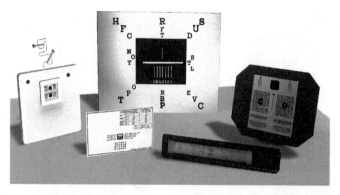

FIG. 13.4. Instruments for clinical measurement of fixation disparity curve parameters include the Disparometer **(left)**, the Woolf **(center)** and Wesson cards **(bottom left)**, the AO Vectographic Adult slide **(bottom right)**, Turville testing, and the Mallett near unit **(right)**. During each of these tests, the majority of the visual field is visible to both eyes and, thus, can be fused. However, a portion of the central field is only visible to one eye or the other, either because of polarized filters or a septum (Turville test).

after opening the eyes. When the lines remain aligned immediately after the eyes have been opened again, the amount of prism that is in place can be prescribed.

Forced Vergence Fixation Disparity Curves

Forced vergence fixation disparity curves can be generated by measuring the fixation disparity through various amounts of vertical prism. When there is a vertical phoria, these measures are typically not curves, but rather are very frequently linear. As a result, the associated phoria measure described above is the clinically used assessment for the majority of patients. Forced vergence curves are useful primarily when contemplating and monitoring a vision therapy program. See Chapter 14 for a complete description of fixation disparity testing and interpretation.

Cyclofixation Disparity

Turville tests show cyclofixation disparity when the letters make an oblique line as the test is done (31). Fixation disparity tests, such as the AO Vectographic Adult slide and the Mallett distance and near tests, show horizontal and vertical fixation disparity and indicate cyclofixation disparity by a tilt of the test targets (32). These tests do not measure the amount of cyclophoria; the amount has to be measured directly by one of the previously described tests. However, a manifest cyclofixation disparity indicates uncompensated cyclophoria; these patients should be questioned closely for symptoms of cyclophoria and treatment instituted as necessary.

Out of Phoropter Testing

Frequently patients with significant cyclovertical heterophoria in the primary position (through the phoropter) tend to tilt or turn their heads to a position that allows more comfortable binocular vision. Trial frame evaluation using the best correction will often give a better evaluation of the patient's habitual binocular status in these cases. If there is a coexisting vertical phoria, correction of it may relieve the cyclophoria and eliminate the symptoms.

TABLE 13.3. *When and how to use diagnostic occlusion*

When:
    Patient has symptoms of vertical heterophoria but
      a. No vertical on clinical testing with
         Maddox rod
         Cover test
         Fixation disparity measures
      b. Apparently good compensation for a small existing cyclovertical deviation
How:
    Occlude the hyperphoric eye for 24 hr based on
      a. Cover testing (including patient reports of phi phenomena movement)
      b. Vertical fixation disparity curves
      c. Reports of vertical instability of the horizontal nonius lines on fixation disparity testing

Diagnostic Occlusion

When occlusion relieves the complaint of the patient, the cause of the complaint is usually some handicap to binocular vision (33). Thus, in cases where a definitive diagnosis cannot be determined using the conventional techniques described above, a trial period of 24 hours of occlusion of the hyperphoric eye should be used diagnostically to determine the effect on the patient's symptoms (34). Table 13.3 lists the considerations that lead to determining when to utilize diagnostic occlusion. The occasionally difficult decision concerning which is the hyperphoric eye is based on cover testing (including patient reports of phi phenomena movement), vertical fixation disparity curves, and reports of vertical instability of the horizontal nonius lines on fixation disparity testing. Following occlusion, vertical prism that neutralizes the vertical fixation disparity (associated phoria) can be prescribed and vertical vergence therapy may also be considered.

Differential Diagnosis

The primary issue in determining the indicated treatment is the etiology of the cyclovertical condition. Newly acquired cyclovertical deviations should be considered to have a serious etiology until proven otherwise. Differential diagnosis of acquired conditions is based on reports of recent onset diplopia, noncomitancy where the deviation changes in various fields of gaze, visual field defects, and recent onset of coexisting ocular health conditions, such as papilledema or retinal disease. Patients with such symptoms or findings should be referred for appropriate systemic, endocrine, or neurological evaluation. Management of the vertical deviation can continue concurrently.

Case Study

Case 13.1: Recent Onset Vertical Diplopia

An 18-year-old male complained of recent diplopia while reading. The diplopia had developed over the previous 2 months and seemed to be increasing in frequency. At the time of the examination, he also reported occasional diplopia on up-gaze. There was an increase in the magnitude and frequency of the diplopia with strenuous exercise. He had been involved in an automobile accident 4 months previously, but denied any dizziness, ataxia, or systemic illness. He also denied taking any medication. He wore no lens correction at the time of the examination.

Examination revealed emmetropia, with 20/15 acuity in each eye. There was no nystagmus. The cover test revealed a 2 Δ left hyperphoria in primary gaze that increased to a 25 Δ left hypertropia in down-gaze. Pupillary reactions were normal; there was no afferent pupillary defect. He had 100 seconds of arc of stereopsis at 40 cm (Randot stereograms). Monocular muscle fields were normal and binocular fields indicated increasing diplopia in down-gaze to the right.

Because of the recent development of vertical strabismus, the patient was referred for neurologic evaluation. Examination findings were consistent with those described above and the patient was scheduled for a magnetic resonance imagery (MRI) evaluation of the posterior fossa. The study revealed the presence of an Arnold-Chiari type I malformation. Surgery was deferred until the summer, between school years. No lens correction was prescribed.

Patients with longstanding congenital deviations generally do not complain of recent onset diplopia; reports of diplopia in patients with congenital cyclovertical deviations have typically been present with varying frequency for a number of years. Further, in contrast to the noncomitancies frequently seen in patients with acquired cyclovertical deviations, many patients with congenital cyclovertical heterophorias have comitant deviations. Patients with congenital deviations are treated using the techniques below.

Treatment

Management of cyclovertical heterophorias follows the same logical sequence as treatment for lateral heterophorias outlined in Chapter 3 of this book (Table 13.4). The initial management step is to provide clear retinal images by prescribing the optimum lens correction. This is followed by additional optical management, which, for cyclovertical deviations, primarily consists of vertical and/or horizontal prism. At times, added plus lenses also play a role if better fusion is gained at near, through a change in alignment or clearer images, in the presence of a coexisting accommodative deficiency. Therapeutic occlusion to eliminate diplopia, by blocking one retinal image, is seldom needed for cyclovertical heterophoria. Usually fusion is well established and only needs to be enhanced. Vision therapy, which can substantially improve alignment and fusion, is considered when a cooperative patient will comply with the prescribed procedures.

Surgery, an important part of management of cyclovertical heterotropias, is needed less often by patients with cyclovertical heterophorias. Consider surgical referral for patients with cyclovertical heterophoria when the vertical angle is larger than 15 Δ or there is a significant noncomitancy.

Refractive Correction

Clear retinal images assist fusion in cyclovertical deviations. As a result, in the presence of hyperphoria, the best lens correction should be determined by retinoscopy and maximum plus

TABLE 13.4. *Sequence of considerations for management of cyclovertical heterophorias*

Occlusion (diagnostic)
Refractive correction
Optical management (usually vertical prism, occasionally near additions if
  accommodative problems or high AC/A)
Occlusion (therapeutic)
Vision therapy
Surgery

TABLE 13.5. *Clinical management of vertical heterophoria*

Vertical	Symptoms	Diagnostic occlusion	Treatment	Estimated patient %
None present	None	No	None	80
Phoria or fixation disparity	None	No	None unless avoiding tasks	3
Phoria and fixation disparity	Yes	No	Prism based on fixation disparity	12
Fixation disparity only	Yes	No	Prism based on fixation disparity	3
None on routine testing	Yes	Yes (1 d over the eye that has the hyperphoria)	Prism based on fixation disparity after diagnostic occlusion	2

binocular refraction. Refractive treatment for cyclophoria depends on the type of cyclophoria. When there is uncorrected oblique astigmatism, lens correction found by binocular refractive techniques will usually eliminate symptoms. Compensatory cyclofusion movements to the natural uncorrected image tilt are made to enhance fusion without spectacle lenses; when the proper correction is in place, the image tilt disappears, there is no need for cyclofusional movements, and the symptoms disappear.

However, there are some patients who are more comfortable without correction of oblique astigmatism. These patients may have aniseikonia caused by the correcting cylinder (27), they may be unable to adjust to vertical prism differences on lateral gaze from the new correction (35), or they may have cyclophoria opposite to the cyclophoria created by fusion of the uncorrected images. For these patients, correction of astigmatism forces the patient to compensate for the cyclophoria, often unsuccessfully (36).

Cyclophoria associated with convergence may cause a change in the near astigmatism axis. This can cause clinically significant symptoms, if the power of the correcting cylinder is large or there is a substantial axis shift. Binocular refraction at distance will give the best refractive correction. If the near cylinder axis shift, as determined by binocular refraction at near, is enough to cause symptoms, separate lens corrections for distance and near may be needed. Careful attention should also be given to correction of associated vertical deviations.

Prism

After prescription of the best lens correction, the next logical consideration, in management of patients with a cyclovertical deviation, is prism. Decisions concerning prescription of prism, for a patient with a cyclovertical heterophoria, are often complicated by the different combinations of symptoms and heterophorias that exist. As illustrated in Table 13.5, when a hyperphoric patient is truly asymptomatic, management is frequently deferred (Table 13.5, row 2). On the other hand, treatment may be indicated if the patient is asymptomatic because of avoidance of symptom-causing tasks.

Case Study

Case 13.2: Symptomatic Cyclophoria

A 35-year-old man had long-standing complaints of headaches over the left eye, eyestrain, and intermittent blurred vision while reading with his glasses. He wore a moderate astigmatic correction. External and internal ocular health was within normal limits. Visual acuity and refraction with cycloplegia were the same as his current correction:

OD: $1.00 - 3.50 \times 95$ 20/15−
OS: $0.75 - 4.00 \times 105$ 20/20+   OU 20/15

There was comitant 3 Δ exophoria at 6 m and 40 cm. There was occasional intermittent suppression of the left eye on Worth dot testing and stereopsis was 40 seconds at 40 cm with Randot circles. There were normal accommodative findings (amplitude = 8 D, lag = +0.25 D, and facility = 10 cpm with ±2.00). There was no fixation disparity at 6 m, but patient reported a torsional disparity of the left eye's target at 40 cm. Near refraction revealed cylinder axes of:

OD: 96
OS: 112

And, although distance vision was blurred, reading with near axes findings allowed comfortable vision with no blurring. Maddox rod testing revealed a 1-degree excyclophoria at 6 m and an 8-degree excyclophoria at 40 cm.

Two pairs of glasses were prescribed—one with the distance axes and the other with the near axes. The patient returned for reevaluation in 2 weeks, with no further symptoms.

Patients who have symptoms and a manifest cyclovertical heterophoria or a vertical fixation disparity are generally more easily managed (Table 13.5, rows 3 and 4) by prescribing prism than by vision therapy. In general, the prism correction that is considered is a vertical prism correction of sufficient amount to relieve the symptoms. However, for certain patients, a horizontal prism prescription will eliminate the vertical associated phoria (30). This type of horizontal correction of vertical deviation is described more completely in the section on fixation disparity.

Criteria for Prescribing

Several techniques have been described that may be used to determine a prism correction for patients having a vertical heterophoria. However, the precise methods used for prescribing the correct amount of prism for vertical heterophoria have not been well defined. In clinical practice, most clinicians base prism prescription decisions on one or more of the following factors: the magnitude of the heterophoria, the vertical or cyclovergence ranges, flip prism tests, or fixation disparity measurements.

Magnitude of the Heterophoria

Clinicians who prescribe based on the magnitude of the vertical heterophoria follow the lead of clinical researchers of the early twentieth century. Unfortunately, the techniques that have been recommended can cause considerable variation in the amount of prism that might be prescribed. For example, Hansell and Reber (37) felt that when a hyperphoria remains after refractive correction, prism power should be prescribed that corrects one third of the hyperphoria. Emsley (38) and Maddox (39) suggested prescribing vertical prism equal to two thirds of the vertical heterophoria. Giles (40) advised correcting three fourths of the vertical heterophoria found at near. Duke-Elder (41) and Peter (42) felt that when the refractive correction has been worn, and over 1 Δ remains, a nearly full correction (or perhaps 0.5 Δ less) should be given for the hyperphoria. Hugonnier et al. (43) recommend complete prismatic correction when the deviation is small.

Thus, many clinicians have relied on rough guidelines or rules of thumb when prescribing prism. For example, Krimsky (44) did not even suggest an amount, but stated that each case should be considered individually and the weakest prism that would relieve symptoms and restore binocularity should be used. An anecdotal method that has been recommended to determine the weakest prism is to place a prism with its base in the appropriate direction in the trial frame with the refractive correction and evaluate the patient's visual acuity or comfort. This lack of standardization and the variety of suggestions imply that other techniques may be superior to use of vertical heterophoria measures and that a more definitive management regimen should be sought.

Prism Vergence

Prism vergence measurement has probably been the method of choice in the management of vertical heterophoria for a majority of optometrists. Methods of determining the amount of prism to prescribe, based on prism vergence ranges, range from that of Tait (45), who recommended prescribing the amount of vertical prism that requires the patient to use one fifth of the vertical fusional amplitude to oppose the deviation, to balancing the vertical vergences (described below). Another recommendation for prescribing vertical prism is to balance the recovery values, when they closely agree with the direction of the heterophoria. Use of the recovery values may yield a prism correction that is more readily accepted subjectively (22).

When prescribing prism based on vertical vergence ranges, the clinician measures vertical vergence reserves after having assessed the vertical heterophoria. Vertical vergence reserves are usually determined using the rotary prisms of the phoropter. The prism vergence test involves increasing the vertical prism power first base-down and then base-up, over one eye, until fusion is interrupted and then recovered. With this technique, patients without a vertical heterophoria will have supravergence and infravergence that are basically equal to each other for each eye. For example, the left infravergence value will equal the right supravergence value. Thus, vergences often need to be measured over only one eye.

The technique of balancing the vertical vergence ranges has probably been used most widely for prescribing vertical prism, particularly before the advent of fixation disparity measurement. The prescribed prism is used to balance the vertical vergence break values; its amount is usually one half to two thirds the actual vertical heterophoria. In the presence of a vertical heterophoria and unequal vertical vergence measurements, the vertical fusional vergence (VFV) break or recovery values can be used to determine the prism power to prescribe. Prism may be determined by the formula:

(Base-down to break base-up to break)/2 = correcting prism
(If resultant is plus, prism is base-down; if minus, base-up.)

For example, if there is 3 Δ right hyperphoria and 6 Δ/3 Δ right supravergence and 4 Δ/2 Δ right infravergence, then 1 Δ base-down OD would equalize the break values [(6 Δ − 4 Δ)/2 = 2 Δ/2 = 1 Δ].

A potential problem with prescribing based on vertical vergence ranges is that vergence ranges are not always useful in determining an appropriate prism amount. There can be substantial variability in the vertical vergence measurements, depending on factors such as the speed the prism disparity is introduced (20), the distance at which the measurement is taken (21), and the actual vertical deviation (22). Numerous researchers have reported that vertical heterophorias and fusional amplitudes are affected by residual tonicity. And, for some patients with vertical heterophoria, the vertical vergence values can be affected by the muscles stimulated first. For example, if the left supravergence is measured first, then the left infravergence value is reduced by tonicity of the first vergence stimulation.

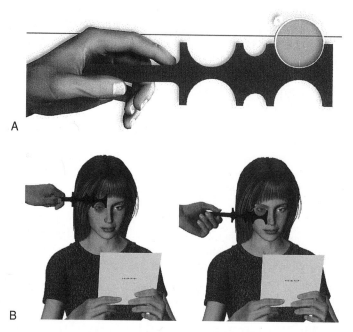

FIG. 13.5. A: A 3 △ prism mounted in a handheld rotatable mount **(A)** can be used to test for vertical deviation and determine the amount of prism to prescribe. **B:** As the patient observes a horizontal row of 0.75 M print, the prism is flipped from base-down to base-up. **C:** The patient observes the vertical separation of the images in each presentation of the prism; the prism to be prescribed is the amount where the vertical separation of the images in each presentation is equal.

Clinically, the problem of altering tonicity is easily circumvented by measuring the compensating fusional reserve and then measuring the opposing fusional vergence on the fellow eye. For example, if a right hyperphoria is present, the right infravergence should be measured first and compared to the left infravergence (e.g., right supravergence). This avoids the effect of residual tonicity on the fusional vergence reserves. Alternatively, assessment of the opposing vergence can be postponed to the end of the examination to allow residual tonic innervation to subside. This will allow measurement of the opposing fusional vergence after some time has elapsed.

Flip Prism

Eskridge (46) suggested that a 3 △ prism in a handheld lens mount could be used for determining the type of hyperphoria and the amount of vertical prism (Fig. 13-5). The prism is flipped from base-down to base-up, and the patient observes the vertical separation of the images in each presentation. The direction of the prism base, where the images are closer, documents the type of heterophoria. Thus, there is a right hyperphoria if the images are closer when the flip prism is base-up before the left eye. The prism power to be prescribed can be determined placing the prism base-down in front of the right eye until the images are equidistant for successive presentations of the flip prism. The sensitivity of the test is high, since bisection tasks are easily done by most patients and the testing procedure approximately doubles small existing vertical heterophorias. The flip prism test measures the deviation while the patient is diplopic. Since fusion causes changes in the vergence adaptive position (47), using the flip prism may overestimate the prism prescription for some patients.

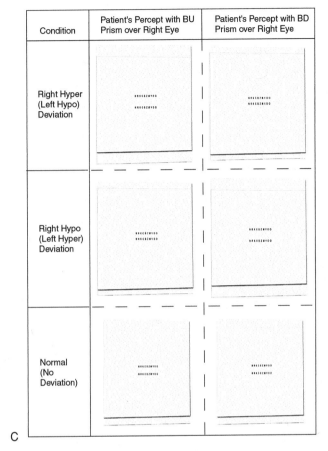

FIG. 13.5. *Continued.*

Fixation Disparity Measurements

Horizontal Prism Corrections

Small amounts of horizontal prism have been shown to reduce a vertical associated phoria to zero in some patients (30). The number of patients with vertical associated phoria who respond in this manner to lateral prism is unknown, since most practitioners prescribe vertical prism for these patients and do not even investigate the effect of horizontal prism. However, when there are small vertical associated phorias (less than 1.5 Δ), the effects of both vertical prism and small amounts of lateral prism should be investigated. When small amounts of horizontal prism (less than 2.5 Δ) are successful in eliminating a vertical associated phoria, the patient is usually better managed by a brief vision therapy program emphasizing horizontal vergence and antisuppression therapy. Such a vision therapy program is almost invariably effective and eliminates the need for any type of prism.

Vertical Associated Phoria–Fixation Disparity

Although there are four types of horizontal fixation disparity curves (see Chapter 14), patients with a vertical heterophoria typically have a linear fixation disparity curve, as their fixation disparity is reduced by a similar amount for each prism diopter of prism added. This linear response pattern was originally reported by Ogle (17), and Rutstein and Eskridge (48,49) suggested that all vertical fixation disparities are linear for patients with normal binocular vision. Petito and Wick (50) confirm the linearity of most vertical fixation disparity curves, but suggest that about 10% of subjects have a clinically significant nonlinearity. Generally, vertical fixation disparity curves are linear enough so that vertical prism may be prescribed in an amount that reduces the disparity to zero (associated phoria).

The assessment of the vertical associated phoria has become the standard method for the prescribing of prism for vertical heterophorias over the past 30 years. Morgan (51) measured the vertical associated phoria by assessing the patient's ability to detect alignment differences of a line of 20/30 letters interrupted by a septum. Over 98% of the 215 patients tested noticed the difference created by a 0.5 Δ prism. Prism was prescribed for 15% of Morgan's patients, based on the perceived vertical misalignment, and over 90% successfully wore the prism. Morgan's results are supported by Elvin (52) and Tubis (53).

Case Study

Case 13.3: Prescribing Vertical Prism Based on Associated Phoria

A 17-year-old male complained of slow reading, loss of place while reading, reading the same line when going back to the beginning of a line, and headaches after approximately 30 minutes of reading (eyelid/brow area). He stated that blinking cleared the near blur. The current spectacle prescription was essentially the same as the refractive findings:

OD: 1.50 diopter sphere (DS)   20/15
OS: 1.75 DS   20/15

All further testing was performed through the habitual spectacle lenses. Cover test and Maddox rod testing revealed 2 Δ of left hyperphoria in all fields of gaze at distance and near. The associated phoria findings were 1.75 Δ left hyper-associated phoria at distance and near. There were no changes in associated phoria response as the patient shifted vision into lateral gaze. Accommodative findings were normal (lag = 0.75 D, amplitude = 14 D, binocular facility = 6 cpm with ±2.00 D flippers at near).

Based on the examination findings, the habitual spectacle correction was judged to be adequate, as were accommodative and fusional abilities. The myopic correction alone and then with the addition of 1.75 Δ base-down before the left eye was placed into a trial frame and the patient was allowed to read for 10 to 15 minutes under both conditions. He expressed a feeling of less eyestrain and more accurate eye movements (easier returning to the next line of letters) with the additional prism, which was then prescribed. With the new prescription, the patient reported a decrease in the frequency of losing his place while reading, and he experienced no symptoms while reading.

Forced Vergence Curves

In the case of vertical deviations, the reduction to zero of the vertical misalignment of the targets, under binocular viewing conditions, is the most accurate and readily accepted method of precise prism prescribing. It also results in the prescription of the least amount of prism that relieves symptoms. The primary clinical value of the forced vergence fixation disparity curve is to monitor vision therapy programs (see later section in this chapter).

Measurement of vertical fixation disparity with the appropriate instrumentation will allow graphing of the data that generates a straight line, although some subjects manifest nonlinear findings (Fig. 13.6A). Figure 13.6B illustrates the linear relationship that is characteristic of most vertical fixation disparities. As increasing amounts of prism are placed over an eye, the fixation disparity is decreased by a similar amount for each prism power increase. This linear relationship occasionally varies in such a way that the associated phoria does not equal the dissociated phoria. Such a difference is easily noted on simple comparison and suggests that vertical vergence therapy will be useful, since there is established prism adaptation evidenced by the nonlinearity. See the prism adaptation discussion in Chapter 15.

Prism Prescriptions for Latent Hyperphoria

Some of the most difficult management decisions in clinical practice arise when the patient has symptoms suggestive of a vertical deviation (Table 13.5), but no vertical heterophoria is evident on routine clinical testing. Small latent vertical phorias can cause patients to be symptomatic. And, just as with some deviations of larger amounts, these vertical deviations only become manifest with prolonged occlusion. We suggest that the patient with latent hyperphoria can be managed successfully by following the procedures listed in Table 13.5, row 5.

Prism corrections can be determined by clinical judgment, based on associated phoria, severity of symptoms, and monocular occlusion. Monocular occlusion is used to unmask the vertical correction by first determining from the fixation disparity curves and dissociated phoria measurements which eye has a tendency to be hyperphoric and then occluding that eye for 24 hours. When the patient returns the next day (still occluded), dissociated phoria measurements are taken at distance and near immediately after removal of the patch and only allowing fusion to occur briefly during the dissociated phoria measurements. Using the prism amount determined during the dissociated phoria testing as the starting prism, vertical fixation disparity measurements are taken in the manner described previously. Thus, prism prescriptions are determined from the prism required to reduce the associated phoria to zero after 24 hours of occlusion.

Case Study

Case 13.4: Latent Hyperphoria

An 11-year-old boy had difficulty reading. He complained of slow reading, loss of place while reading, reading the same line when going back to the beginning of a line, headaches after approximately 30 minutes of reading (eyelid/brow area), and blurring of material after the onset of headaches. He stated that blinking cleared the near blur. The current spectacle prescription was essentially the same as the refractive findings:

OD: −2.50 DS   20/15
OS: −2.25 DS   20/15

All further testing was performed through the habitual spectacle lenses. Cover test and Maddox rod testing revealed 1 Δ of exophoria in all fields of gaze at distance and near. The associated phoria findings were orthophoria/isophoria at distance and an unstable 0.75 Δ left hyper-associated phoria at near that increased with time. There were no changes in associated phoria response as the patient shifted vision into lateral gaze. Accommodative findings were normal (lag = 0.75 D, amplitude = 14 D, binocular facility = 6 cpm with ±2.00 D flippers at near). Vertical vergence ranges were symmetrical at distance and near.

Based on the examination findings, the habitual spectacle correction was judged to be adequate, as were accommodative and fusional abilities. Instability and variability of the vertical associated phoria measurement suggested a latent left hyperphoria, and it was decided that diagnostic occlusion would be useful for further assessment. The patient was instructed to patch the left eye constantly 24 hours before a follow-up examination. During the follow-up examination, the patch was removed and fusion was prevented until associated phoria measurements were taken. Cover test at distance revealed 2 Δ left hyperphoria. Associated phoria testing at distance revealed 2.75 Δ left hyperphoria.

The myopic correction alone and then with the addition of 2.75 Δ base-down before the left eye was placed into a trial frame and the patient was allowed to read for 10 to 15 minutes under both conditions. He expressed a feeling of less eyestrain and more accurate eye movements (easier returning to the next line of letters) with the additional 2.75 Δ base-down, which was then prescribed. With the new prescription, the patient initially experienced mild discomfort that subsided in less than 30 minutes. At this visit and for at least 1 year (the latest follow-up), the patient reported a decrease in the frequency of losing his place while reading, and he has experienced no symptoms while reading. Associated phoria measurements continued to indicate that approximately 3 Δ base-down was required before the left eye to reduce the left hyperfixation disparity to zero. All other findings remain within normal limits.

Prism Adaptation

When vertical prism is placed before one eye of a patient with normal binocular vision and no cyclovertical heterophoria, remeasurement of the induced vertical deviation after 15 minutes will indicate that the resultant deviation is less than the amount of prism placed before the eye. This adaptation to vertical prism has been shown by Rutstein and Eskridge (54) and others (55,56), and individual differences in the rate and amount of prism adaptation have been observed (57). Nearly 80% of patients adapt to vertical prism (58). However, symptoms generally are not reported by subjects who completely adapt to vertical prism (59). In addition, Schor (60) has demonstrated that patients who do not adapt adequately to prism are most likely to be symptomatic. These factors suggest that patients who have reduced ability to adapt to prism are those who manifest symptoms.

Lie and Opheim (61) used prism to correct heterophoric patients with long-standing severe visual symptoms. They reported that a small vertical deviation was present in most of these cases. Furthermore, in 80% of their cases, prism corrections needed to be increased over a period of time before the full deviation that eliminated symptoms was determined. Clinical reports by Surdacki and Wick (62) also suggest that patients may require multiple prism corrections before a latent vertical deviation is completely compensated.

Based on basic and clinical research, we suggest that the prescription of vertical prism for symptomatic patients does not lead to adaptation to the prisms. Increases in the prism required are probably not adaptation in the classic sense, but rather are similar to that seen in latent hyperopia, where the increase in plus is not adaptation, but rather occurs because the entire correction was not prescribed initially.

Patient Counseling

Frequently, symptoms associated with cyclovertical heterophorias can be minimized by proper patient counseling. After prescription of the best refractive correction and any necessary prism, patients who have increased cyclovertical heterophoria, in a certain direction of gaze, can be

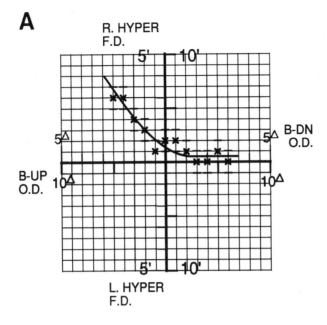

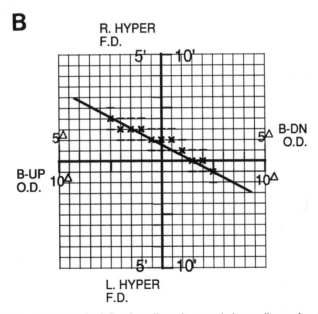

FIG. 13.6. A: Although the vertical fixation disparity graph is nonlinear for 15% of patients, only about 5% have a clinically significant nonlinearity. **B:** The vertical fixation disparity graph is typically linear for about 85% of patients tested. As a result, the prism indicated by the associated phoria measure (prism to reduce fixation disparity to zero) can be prescribed in virtually all cases.

TABLE 14.1. *Instruments for measuring associated phoria*

Distance	
Instrument:	Available from:
Mallett unit	Bernell Corporation
American Optical	American Optical Company
Vectographic chart	
Bernell lantern	Bernell Corporation
Near	
Instrument:	
American Optical Near	American Optical Company
Vectographic cards	Available from:
Borish card	
Mallett near unit	Bernell Corporation

Available Instrumentation

Associated Phoria Measuring

Vertical and horizontal associated phoria can be measured at distance and near, neutralizing any reported misalignment of the lines with appropriate prism using instruments listed in Table 14.1.

Fixation Disparity Curve and Associated Phoria Measuring

Vertical and horizontal fixation disparity curves and associated phoria can be measured at distance and near, using several instruments. For distance, there is the *Woolf card[a]*; for near, the *Disparometer[b]* (Fig. 14.4) or *Wesson card.[c]* The Wesson card is the most commonly used instrument for clinical measurement of fixation disparity curve parameters. Other instruments include the Woolf and Wesson cards. The most affordable readily available clinical instrument is the Wesson card.

The Disparometer consists of two 1.5-degree circular targets, each containing two oppositely polarized lines. The circle provides the fusion lock. The upper circle is used for vertical

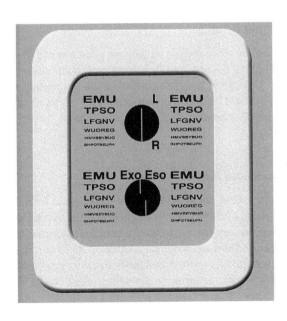

FIG. 14.4. The Disparometer consists of two 1.5-degree circular targets, each containing two oppositely polarized lines. The circle provides the fusion lock. The upper circle is used for vertical fixation disparity measurement; the left line is seen by the left eye. The lower circle allows analysis of horizontal deviations; the lower line is seen by the left eye. A wheel with a knob at the back can be rotated to present various vernier offsets. The patient's task is to judge which of the pairs of vernier lines is vertically aligned.

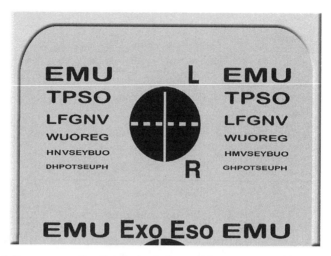

FIG. 14.5. The letters surrounding the circles help provide accurate stable accommodation and modification of the instrument. Using thin strips of black tape on the plastic protector (over sections of the nonius lines) further aids in keeping accommodation at the plane of regard. (From Schor CM. The influence of rapid prism adaptation upon fixation disparity. *Vision Res* 1979;19:757–765, with permission.)

fixation disparity measurement; the left line is seen by the left eye. The lower circle allows analysis of horizontal deviations; the lower line is seen by the left eye. The letters surrounding the circles help provide accurate stable accommodation, and modification of the instrument using thin strips of black tape on the plastic protector over sections of the nonius lines (Fig. 14.5) further aids in keeping accommodation at the plane of regard (14). Suppression is evident when there is disappearance of an entire line. To generate forced vergence fixation disparity curves at 40 cm using the Disparometer or Woolf/Wesson cards, use the following steps (pages 432–436) (3).

Phoropter Setup

Place the test instrument (Disparometer, Woolf, or Wesson card) on the near point rod with the target plane at 40 cm and aim the overhead light at the test card. Set the proper interpupillary distance (IPD) and desired lens correction. Utilize the polarizing filters in the phoropter or have the patient wear polarizers. Position the patient behind the phoropter with Risley prisms set at zero in front of each eye. When using the Disparometer, set the disparity reading to zero with the knob on the back of the instrument.

Vertical Associated Phoria

Patients with vertical vergence anomalies often show steep slopes of their horizontal forced vergence fixation disparity curves (19). For some of these patients, vertical prism corrections can cause the lateral forced vergence fixation disparity curve to have a flatter slope, smaller associated phoria, and smaller fixation disparity. Because vergence adaptation is slower and often incomplete for vertical vergence (20), vertical prism correction is often readily accepted. Prism correction based on vertical associated phoria measures is generally considered to be the treatment of choice (21). See Chapter 13 for a more complete description of the technique to assess the vertical associated phoria.

When a vertical and lateral deviation are both present, we recommend evaluation and correction of any existing vertical deviation before corrective measures are instituted for the lateral deviation (19). When vertical prism is indicated, place it in front of the appropriate eye. When more than 2 Δ of vertical prism is needed, use equal amounts of prism in front of each eye. Loose vertical prisms may be taped on the phoropter at the front of the lens well, Fresnel prism used, or the patient can wear the correct prism in eyewear or a trial frame. It is often desirable to make lateral fixation disparity measurements with and without any indicated vertical prism correction to analyze the value of an indicated vertical correction (19).

Horizontal Fixation Disparity Curve

Measurement

Return the Risley prisms to the horizontal position and zero them in front of each eye. When using the Woolf/Wesson cards, the amount and direction of disparity is read directly from the card (Fig. 14.6). For example, when the patient reports that the top arrow is to the left, there is a right exofixation disparity.

When using the Disparometer to measure fixation disparity parameters, use the knob at the rear of the Disparometer and offset the vertically oriented nonius lines to approximately 10 seconds exodisparity. Have the patient report the relative placement of the upper line. If it appears to the right, reduce the exodisparity in 2-second steps until alignment is reported. Note the disparity in the window and continue to reduce the exo (or increase eso) until misalignment is noted in the opposite direction. Measurements should be made within 15 seconds to minimize vergence (prism) adaptation (22). The actual fixation disparity measurement is the midpoint of the range between reported alignment in one direction and reported alignment in the other.

> **Example 14.1** The patient reports that the lines are misaligned to the left when the lines are set at 10 seconds exodisparity. When the exodisparity is reduced in 2-second steps, misalignment is still reported at 4 seconds, and first reported alignment occurs at 2 seconds of exodisparity is continually reduced in 2-second steps and the first reported eso-misalignment occurs at 4 seconds of esodisparity. This point represents the other end

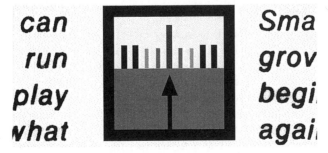

FIG. 14.6. When the Wesson cards are used, the amount and direction of disparity are read directly from the card. For example, when the patient reports that the top arrow is to the left, there is a right exofixation disparity.

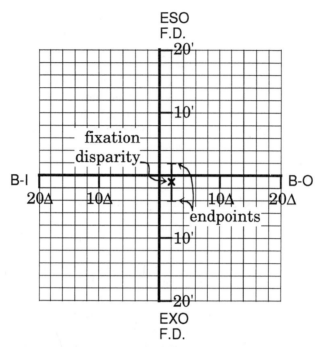

FIG. 14.7. If misalignment is still reported at 4 seconds and first reported alignment occurs at 2 seconds of exodisparity, this point is marked on the graph as one end of the range. The disparity is reduced in 2-second steps, and the first reported eso-misalignment occurs at 4 seconds of esodisparity. This point represents the other end of the range. These endpoints are plotted with horizontal lines and the midpoint of the limits (marked with an "X") represents the actual fixation disparity.

of the range. Figure 14.7 indicates these endpoints with horizontal lines. The midpoint of the limits (marked with an "X") is a 1-second esodisparity, which represents the actual fixation disparity.

Introduce prism with Risley prisms to measure binocular responses at other vergence demands. When the test is conducted at 40 cm, vergence demand is introduced in 3 Δ steps, first placing 3 Δ base-in before the dominant eye and subsequently alternating base-in and base-out. When testing at 6 m, the vergence demand is introduced in 2 Δ steps for base-in vergence and 3 Δ steps for base-out vergence, again alternating base-in and base-out prism demands. The patient should be instructed to close his or her eyes for approximately 15 seconds between measurements. Diplopia or suppression marks the endpoint of the curve. When there is instability, it often helps to cover one nonius line and briefly expose ("flash") it periodically during each setting until the patient reports alignment.

Often there will be diplopia for base-in vergence when the patient can still fuse base-out vergence demands. In addition, if vergence demands are always given in the same direction, the curve shape may be artificially altered, due to prism adaptation (14). If diplopia occurs prematurely, vergence demands are alternated between the appropriate base-out demand and a base-in demand that the patient can just fuse. The base-out demands are graphed, and the last base-in demand to be graphed is the one before fusion was lost. This measurement technique is used to give alternating vergence demands and helps to maintain the curve shape. After all measurements are complete, the results are graphed.

Measurement in Free Space

Free-space measurements permit the clinician to test in different positions of gaze, especially down-gaze, using a prism bar before one eye. This is generally acceptable, despite the asymmetric vergence demand. The position of gaze and distance tested are recorded, along with a notation of the correction worn. When free-space curves are measured, frequently a modified curve can be generated.

Modified Curve Generation

Measurements are made at zero demand and then alternated between 3 Δ base-out and base-in and then 6 Δ base-out and base-in. A prism bar or prism flippers may be used for convenience. When time is limited during a binocular vision analysis, the modified curve can also be generated through the phoropter using vergence demands of zero, 3 Δ base-in and base-out, 6 Δ base-in and base-out, and 12 Δ base-out. These measurements will allow rapid determination of the basic curve shape, fixation disparity, associated phoria, and slope. Clinical experience indicates that these parameters are frequently all that are required to design an appropriate prism correction.

EXAMPLE 14.2 Figure 14.8 documents the modified curve generated using vergence demands of zero, 3 Δ base-in and base-out, 6 Δ base-in and base-out, and 12 Δ base-out.

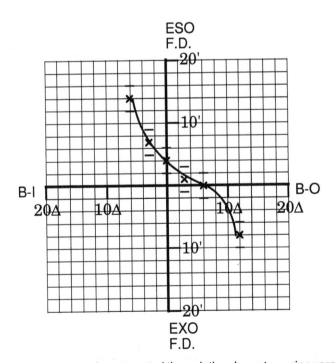

FIG. 14.8. A modified curve can be generated through the phoropter, using vergence demands of zero, 3 Δ base-in and base-out, 6 Δ base-in and base-out, and 12 Δ base-out. These measurements allow rapid determination of the basic curve shape (type I), fixation disparity (4 minutes arc eso), associated phoria (6 Δ base-out), and slope.

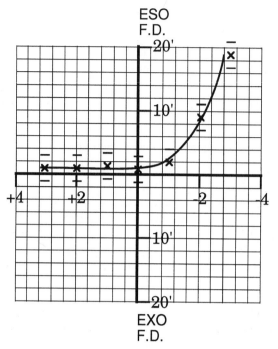

FIG. 14.9. Plotting the change in fixation disparity against the change in lens power of 0.50 D to 1.00 D allows representation of the lens fixation disparity curve.

As seen on the graph, these measurements allow determination of the curve shape, fixation disparity, associated phoria, and slope.

Lens-generated Fixation Disparity Curves

Changes in lens power can also alter fixation disparity responses. Graphical representation allows generation of the lens fixation disparity curve (6) (Fig. 14.9). Plus power is recorded on the left side of the y-axis and minus on the right, using 0.50 D to 1.00 D steps. First make measurements through plus, then through minus, in the approximate range of +2.00 to 3.00 D or the individual patient's limit.

The lens-generated fixation disparity curve can be combined with the prism curve to yield a binocularly derived AC/A (6,23) (Fig. 14.10). This binocularly derived AC/A includes interactions of convergence accommodation (CA/C) and may help direct more accurate prescription of near additions for pre-presbyopic patients.

GRAPHING FINDINGS

When graphing forced vergence fixation disparity findings, eso is above the horizontal and exo is below; base-out is to the right and base-in is to the left. Using graph paper designed for fixation disparity curves, mark the midpoint of the interval where the patient reported alignment on the y-axis with an "x" or a dot and mark the interval ranges with horizontal slashes (refer to Fig. 14.8). Make sure to note the interval ranges, as they may change with training. Record the y-intercept, x-intercept, and slope on the top of the record. The y-intercept is the fixation disparity, while the x-intercept is the associated phoria measurement (prism

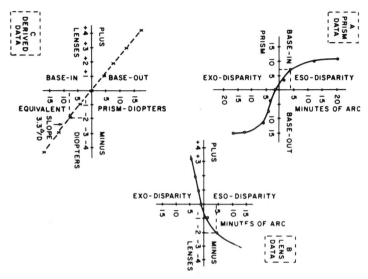

FIG. 14.10. A binocularly derived AC/A can be determined by combining the lens-generated fixation disparity curve data with the prism curve data. This binocularly derived AC/A includes interactions of convergence accommodation and helps direct more accurate prescription of near additions for pre-presbyopic patients.

required to reduce fixation disparity to zero). The slope is most frequently measured about the y-intercept (between 3 Δ base-in and 3 Δ base-out), since that is considered to reflect the vergence posture where the patient habitually functions. Measure and record the slope as the change in minutes of arc per 6 Δ (3 Δ BI to 3 Δ BO); see Example 2, Fig. 14.8. The slope between the y- and x-intercepts may also be useful.

INTERPRETATION

With a small amount of practice, forced vergence fixation disparity curves are easily interpreted. The major important parameters are the curve type, slope, fixation disparity, and associated phoria. All factors should be viewed together, rather than considering only one in isolation. For example, used by itself, the associated horizontal phoria may give little additional clinically useful information. However, when considered with other fixation disparity parameters, a great deal of useful patient care information is gained.

CLINICAL USEFULNESS PRESCRIBING

Forced vergence fixation disparity curves can be used to design prism prescriptions and modify spherical prescription power and they are useful in monitoring the progress of vision therapy. The curves generally flatten as therapy is successfully completed. Usually there will be a small residual fixation disparity when the patient is tested with an instrument designed to measure fixation disparity (24).

Prism Correction Design

Lateral Prism

A carefully designed prism correction reduces the need for corrective fusional movements and minimizes adverse interactions between convergence accommodation (25) and accommodative

438 III. MANAGEMENT

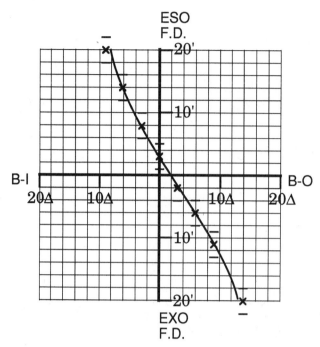

FIG. 14.11. There is a relatively steep slope and a comparatively narrow range of fusion, as documented by the diplopia endpoints of the curve at 9 △ base-in and 12 △ base-out. Prescription of 2 △ base-out for distance vision will locate the center of symmetry about the y-axis.

vergence. The area of most rapid adaptation to changing vergence stimuli is represented by the flattest portion (center of symmetry) of the fixation disparity curve. Prism is prescribed to move the center of symmetry toward, or more nearly centered about, the y-axis.

> **EXAMPLE 14.3** The fixation disparity curve shown in Fig. 14.11 has a relatively steep slope and the patient demonstrates a comparatively narrow range of fusion, as documented by the diplopia endpoints of the curve at 9 △ base-in and 12 △ base-out. Patients who demonstrate this type of pattern are typically esophores who benefit from prescription of prism that locates the center of symmetry about the y-axis. The patient depicted in Fig. 14.11 was prescribed 2 △ base-out for distance vision, which eliminated his symptoms of discomfort while driving and watching television. Calculation of Sheard's criteria for the same patient suggested a need for substantially more prism (5 △ base-out).

When the forced vergence fixation disparity curve has a large flat slope, there is rapid vergence adaptation over a large area of vergence stress. Prism can be prescribed to shift the curve so that the flat (vergence adaptation) portion begins as close as possible to the y-axis. This allows the patient to maintain binocular vision in the area of maximum vergence adaptation, minimizing the amount of prism required. The prism prescribed is the minimum amount of base-out prism (for esofixation disparity/associated phoria) or base-in (for exofixation disparity/associated phoria) that allows the flat portion of the curve to first cross the y-axis.

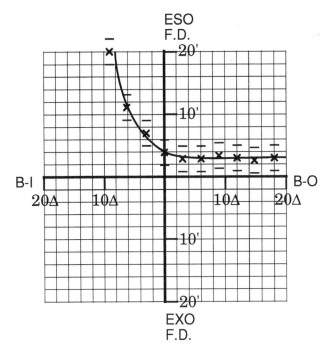

FIG. 14.12. The fixation disparity curve shows a large flat area and a wide range of fusion from 9 △ base-in and 20 △ base-out, with no center of symmetry. Prescription of 2.5 △ base-out for distance vision shifts the curve so that the flat portion begins as closely as possible to the y-axis.

EXAMPLE 14.4 The fixation disparity curve in Fig. 14.12 has a large flat area, and the patient demonstrates a wide range of fusion from 9 △ base-in to 30 △ base-out. Often there is no center of symmetry for these patients. Patients who demonstrate this type of pattern are typically esophores. They are often made more comfortable by prescription of prism that shifts the curve so that the flat portion begins as closely as possible to the y-axis. The patient depicted in Fig. 14.12 was prescribed 2.5 △ base-out for distance vision, which eliminated his symptoms of occasional diplopia while playing tennis. Calculation of Sheard's criteria for the same patient suggested a need for 7 △ base-out.

When patients have a steep curve, there is very little vergence adaptation and often no center of symmetry. Prism can be prescribed to reduce the fixation disparity to zero (associated phoria) or vision therapy can be prescribed to develop increased vergence adaptation. Complete correction of the associated phoria of patients with steeply sloped fixation disparity curves simplifies correction of binocular disorders and reduces the need to consider often complex CA/C and AC/A interactions (3,25).

EXAMPLE 14.5 The fixation disparity curve in Fig. 14.13A has a steep slope, and the patient demonstrates a narrow range of fusion from 6 △ base-in to 9 △ base-out. There is no center of symmetry because there is no obvious vergence adaptation. Patients who demonstrate this type of pattern may be more comfortable after prescription of prism that shifts the curve so that the associated phoria is corrected; 2 Δ base-out was prescribed for this patient. However, it is generally superior management to prescribe vision therapy to develop more complete vergence adaptation. Vision therapy (which was prescribed for this patient to minimize suppression, expand fusional ranges, and enhance vergence accuracy) successfully eliminated his symptoms of reading distress. His fixation disparity curve after therapy is seen in Fig. 14.13B.

Figure 14.14 shows the distance fixation disparity curve of a myopic pre-presbyopic patient with a large distance esophoria and a small near esophoria (divergence insufficiency). This type II curve does not cross the x-axis, which is typical for patients with large esophorias. Generally, prism prescriptions for patients who have this curve type should contain enough power so that the flat portion of the curve starts before the x-axis. For example, contrast this with the discussion of the patient portrayed in Example 14.4.

Figure 14.15 shows a near fixation disparity curve for a patient with an equal esophoria at distance and near. This steep curve has essentially no central flat portion. There is a small associated esophoria. When there is a steep curve, prism that reduces fixation disparity to zero (associated phoria) provides the smallest prism correction that gives relief of symptoms. For this patient, 2 Δ base-out will move the associated phoria to the zero point and should eliminate symptoms. Comparing this curve with the curve for the divergence insufficiency patient (Fig. 14.14), illustrates the errors that can arise when only the associated phoria is used to determine prism corrections. Frequently, an indicated prism correction may not be appropriate when there is a type II or type III forced vergence fixation disparity curve that does not cross the y-axis. In general, vision therapy should be the initial therapy for these patients, with supplemental prism as needed.

Vertical Prism

Proper management of lateral heterophorias often requires decisions as to whether a coexisting vertical heterophoria requires correction. Prism prescription design for vertical heterophoria requires clinical judgment, using any of the various techniques that have been recommended for prescription design: equating vergence ranges, flip prism techniques (26), and fixation disparity (27).

For patients who give accurate responses, tests based on vertical fixation disparity measurements and reducing the vertical fixation disparity to zero are the techniques of choice for vertical prism prescription design. Vertical associated phoria tests indicate the vertical prism required. Nearly all patients will notice a difference of 0.5 Δ on vertical fixation disparity testing (27), and most symptomatic patients with vertical associated phoria measurements of 0.75 Δ or more benefit from vertical prism corrections or vertical vergence therapy. Refer to Chapter 13 for a more complete description of the decision processes involved in determining the amount of vertical prism to prescribe.

SPHERE MODIFICATION

Near Addition Determination

Therapy techniques for most binocular disturbances are based on the application of lenses, prisms, and/or vision therapy. For example, near plus additions are frequently helpful during management of patients with vergence and/or accommodative anomalies. For symptomatic esophoric patients, an approximate near addition is often easily determined by finding the plus

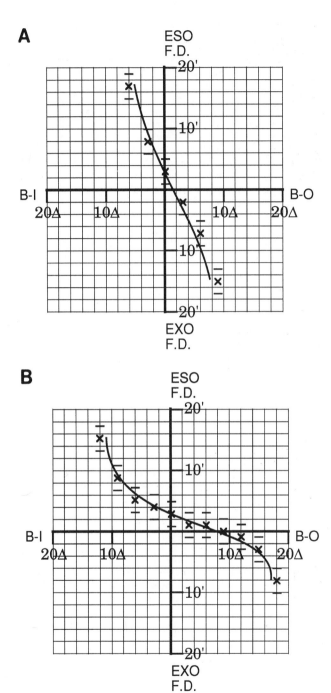

FIG. 14.13. A: The fixation disparity curve has a steep slope, and the patient demonstrates a narrow range of fusion from 6 △ base-in to 9 △ base-out. There is no center of symmetry because there is no obvious vergence adaptation. **B:** Vision therapy (which was prescribed for this patient to minimize suppression, expand fusional ranges, and enhance vergence accuracy) successfully eliminated his symptoms of reading distress. Although the fixation disparity remained the same, there was a flattening and expansion of the flat portion of the fixation disparity curve.

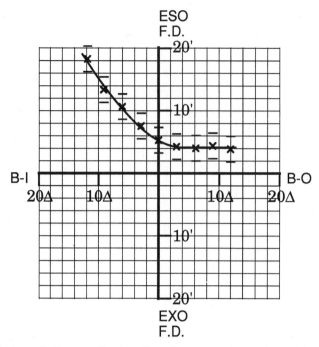

FIG. 14.14. This type II distance fixation disparity curve of a patient with a large distance esophoria does not cross the x-axis. Generally, prism prescriptions for patients who have this curve type should contain enough power so that the flat portion of the curve starts before the x-axis, about 3 △ base-out for this patient.

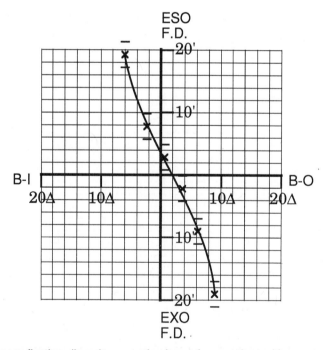

FIG. 14.15. A near fixation disparity curve is shown for a patient with an equal esophoria at distance and near. This steep curve has essentially no central flat portion. There is a small associated esophoria. For this patient, 2 △ base-out will move the associated phoria to the zero point.

lens addition that reduces an existing esofixation disparity to zero. If desired, forced vergence prism curves can be determined through the tentative near addition to verify the efficacy.

EXAMPLE 14.6 A patient has orthophoria at 6 m and a 6 Δ esophoria at 40 cm, measured with prism dissociation. An esoassociated phoria is measured at 40 cm through the distance refractive correction. To determine a near addition power with fixation disparity testing, plus lenses are added in +0.25 D steps, over the distance refractive correction, until the patient reports alignment of the nonius lines (a zero associated phoria at near). The fixation disparity technique suggested a need for a near addition of +0.75. This prescription successfully eliminated his symptoms of blur and tired eyes after 20 minutes of reading.

Distance Sphere Modification

For divergence excess patients under the age of 15, minus power greater than the distance refractive findings may be combined with a near add and used to enhance fusion when an active vision therapy program is not feasible. Usually only a small amount of additional minus power (a maximum of 1.00 to 1.50 D) is needed over the distance refractive findings. For selected patients, up to 3 D (or occasionally 4 D) of distance minus lens overcorrection may be necessary. Because of the frequent symptoms of accommodative asthenopia, overcorrections of large magnitude should be used as an adjunct to vision therapy and generally be reserved for part-time wear during therapy rather than full-time wear.

Before fixation disparity curves were used to measure binocular vergence responses to lens intervention, the amount of distance over minus correction had to be determined empirically. However, fixation disparity curves may be used to determine the amount of distance overcorrection to prescribe and to help determine the amount of the near addition. The amount used is just enough to facilitate convergence and fusion.

EXAMPLE 14.7 Figure 14.16A illustrates fixation disparity curves for a 10-year-old divergence excess patient. There is a type III curve; this is typical for patients with large exophorias. An exact associated exophoria cannot be determined for distance, although it is obviously exophoric. Figure 14.16B shows the response curves to added minus lens powers. Almost −2.00 D of minus lens power is required to allow the distance curve to cross the x-axis. Less than −1.00 D of added minus power causes the near curve to cross the x-axis. Thus, according to the data presented in these curves, if lens management alone is desired, a −2.00 D distance overcorrection is required. However, the −2.00 D distance overcorrection would create an esofixation disparity and esoassociated phoria at near. Consequently, if a distance over minus correction is used, a near addition of +1.00 to +1.50 D will be needed to allow both curves to cross the x-axis at about the same point.

Planning and Monitoring Vision Therapy Programs

Using fixation disparity data (which includes the effects of vergence adaptation ability, tonic vergence, and accommodation/convergence interactions), vision therapy programs can be

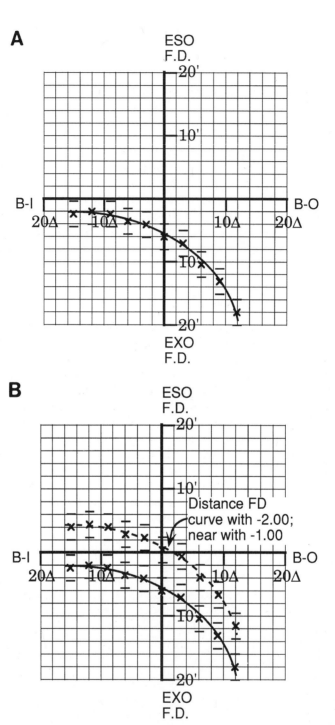

FIG. 14.16. A: A 10-year-old divergence excess patient shows a type III curve; this is typical for patients with large exophorias. An exact associated exophoria cannot be determined for distance, although it is obviously exophoric. **B:** Almost 2.00 D of minus lens power is required to allow the distance curve to cross the x-axis. Only 1.00 D of added minus power causes the near curve to cross the x-axis. If lens management alone is desired, a 2.00 D distance overcorrection is required. However, the 2.00 D distance overcorrection would create an esofixation disparity and esoassociated phoria at near. Thus, if a distance overminus correction is used, a near addition of +1.00 to +1.50 D will be needed to allow both curves to cross the x-axis at about the same point.

modified so that training is specifically directed toward improving the deficient skill. Patients who have transient accommodative-based symptoms and high CA/C ratios respond best to vision therapy techniques that train rapid large magnitude responses to lenses (accommodative rock therapy) and incorporate a moderate amount of prism training (some jump vergence therapy). Patients with large heterophorias (tonic vergence disorders) respond best to vision therapy techniques that include rapid large vergence changes to prisms (primarily jump vergence therapy) and some lens therapy (accommodative rock therapy). Patients with reduced vergence adaptation (steep curves) require vision therapy that develops rapid sustained responses combined with some adaptive vergence training (isometric exercises) (28). Patients with both reduced vergence adaptation (steep slope) and abnormal CA/C and AC/A interactions are treated by adaptive vergence training (isometric exercises) and training that emphasizes rapid responses to moderate magnitude stimuli (jump and smooth vergence training plus accommodative rock).

EXAMPLE 14.8 Figure 14.17A,B illustrates distance and near fixation disparity curves for a convergence insufficiency patient with associated accommodative problems. The near curve is irregular, with each measurement point having a large range where alignment was reported. Irregular curves with large ranges of alignment frequently result from accommodative inaccuracy, causing convergence problems. The patient inappropriately uses accommodation to assist convergence and the result is a forced vergence fixation disparity curve that is irregular in shape with large ranges of error for each measurement point. The near curve for the same patient after accommodative therapy is shown in Fig. 14.17B. Each measurement point is more accurate (the curve is smoother) and there is a smaller fixation disparity (closer to the intercept). This illustrates an example of the use of fixation disparity curves to monitor progress of vision therapy for a patient who underwent accommodative therapy. As therapy is successfully completed, the curves generally flatten and often smooth out. Usually a small fixation disparity remains when the patient is tested with an instrument designed to measure fixation disparity (24).

CONCLUSION

There are many elaborate factors that combine, through a series of complex interactions, to result in single binocular vision. Many of these factors can only be adequately analyzed diagnostically using techniques that test under binocular conditions. Fixation disparity measures of ocular alignment responses to vergence and/or accommodative stress provide a useful technique for accurate assessment of many of these factors. With fixation disparity testing, it is not necessary to assume that a measured latent neuromuscular bias (heterophoria) is operative under binocular conditions. Rather, residual misalignment can be directly measured, along with assessment of the ability to adjust to induced external vergence and accommodative demands.

With fixation disparity data, treatment techniques can be designed using lenses, prisms, or vision therapy. Effects on performance when the sphere power of the prescription has been modified to include plus additions for near and/or minus overcorrections for distance can be monitored. Prism therapy can be easily designed to be appropriate for distance and near a task that is frequently difficult using conventional analysis techniques. Vision therapy progress can also be monitored using forced vergence fixation disparity curves.

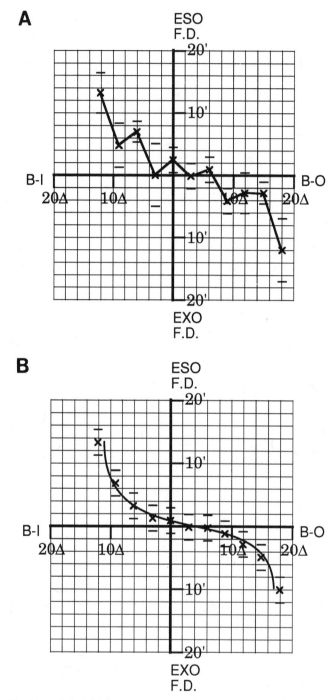

FIG. 14.17. A: The curve is irregular, with each measurement point having a large range where alignment was reported. Irregular curves with large ranges of alignment frequently result from accommodative inaccuracy, causing convergence problems. **B:** After accommodative therapy, each measurement point is more accurate (the curve is smoother) and there is a smaller fixation disparity (closer to the intercept). This illustrates an example of the use of fixation disparity curves to monitor progress of vision therapy for a patient who underwent accommodative therapy.

STUDY QUESTIONS

1. Describe how the characteristics of the four types of horizontal fixation disparity curves relate to the type of phoria the patient has.
2. What factors might lead to a different type of horizontal fixation disparity curve at distance and near?
3. What is the difference between associated and dissociated phoria?
4. How do the concepts of center of symmetry, associated phoria, and fixation disparity influence prism prescription decisions?
5. Why can't determination of the fixation disparity curve be done at distance with the Vectographic adult slide?
6. Why can the basic shape of a fixation disparity curve be determined with only six measures (6 Δ BI and BO, 3 Δ BI and BO, and zero)?
7. What changes might be expected in the shape of the forced vergence fixation disparity curve after vision therapy?
8. How can an AC/A ratio be determined with fixation disparity testing? Why might it be useful to differentiate the associated AC/A from the dissociated AC/A?
9. Why is it often difficult to determine the amount of base-out prism to prescribe, based on associated phoria measures alone?
10. How little prism might be useful in treatment of vertical phoria? How would you determine this amount in a patient with good binocular vision and no suppression?

SOURCES OF EQUIPMENT

a. Available from author (B.W.), University of Houston College of Optometry, 4901 Calhoun, Houston, TX.
b. Not current commercially available; used instruments may be available from time to time.
c. Available from Michael Wesson, OD, University of Alabama, Birmingham, College of Optometry, University Station, Birmingham, AL.

REFERENCES

1. Ogle KN. *Researches in binocular vision.* New York: Hafner, 1962:69–93.
2. Sheedy JE, Saladin JJ. Association of symptoms with measures of oculomotor deficiencies. *Am J Optom Physiol Opt* 1978;55:670–676.
3. Wick B. Horizontal deviations. In: Amos J, ed. *Diagnosis and management in vision care.* Boston: Butterworth-Heinemann, 1987:474–476.
4. Wick B. Nearpoint symptoms associated with a change from spectacle lenses to contact lenses. *J Am Optom Assoc* 1978;49:1295–1297.
5. Remole A. Fixation disparity vs. binocular fixation misalignment. *Am J Optom Physiol Opt* 1985;62:25–34.
6. Ogle KN, Martens TG, Dyer JA. Oculomotor imbalance. *Binocular vision and fixation disparity.* Philadelphia: Lea & Febiger, 1967.
7. Fry GA. An analysis of the relationships between phoria, blur, break and recovery findings at the near point. *Am J Optom Arch Am Acad Optom* 1941;18:393–403.
8. Lesser SK. *Introduction to modern analytical optometry.* Duncan, OK: Optometric Extension Program Foundation, 1969.
9. Morgan MW. Analysis of clinical data. *Am J Optom Arch Am Acad Optom* 1944;21:477–491.
10. Carter DB. Studies of fixation disparity—historical review. *Am J Optom Arch Am Acad Optom* 1957;34:320–329.
11. Sheedy JE, Saladin JJ. Exophoria at near in presbyopia. *Am J Optom Physiol Opt* 1975;52:474–481.
12. Wick B. Forced vergence fixation disparity curves at distance and near in an asymptomatic young adult population. *Am J Optom Physiol Opt* 1985;62:591–599.
13. Carter DB. Fixation disparity with and without foveal contours. *Am J Optom Arch Am Acad Optom* 1964;41:729–736.
14. Schor CM. The influence of rapid prism adaptation upon fixation disparity. *Vision Res* 1979;19:757–765.

15. London R. Fixation disparity and heterophoria. In: Baresi BJ, ed. *Ocular assessment: the manual of diagnosis for office practice*. Boston: Butterworth-Heinemann, 1984:141–150.
16. Schor CM. Analysis of tonic and accommodative vergence disorders of binocular vision. *Am J Optom Physiol Opt* 1983;60:114.
17. Wick B. Clinical factors in proximal vergence. *Am J Optom Physiol Opt* 1985;62:118.
18. Mallett RFJ. The investigation of heterophoria at near and a new fixation disparity technique. *Optician* 1964;148:547–551, 574–581.
19. Wick B, London R. Vertical fixation disparity correction; effect on the horizontal forced vergence fixation disparity curve. *Am J Optom Physiol Opt* 1987;64:653–656.
20. Eskridge JB, Rutstein RP. Clinical evaluation of vertical fixation disparity. Part I. *Am J Optom Physiol Opt* 1983;60:688–693.
21. Eskridge JB, Rutstein RP. Clinical evaluation of vertical fixation disparity. II. Reliability, stability, and association with refractive status, stereoacuity, and vertical heterophorias. *Am J Optom Physiol Opt* 1985;62:579–584.
22. Schor CM. The relationship between fusional vergence eye movements and fixation disparity. *Vision Res* 1979;19:1359–1367.
23. Hebbard FW. Foveal fixation disparity measurements and their use in determining the relationship between accommodative convergence and accommodation. *Am J Optom Arch Am Acad Optom* 1960;37:326.
24. Schor CM. Fixation disparity and vergence adaptation. In: Schor CM, Ciufreda KJ, eds. *Vergence eye movements: basic and clinical aspects*. Boston: Butterworth-Heinemann, 1983:465–516.
25. Schor CM, Narayan V. Graphical analysis of prism adaptation, convergence accommodation, and accommodative vergence. *Am J Optom Physiol Opt* 1983;60:774–784.
26. Eskridge JB. The flip prism test for vertical phoria. *Am J Optom Arch Am Acad Optom* 1961;38:415–421.
27. Morgan MW. The Turville infinity balance test. *Am J Optom Arch Am Acad Optom* 1949;26:231–239.
28. Vaegan. Convergence and divergence show large and sustained improvement after short isometric exercise. *Am J Optom Physiol Opt* 1979;57:23–33.

PART IV

Advanced Diagnostic and Management Issues

15

Interactions Between Accommodation and Vergence

Binocular vision dysfunctions occur because of excessive tonic vergence, abnormal interactions of vergence, proximal vergence, and accommodation (1), and/or deficient vergence (prism) adaptation (2). Recent analysis of tonic vergence disorders (3) and accommodation/vergence interactions (2) suggests that classical analysis techniques are often not sufficient. More than one analysis system has traditionally been needed to determine whether existing binocular deficiencies are related to existing symptoms (4). Because of the deficiencies in current analysis techniques, we have introduced integrative analysis in Chapter 2 of this book.

Although many areas remain to be fully explored, in this chapter we discuss binocular vision from a theoretical and practical clinical viewpoint to introduce the concepts behind integrative analysis. Effects of the magnitude of proximal vergence and the influence of the depth of focus of the eye, lag of accommodation, and tonic vergence are considered and related to a dual interactive model of accommodation and vergence. We discuss many of the tests of binocular function that are currently performed clinically and relate them to the model. In addition, we suggest new tests that may be used in the future to provide diagnostic information [e.g., measurement of the convergence accommodation to convergence (CA/C) ratio and/or proximal vergence].

ANALYSIS APPROACHES

Traditional Analysis Techniques

Three techniques have been used for analysis of examination data to determine whether vergence or accommodative deficiencies exist in sufficient magnitude to result in symptoms. The graphical method of analysis (5) emphasizes the role of the vergence system in the etiology of symptoms. The analytical method emphasizes the role of accommodation (6) and the normative method is not selective (7).

Graphical Analysis

Graphical analysis is based on the hierarchy of vergence mechanisms originally described by Maddox. Graphical analysis is designed to predict how tonic, accommodative, and fusional/disparity vergence (8) respond to result in the final eye position. Proximal vergence is generally not represented graphically (9).

Conventional graphical analysis is based on the:

Distance dissociated heterophoria
AC/A
Positive relative convergence
Negative relative convergence
Amplitude of accommodation

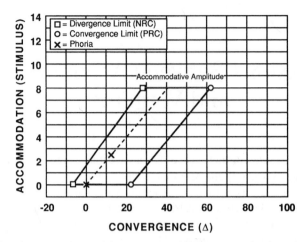

FIG. 15.1. By using the parameters of distance dissociated heterophoria, AC/A, positive relative convergence, negative relative convergence, and amplitude of accommodation, the zone of clear single binocular vision is graphed to visually represent the ranges of stimulus values through which the accommodative and/or vergence system can maintain binocular vision.

Using these parameters, the zone of clear single binocular vision is graphed (10) to visually represent the ranges of stimulus values through which the accommodative and/or vergence system can maintain binocular vision (Fig. 15.1).

The relationship of the heterophoria and AC/A to relative vergence measurements is used to determine visual efficiency and, subsequently, to plan therapeutic intervention. In classical methods, the vertical lines of the zone are the reciprocal of the stimulus AC/A and represent the vergence limits of clear single binocular vision (10). Proponents of graphical analysis imply that deficits or excesses of tonic and accommodative vergence are compensated by disparity (fusional) vergence and excessive demands on disparity (fusional) vergence cause asthenopic symptoms (11). Diagnostic criteria, such as those of Sheard (12), and Percival (13), have been adopted to determine lens or prism corrections that sufficiently reduce the disparity (fusional) vergence demand. Unfortunately, using graphical analysis, it is sometimes difficult to identify the underlying problem when a purely accommodative dysfunction exists.

Analytical Analysis

The physiologic basis of analytical analysis is that faulty accommodation forces the visual system to compensate, resulting in development of a vergence dysfunction (14). The aspect of accommodation emphasized in this analysis is posture (lag). Aspects such as facility, sustaining ability, velocity, and amplitude are not typically considered. Further, nearly all anomalies (up to 95%) are given an accommodative basis when other causes often seem equally or, in some cases, even more likely.

Normative Analysis

Normative analysis involves determination of how individual test results (phorias, vergence and accommodative amplitudes, accommodation/vergence interactions) deviate from clinical norms (15). Normative analysis, which is most accurate when diagnosing a single problem, is not as accurate for diagnosis when there is excessive tonic vergence combined with abnormal vergence/accommodation interactions. Multiple interactions can be analyzed using a mechanistic approach (16) with partial success.

KEY CONCEPTS

The flaw with current systems that are used to analyze results of binocular visual function tests is that many important accommodation and vergence interactions can only be adequately evaluated under binocular conditions. For example, demands on disparity (fusional) vergence during binocular viewing may be dramatically different from predictions of stress on sensory and motor fusion based on measures of the dissociated heterophoria (17). Variations between results, determined using monocular and binocular testing, may be caused by two components neglected in the Maddox hierarchy—vergence (prism) adaptation (2) and CA/C—and an additional one not usually considered in any analysis, proximal vergence.

Dissociated Versus Associated Testing

Binocular testing provides a more complete picture of the interactions between binocular components than traditional systems that compare various monocular (dissociated) measures. The fixation disparity curve, measured at distance as well as near fixation distances, provides a binocular test that allows the clinician to determine a treatment that results in optimal binocularity. With the fixation disparity testing described in Chapter 14, residual misalignment can be directly determined; it is unnecessary to assume that a measured latent neuromuscular bias (heterophoria) also exists and causes symptoms noted during binocular viewing. These tests are useful clinically to determine prism prescriptions for patients who have eso- or hyperphorias and as a means to monitor vision therapy programs.

Theoretical Interactions

A previously published representation (18) of the interactions of accommodation and vergence is shown in Fig. 15.2. The lower block diagram represents the components that describe vergence responses and the upper section represents the accommodative system. The convergence and accommodative systems interact through separate crosslinks of CA/C and accommodative vergence. Because of these crosslinks, innervation to convergence drives accommodation through CA/C, just as innervation to accommodation drives convergence through the AC/A. Proximal effects are input into each section of the system before the crosslinks.

The model in Fig. 15.2 has significant implications about normal binocular vision, and we have considered these in developing the integrative analysis system (Chapter 2). In designing integrative analysis, we have incorporated implications about interactions between accommodation and convergence described by the model in Fig. 15.2, tonic vergence, the depth of focus and lag of accommodation, and recent research implications concerning the influences of proximal vergence (19). Certain assumptions must be made about the model so that predictions about the accommodative and vergence system can be made. For example, at this time, considerations are limited to static situations where constant stimuli are held at a fixed position. This makes the potentially complex interactions somewhat less complicated. However, even with these limitations, the results apply to a large number of clinical and real life situations.

Application of the model to measurement of heterophorias, fixation disparity, associated phoria, and the zone of clear single binocular vision helps explain many binocular vision responses seen during clinical patient care, including why presbyopic patients are generally asymptomatic despite loss of accommodative vergence. In the following sections, we describe

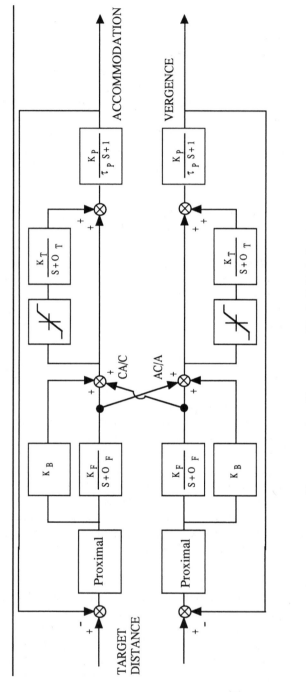

FIG. 15.2. The lower block diagram represents the components that describe vergence responses and the upper section represents the accommodative system. The convergence and accommodative systems interact through separate crosslinks of convergence accommodation (CA/C) and accommodative vergence. Proximal effects are input into each section of the system before the crosslinks. Innervation to convergence drives accommodation through CA/C, just as innervation to accommodation drives convergence through the AC/A.

how the model applies to many of the examination and diagnostic techniques we suggest in Chapter 1. Additionally, we discuss areas where further clinical research needs to be performed and how the model might direct such research.

TONIC VERGENCE

Tonic vergence represents the eye position that results in the absence of disparity, blur, and proximal stimuli. Tonic vergence can be measured directly by incorporating pinhole apertures during distance von Graefe phoria testing. The disparity and accommodative systems are open loop,[1] and proximal input is absent because fixation is at distance. Repeatable measures can be made, due to the stable nature of tonic vergence.

Testing tonic vergence is typically not done in a clinical setting, and, for most patients, there is probably little need to add this testing. In normal adults, tonic vergence is only approximately 2 Δ more convergent than the distant phoria and the distribution of tonic vergence is similar to the leptokertotic distribution of the distance phoria where the peak is 1 Δ exo ±2. Thus, for normal adults, tonic vergence outside the range of 2 Δ exophoric or 1 Δ esophoric is abnormal. As will be seen in subsequent discussions, the model in Fig. 15.2 suggests that significant tonic vergence has a major effect on interactions between accommodation and vergence (20). For patients who have large esophorias at distance, assessment of tonic vergence may yield some useful diagnostic information. For example, a substantial difference between the distance phoria and the tonic measure would suggest a need to increase the amount of base-out prism incorporated in the prescription.

Depth of Focus and Lag of Accommodation

Determination of the role played by accommodation requires knowledge of the amount of accommodation (or accommodative effort) used (21). To maximally relax accommodation at distance, refraction is generally done to achieve best visual acuity with the maximum plus (or least minus) lenses possible. The maximum plus refraction places distant objects at the farthest focus point from the retina. Because of the refractive technique and the depth of focus of the eye, small accommodative stimuli do not affect accommodative activity (22) with distance fixation. As an object is moved closer, the blur circle moves through the limits of the depth of focus and no change in accommodation occurs because no appreciable blur results until the object focus goes beyond the depth of focus of the eye.

Clinicians typically think in terms of the stimulus rather than the response to accommodation. However, the preceding discussion suggests that the accommodative response is generally significantly smaller than the stimulus. For approximately the first 0.75 D of accommodative stimulus, there is no accommodative change due to the refraction and the depth of focus of the eye (22). The distance depth of focus, combined with the normal lag of accommodation of 0.50 D or more when accommodating on near objects (23), causes only approximately 1.50 D of accommodative change when fixation is changed from distance to 40 cm (24) (Fig. 15.3). This is significantly less than the 2.5 D accommodative stimulus.

---

[1] "Opening the loop" is done using any technique that eliminates feedback from either the vergence or accommodative system. For example, occlusion prevents fusion and opens the disparity loop because feedback about binocular eye alignment is prevented by the occluder. The vergence loop can also be opened by having the subject view a long horizontal line that has no fusion contours. In contrast, pinholes eliminate blur feedback and open the accommodative loop. Alternative methods of opening the accommodative loop include Difference of Gaussian (DOG) targets or dim illumination, both of which render blur-driven accommodation ineffective.

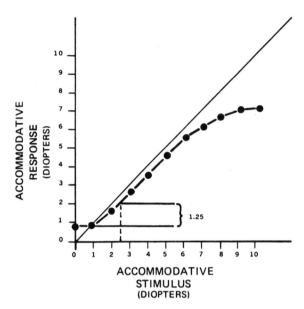

FIG. 15.3. The distance depth of focus, combined with the normal lag of accommodation of 0.50 D or more when accommodating on near objects, causes only approximately 1.50 D of accommodative change when fixation is changed from distance to 40 cm. (From Wick B. Clinical factors in proximal vergence. *Am J Optom Physiol Opt* 1985;62:119, with permission.)

The average lag of accommodation is between 0.25 and 0.50 D for children and young adults. Determination of the accommodative lag is done routinely in clinics using monocular estimation method (MEM) retinoscopy. MEM retinoscopy is very useful for evaluating the accommodative response of patients who complain of near blur or other symptoms of accommodative dysfunction. A finding of a high lag of accommodation during MEM retinoscopy suggests a tentative power for a near addition and/or a need to prescribe accommodative therapy. An excess of accommodation on MEM retinoscopy (lead of accommodation) directs treatment to techniques that maximally relax accommodation, such as the prescription of near plus additions, which reduce accommodative demand to zero, and/or vision training emphasizing plus acceptance. Integrative analysis routinely includes MEM retinoscopy and, thus, incorporates many of the effects of accommodative lag and the depth of focus of the eye.

Proximal Vergence

Proximal vergence contributes up to 70% of the vergence demand for near tasks (25) and is greater when measured under binocular conditions (24,26). Measurements of proximal vergence velocity using infrared limbal sensing have found that the mean peak velocities for proximal convergence and divergence (66 and 39 degrees per second, respectively) are substantially faster (27) than disparity vergence velocities of 14 and 10 degrees per second (28). The magnitude and velocity of proximal vergence responses suggest that this component is a major contributor to the total vergence response when looking from distance to near. Proximal effects are included as the initial entry in the vergence/accommodation interactive model shown in Fig. 15.2.

Disparity vergence has been shown to have a shorter latency and more rapid course than accommodative vergence (29). As a result, most clinicians feel that disparity vergence initiates the near vergence response. However, there are a number of situations where disparity cannot serve as the initiator of near vergence. For example, if a near object located so that it is seen by only one eye is to be fixated, an eye movement and a head movement will be required for bi-foveal fixation. In this situation, knowledge of the object location and "awareness of nearness" (proximal vergence) probably provide the initial vergence and accommodative component. Another frequent situation involves copying from a blackboard in school. The images of the object are frequently located so far in the peripheral retina that disparity cues are not applicable (30) and, again, proximal vergence is more likely to be the initial vergence component. Since binocular proximal effects make up a large portion of the near demand (24), they can move the system within the ranges of foveal vision, where disparity vergence and blur-driven accommodation can "fine-tune" the response.

Proximal vergence can be measured clinically by incorporating pinholes (to eliminate accommodative vergence) and measuring the heterophoria at different distances using the von Graefe technique (to eliminate disparity vergence). Changes in the proximal stimulus are introduced using targets located at 2.0, 1.0, 0.5, and 0.25 m. The change in angle that is measured provides an estimate of proximal vergence. For an optimal stimulus to proximal vergence, the patient must be fully aware of the target location. This is accomplished by having the patient view the targets under natural viewing conditions before recording the measurements and by having him or her hold the target during the nearer measurements. Although these proximal measures are not currently utilized in routine clinical testing, they may provide useful information for clinical management. For example, in preliminary studies, deficient proximal vergence has been linked to the prolonged blur that some patients report after reading (31).

Binocular Vergence Interactions

The relationships considered in the preceding section become somewhat more complicated when considering interactions between vergence and accommodation. For example, consider the situation in which no output is needed from accommodation (such as when a pinhole is placed in front of the eyes to greatly increase the depth of field). This eliminates the effects of accommodative lag and depth of focus and reduces accommodation due to blur to zero. Thoughtful clinicians will recognize that accommodation due to blur is also zero in a common physical condition—absolute presbyopia when there is physiologically no accommodation. Analysis of the situation, where there is no blur-driven accommodation using the model described in Fig. 15.2, helps explain why presbyopic patients are routinely asymptomatic when classical analysis systems frequently predict binocular distress (32). The effects of interactions between accommodation and vergence are often deleterious; presbyopia removes this interactive problem, and patients are commonly asymptomatic.

Convergence Accommodation

Measurement of the CA/C ratio provides information concerning the strength of the crosslink from the vergence system to accommodation. The model of Fig. 15.2 shows why interactions between vergence and accommodation, via the CA/C ratio, complicate findings of classical graphical analysis. For example, suppose that vergence measures were made in a patient with a zero CA/C ratio (so that changes in vergence did not affect accommodation), while proximal vergence was held constant. Clinically, this measurement is called relative vergence or "vergence free of accommodation." Under these conditions, graphical analysis techniques suggest that disparity vergence equals the dissociated phoria. However, except in presbyopia, the CA/C is seldom zero, and changes in vergence are accompanied by changes in

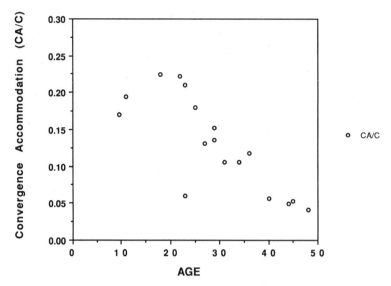

FIG. 15.4. The convergence accommodation (CA/C) is inversely related to age. For young adults, the average CA/C ratio is about 0.5 D per meter angle (a meter angle is determined by dividing the interpupillary distance (IPD) by 10 and expressing the value in prism diopters). For clinical purposes, the average value is about 6 MA.

accommodation, forcing reflex accommodation to change to compensate for vergence accommodation. As a result, the relationship between the dissociated phoria and disparity vergence is not adequately predicted by classical methods of analysis.

Clinical research on the CA/C ratio indicates a linear relation, although, as extremes of the vergence stimulus are reached, the range becomes nonlinear—possibly due, in part, to the decrease in pupil size and increased depth of focus that accompanies increased vergence (33). Because there is generally very little difference between the vergence stimulus and the vergence response, there is very little difference between the stimulus and response CA/C ratio. For young adults, the CA/C ratio is about 0.5 D per meter angle [a meter angle is determined by dividing the IPD, in millimeters, by 10 and expressing the value in prism diopters (see Chapter 1)]; for clinical purposes, the average value of a meter angle is about 6 Δ. The CA/C is inversely related to age (Fig. 15.4).

The CA/C ratio can be measured clinically using pinholes before each eye or using a "blurfree" grating target (DOG or difference of Gaussians) (Fig. 15.5). These techniques open the accommodative system loop so that stimulation of accommodation by vergence is completely effective. The clinician who wishes to assess the CA/C can use a Wesson DOG card (34) and perform MEM retinoscopy, with bifixation on the central bright target region, while the patient fuses disparity stimulation of 12 Δ base-in (BI), 0 Δ, and 12 Δ base-out (BO). The MEM findings can be determined at each vergence level, the change averaged (assuming linearity), and the CA/C ratio computed.

Although not yet commonly assessed clinically, measurement of the CA/C ratio has implications concerning the treatment of patients with greater exo at distance than at near (divergence excess exodeviations). When the divergence excess patient converges to fuse at distance, there will usually be excess accommodation stimulated, due to CA/C. For divergence excess patients who cannot inhibit this extra accommodation, small amounts of added minus lens power, over and above the distance monocular subjective findings, may help maintain clear single binocular

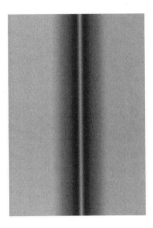

FIG. 15.5. The convergence accommodation ratio can be measured clinically using pinholes before each eye or using a "blurfree" grating target (DOG or difference of Gaussians).

vision. This becomes less of a problem as the patient ages and the CA/C decreases. This may explain why some intermittent exotropia patients have increased binocular skills with age, even though they have had no therapeutic intervention other than wearing a refractive correction (35).

AC/A Ratio

Measurement of the AC/A ratio, which provides insight into the relative strength of the crosslink from the accommodative system to vergence, is one of the most common clinical evaluations. In most clinical tests, the stimulus AC/A ratio is determined and the accommodative response is often simply assumed to equal the accommodative stimulus. However, the response AC/A ratio can be determined using MEM retinoscopy in the clinic, or a research optometer in the laboratory, and determining both the change in vergence and the accommodative response. In normal patients, the response AC/A ratio is about 10% greater than the stimulus AC/A because the accommodative response is typically slightly less than the accommodative stimulus (23). In patients with abnormal binocular vision, such as those with divergence excess strabismus, this difference may be substantially greater. For young adults, the AC/A ratio is about 4.0 per diopter (36). The AC/A remains about the same, until the onset of presbyopia (37) (Fig. 15.6).

To measure the stimulus AC/A ratio, the disparity or fusional vergence system is made open loop, either by occlusion or introduction of a vertical dissociating prism before one eye. As described in Chapter 1, the stimulus to accommodation is altered in the fellow eye using negative lenses at a fixed near target distance (gradient technique) or by making the measurements at distance and near and calculating the AC/A (calculated method).

With the gradient technique, the patient is dissociated with prism and a detailed target is provided to the fixating eye. The heterophoria is measured with the distance prescription and with an additional 1.00 and 2.00 D. To determine the AC/A ratio, the accommodative convergence measured at each stimulus level can be averaged, since the AC/A is generally linear. When measuring the AC/A ratio using the distance/near heterophoria method, a detailed target is presented at distance and then at near. The heterophoria is assessed at these two distances and the AC/A ratio is calculated, as described in Chapter 1. With either technique, multiple measurements should be obtained at each stimulus level and averaged.

The AC/A is routinely measured by virtually all clinicians. However, there are some important points that vision research has developed concerning measurement and use of the stimulus AC/A ratio. First, use of minus lenses is preferred when determining the AC/A using the near gradient technique. Minus lenses stimulate within the linear region of the accommodative

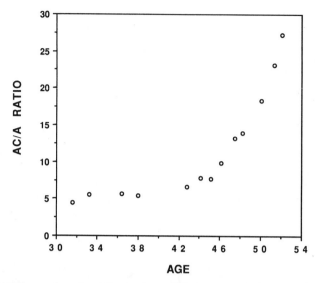

FIG. 15.6. The AC/A remains about the same until the onset of presbyopia. For young adults, the average AC/A ratio is about 4.0 per diopter. (From Eskridge JB. The AC/A ratio and age—a longitudinal study. *Am J Optom Physiol Opt* 1983;60:911–913 and Morgan MW. Clinical measurements of accommodation and vergence. *Am J Optom* 1944;21:301–313, with permission.)

stimulus/response function (Fig. 15.3), making stimulation of accommodation more effective than relaxation for obtaining a realistic measure of blur-driven accommodation. Of course, measures can also be made to determine the effect of plus lenses on the near heterophoria, patient comfort, relative vergence, and accommodation ranges. Second, for diagnostic and management purposes, the calculated method, in which distance is used to alter the stimulus,

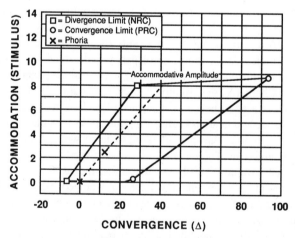

FIG. 15.7. At the limits of fusion, the proximal-based interactive model predicts that the boundaries of the zone of clear single binocular vision should be two straight, but not parallel, lines. In contrast to Fig. 15.1, the convergence side of the zone is more slanted than the divergence side, especially at maximal levels of accommodation, as more proximal vergence is introduced via increased "nearness." In addition, the top of the zone is not parallel to the bottom, due to increased accommodation from convergence driven accommodation.

TABLE 15.1. *Delineation of phoria predictors*

	Strabismus		Heterophoria								
			Low AC/A (16%)			Normal AC/A (68%)			High AC/A (16%)		
	Esophoria	Exophoria	Tonic vergence			Tonic vergence			Tonic vergence		
			Low (3%)	Norm (94%)	High (3%)	Low (3%)	Norm (94%)	High (3%)	Low (3%)	Norm (94%)	High (3%)
Expected per 100	3−	2+	1−	14	1−	2+	64	2+	1−	14	1−
Category			Convergence insufciency		DI	BExo	Norm	BEso	DE	Convergence excess	

DI, divergence insufficiency; BExo, basic exo; BEso, basic eso; DE, divergence excess.

is preferred over the gradient technique, in which lenses are used to alter the accommodative stimulus. The calculated method includes influences of proximal vergence in the measure and provides a more useful AC/A estimate, since proximal effects are present in all normal seeing conditions.

The AC/A ratio has a normal distribution (Fig. 15.7). When combined with the leptokertotic distribution of the distance phoria, the two measures (Fig. 15.7) can be used to roughly predict the numbers of patients who will be seen with any given distance and near phoria combination. Table 15.1 delineates these relations. The numbers suggest that there will be few patients with basic eso- or exophoria, and relatively more will be seen who have convergence insufficiency and convergence excess. These predictions are similar to recent findings by Scheiman et al. (38) on grade school children and Porcar and Nartinez-Palomera (39) on university students.

Relationship Between Convergence Accommodation and AC/A

In general, the interactive model in Fig. 15.2 predicts that disparity vergence and accommodative vergence change in opposite directions when the stimulus to accommodation is held constant. When disparity vergence increases, accommodative vergence decreases. The reason for the reciprocal action can be traced to the negative feedback system. When the accommodative stimulus is constant, a change in vergence causes an opposite change in accommodation, due to interactions between vergence and accommodation and the negative feedback loop in the accommodative system.

Disparity vergence and the dissociated heterophoria are influenced by the response AC/A and the response CA/C. Assuming that proximal vergence is held constant in the measurements, consider two situations:

1. When CA/C and AC/A are weakly related, the amount of disparity vergence required will be much larger than predicted from measures of the dissociated heterophoria. As an example, consider the situation of an exophoric patient when an occluder is removed from one eye. Initially disparity vergence and increased proximal vergence with binocular viewing help bring the eyes to the appropriate binocular position. However, this change in vergence causes an increase in accommodation due to vergence accommodation, which means that reflex accommodation must be changed to compensate if clear vision is to be maintained, since the accommodative stimulus remains constant. This, in turn, decreases accommodative vergence and more accommodative vergence is required. Consequently, except for the fact that proximal vergence is larger under binocular conditions as a partial compensation, the

final amount of the disparity vergence would be larger than predicted from measures of the dissociated heterophoria.

2. When the AC/A and CA/C are strongly related, the disparity vergence used may, in fact, be in a direction opposite to the dissociated heterophoria. To understand this, consider another exophoric patient. Suppose that to regain fusion after an occluder is removed, proximal vergence increases under binocular conditions and disparity vergence converges the eyes to enable fusion to be regained. Just as in the previous case, accommodation is stimulated and reflex accommodation must be inhibited. However, the effect of accommodative interactions may be larger than disparity vergence and, consequently, the eyes may overconverge. When the eyes finally reach the target, disparity vergence must be in the opposite direction to the initial dissociated heterophoria. This prediction helps explain why near plus additions are clinically useful to improve binocular responses of some exophoric patients, contrary to classical predictions. The prediction also explains why esofixation disparity and esoassociated phoria are seen during clinical measurement of some exophoric patients (40).

The relationship between the CA/C and AC/A critically determines the binocular responses described above. When the ratio becomes about 1.00, the model suggests an unstable relationship and compromised binocularity (41). Clinically, this occurs most frequently in the presence of a high AC/A ratio, where the demands on fusional vergence are underestimated when predicted from monocular heterophoria measures. This may explain why full correction of the angle of strabismus with prism is frequently necessary in esotropia with normal correspondence before binocularity can be enhanced with vision therapy.

CLINICAL TESTING

In the preceding sections, current research findings were discussed to clarify tonic, accommodative, and proximal vergence. In the following section, the model and current research will be considered with respect to the typical examination done by many clinicians.

Near Point of Convergence

The far point of convergence is represented by the intersection of the lines of sight when the eyes are in a position of minimum convergence, usually within a few minutes of arc of infinity. Assessment of the near point of convergence stimulates accommodative, disparity, and proximal vergence maximally, and interactions of all of these are included in the ultimate result. In normal persons, the amplitude of convergence is approximately 120 Δ (about 20 meter angles).

Repeated or sustained measures of the near point of convergence stimulate tonic vergence in some patients, evidenced by a transient convergent shift in the distance heterophoria. For patients who complain of transient blur or diplopia when shifting gaze from distance to near, sustained measures of the near point of convergence may help identify whether the accommodative or vergence system is at fault. If vergence is at fault, the model predicts that distance diplopia will occur without blur, while, if the accommodative system is implicated, distance blur will occur either alone or with diplopia. This is consistent with observations that patients with intermittent vertical strabismus typically only report diplopia; no accommodative component is present in vertical strabismus.

Relative Fusional Vergence

During patient examinations, fusional vergence measurements are performed at distance and near using loose or rotary prisms in free space and/or through a phoropter. Loose prism measurements, which are presented in discrete steps, provide a useful indication of fusional ranges as well as recovery ability. Rotary prism measurement of vergence ranges through the phoropter can frequently be eliminated from the test sequence when forced vergence fixation disparity curves are measured.

When testing fusional vergence, the vergence stimulus is gradually changed while the accommodative stimulus remains constant. To maintain target clarity, the model suggests that accommodation driven through the CA/C ratio must be inhibited. For example, assume that the patient bifixates a target. Introducing base-out prisms forces the eyes to increase convergence to maintain fusion. Concurrently, the accommodative response increases due to increased vergence accommodation, with the magnitude related to the CA/C ratio. Thus, vergence-driven accommodation increases and blur-driven accommodation must be inhibited to maintain clear vision. According to the model in Fig. 15.2, the blur limit of the test is reached when blur-driven accommodation can no longer be inhibited. As disparity is increased beyond the blur limit, diplopia results when fusion is no longer possible.

Prism Flipper

Prism flippers are related to relative vergence range testing. However, rather than gradually increasing disparity, the prism flipper introduces comparatively large disparity steps (e.g., 12 Δ BO and 6 Δ BI). During testing, there are changes in the vergence stimulus, vergence response, and accommodative response as described previously. However, the prism flipper is a dynamic test in which frequency of the change is assessed over time, allowing inferences regarding dynamic aspects of vision (e.g., copying from the blackboard). Additionally, the large disparity steps of the prism flipper may "stress" an abnormal vergence system more than the gradual changes in vergence demand used in the fusional vergence measurement. As a result, the prism flipper may have greater diagnostic capabilities for patients who complain of problems when changing fixation distances.

Accommodative Vergence

Because of the interactions between the accommodative and vergence systems shown in Fig. 15.2, the conclusions made when discussing the vergence system also relate to the accommodative system. When looking from distance to near, the convergence required to bifoveally fixate a target causes an amount of accommodation determined by the convergence demand and the CA/C ratio (due to the crosslinkage between the vergence and accommodative systems). When the CA/C has an "average" (0.50 D/MA 42) magnitude, the amount of accommodation generated by convergence is about 1.25 D.[2] Because of the refractive technique, depth of focus of the eye, and lag of accommodation at near, the amount accommodation changes when looking from distance to near is also approximately 1.25 to 1.50 D (Fig. 15.3). Thus, accommodation caused by convergence makes up a large portion of the accommodative response so that the system is within the ranges where blur-driven accommodation can "fine-tune" the response.

When the CA/C is greater than 0.5 D/MA, as it frequently is for young (grade school age) children (18), there may be more accommodation than needed for near tasks. This could require inhibition of the excess—possibly seen as a lead of accommodation if there is no inhibition, accommodative instability, or as an excessively high lag at near if the excess accommodation is overinhibited. When excess accommodation is not appropriately inhibited, there could be a

---

[2]Determined by multiplying convergence accommodation by the convergence demand: 0.50 D/6 Δ × 15 Δ = 1.25 D.

convergent shift after prolonged near work. These factors may partially explain the apparently accommodation-based asthenopic symptoms frequently seen in the school age group. The model in Fig. 15.2 suggests that small amounts of plus at near would be beneficial as a preventative measure, if prescribed prior to the development of accommodative excess. The plus lenses would counteract the adverse relationship of CA/C interactions with accommodation, allowing more accurate use of the lag of accommodation for clear near vision. Integrative analysis can be used to determine these relationships (Chapter 2).

Accommodative Parameters: Lag, Depth of Focus

According to usual convention, accommodative response is considered to be zero when the refractive error is fully corrected and the retina is conjugate to optical infinity. However, the accommodative response must be considered with respect to actual clinical findings. The refractive technique, influenced by the depth of focus of the eye and tonic accommodation, allows a residual accommodative activity and therefore the actual accommodative response is greater than the stimulus at distance (Fig. 15.3). Clinical measurements at near indicate that the typical lag of accommodation is approximately 0.25 to 0.50 D (42). The aggregate of these findings often causes the total accommodative response to be only about one half of the accommodative stimulus. Clinical findings on symptomatic patients can indicate a much higher lag of accommodation, even up to 1.50 D in young patients, which is occasionally seen (42). Integrative analysis routinely requires assessment of the actual lag of accommodation so that application of interactive models of accommodation and convergence can be made to clinical findings.

Binocular Amplitude of Accommodation

The binocular amplitude of accommodation represents the dioptric range between the farthest and the nearest point of clear vision under normal fused viewing. For simplicity, the far point of accommodation is assumed to be at infinity (the approximately 0.5 D normal depth of focus is ignored). During measurement, the stimulus is brought progressively closer to the patient until the first sustained blur is reported. This value is approximately 0.5 D greater than the monocular accommodative amplitude. The model suggests that this increase is due to added vergence drive to the accommodative system (CA/C).

Relative Accommodation

In evaluation of relative accommodation, the binocular stimulus to accommodation is systematically altered while maintaining a constant vergence stimulus. The clinician binocularly introduces either plus negative relative accommodation (NRA) or minus positive relative accommodation (PRA) lenses in 0.25 D steps. This alters the accommodative response, while vergence (fusion and fixation disparity) is maintained within Panum's area. Small changes in apparent target distance may also slightly alter the proximal effects. Testing of relative accommodation assesses the flexibility in the linkage between accommodation and vergence.

To clinically measure relative accommodation requires the patient to bifixate a detailed target. Upon introduction of, say, minus lenses, the eyes are transiently driven to converge by the increased accommodation and corresponding accommodative vergence. To maintain fusion and return the target to the center of Panum's fusional area requires an immediate compensatory stimulus to negative fusional vergence (NFV) to place the target back toward the center of Panum's area, but there is a relative increase in esofixation disparity. In the absence of the compensatory vergence response, this relative increase in convergent error would become progressively larger with additional minus lenses, until diplopia resulted (although most patients without a very high AC/A ratio maintain fusion and report a blurred image). Thus, as the model in Fig. 15.2 suggests, the blur point on relative accommodation testing indicates the amount that vergence can be inhibited, while maintaining clear vision as accommodation is stimulated. The magnitude of the relative accommodation finding is determined by the vergence range and the AC/A ratio.

Under clinical test conditions, interactions between accommodation and vergence are assessed simultaneously; the disparity vergence response is not determined in isolation from accommodative vergence. However, this has been performed experimentally by measuring fixation disparity curves through pinholes so that blur feedback was not available and only the disparity vergence system responded. Accommodative interactions account for up to 50% of the measured fixation disparity found under normal viewing conditions. These findings support the theory that accommodative abnormalities can contribute to vergence dysfunction.

Clinical testing in the future might incorporate assessment of forced vergence fixation disparity curves with and without pinholes. Such testing would allow the clinician to differentiate the contribution of accommodation from that of disparity in the vergence response. Treatment might then be more specifically tailored toward one system rather than the other.

Lens Flipper

The lens flipper test is related to relative accommodation testing. However, rather than introducing small sequential steps of defocus, the flipper test introduces large changes, typically ±2.00 D (a total of 4 D). During lens flipper testing, there are changes in the accommodative stimulus, accommodative response, and vergence response. As with the prism flipper, the lens flipper is a dynamic test where the frequency of the stimulus and system response change is assessed over time so that inferences regarding sustained clear near vision can be made. Lens flipper ability gives an accurate assessment of relative accommodative ability at high demand levels. The model in Fig. 15.2 predicts that the lens flipper test produces considerable vergence "stress." As a result, it may have particularly useful diagnostic capabilities. The flipper test is an integral part of integrative analysis (Chapter 2).

Zone of Single Binocular Vision

Determining the maximum convergent and divergent disparity that the system can handle gives a situation that drives the vergence system to its limit. At the limits of fusion, the proximal-based interactive model predicts that the boundaries of the zone should be two straight, but not parallel, lines. The convergence side of the zone is more slanted than the divergence side, especially at maximal levels of accommodation, as more proximal vergence is introduced via increased "nearness" (Fig. 15.7). As convergence stimulation increases, accommodation increases due to CA/C, causing a convergence "spike" at maximum accommodation. Due to influences of CA/C, there should also be a divergence "spike" at zero accommodation (43).

Similarly, accommodation can be driven to its limit, represented by a line with a slope equal to the CA/C ratio. This represents the top of the zone of clear single binocular vision. However, there is a difference between this zone and the classical zone. In the classical zone, the top portion is represented by a flat line, the location of which is determined by the accommodative amplitude. The model discussed here represents the top portion of the zone by a tilted line that is determined by the binocular accommodative amplitude, which is, in turn, related to the value of the stimulus CA/C ratio. Of course, the upper limit of the two zones becomes similar, as the patient ages and the CA/C ratio approaches zero.

Vergence Adaptation

The stimulus to disparity vergence is the difference in image disparity between the angle subtended by the fixation target and the angle of convergence of the eyes after proximal vergence has brought the eyes nearly to binocular fixation. Vergence adaptation is stimulated by the effort of the disparity vergence system (44). Within one second, proximal vergence and disparity vergence reduce retinal image disparity to less then 28 seconds of arc (26). Vergence adaptation occurs well after this and serves to reduce the demand on disparity vergence to a minimum by resetting the "zero point" so that less vergence is required to maintain fusion. Asymmetries in vergence adaptation—to different prism stimuli (base-in or base-out)—cause different fixation disparity curve types (45), and the same asymmetries also cause symptoms of binocular discomfort when binocularity is insufficient.

Stimulating disparity vergence for several minutes with prism often results in prolonged alteration of the heterophoria in the direction of the prism stimulus (20). Changes in the heterophoria with prism stimulation have been proposed as evidence of a slow-acting fusional vergence change known as vergence adaptation, which exists under binocular viewing conditions (45). A clinical estimate of the magnitude of vergence adaptation can be obtained by assessing the change in tonic vergence (distance heterophoria) immediately after a period of sustained near vision. Although this information is not routinely gathered clinically at the present time, it may prove useful in the future after further research.

The model in Fig. 15.2 suggests that adaptation of disparity vergence would not be stimulated during measurement of the near point of convergence, since there has been no sustained bifixation at a fixed near distance. However, repeated measurement of the near point of convergence does transiently affect tonic vergence in some individuals. In symptomatic patients with a receded near point of convergence, the increased effort to converge and maintain fusion seems to be sufficient to elicit a vergence adaptive response. This suggests that these patients have very rapid adaptive responses. As such, assessment of distance tonic vergence of these individuals may be important diagnostically.

Fixation Disparity

Fixation disparity is the result of an incomplete vergence response to the stimulus. Although the eyes are brought within Panum's area, they may not maintain exact bifoveal alignment; the remaining residual misalignment is termed fixation disparity. Schor (45) proposed that the fixation disparity is a steady-state error that enables disparity vergence to maintain fusion. In this view, fixation disparity serves as a control for the vergence system and acts to stimulate continued vergence to maintain binocular alignment.

A fixation disparity is usually of the magnitude of 6 seconds of arc and is virtually never greater than 30 seconds of arc (46). In general, fixation disparity is in the direction of the heterophoria, but, for some patients seen clinically, the fixation disparity will be in the opposite direction of the heterophoria (40). This may result from an abnormal relationship between CA/C and AC/A. The model in Fig. 15.2 predicts that fixation disparity will change nonlinearly with alteration in the vergence demand. These nonlinearities, which are caused by CA/C (47) and vergence adaptation (40), are represented by the four different shapes of fixation disparity curves (Fig. 15.8). Persons who have more vergence adaptation to base-out prism have type II curves and persons who have type III curves have more adaptation to base-in prism (46).

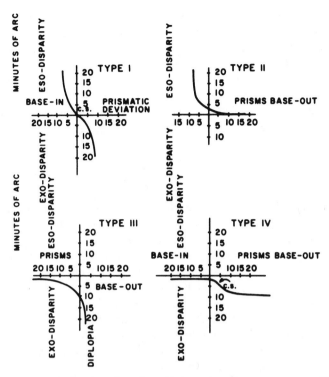

FIG. 15.8. Nonlinearities in fixation disparity with forced vergence are caused by convergence accommodation and vergence adaptation. These nonlinearities are represented by the four different shapes of fixation disparity curves.

Clinical studies (48) indicate that analyzing binocular vision, using forced vergence fixation disparity techniques, is useful for detecting patients likely to have binocular symptoms and results in appropriate prism prescriptions with good prognosis for relieving binocular symptoms. Curves with steep slopes, high associated heterophorias, and large fixation disparities are found more frequently when testing symptomatic patients (4). Asymptomatic patients usually have type I curves. Other curve types are frequently associated with patients who have large heterophorias (type II eso, type III exo). For pre-presbyopic patients, type IV curves are considered to be associated with symptoms and caused by unstable binocularity due to abnormal CA/C interactions. Presbyopic patients, who have type IV curves more frequently, do not have CA/C and therefore do not have the associated symptoms (32). Fixation disparity curves are assessed in integrative analysis to help design prism prescriptions for patients with esophorias and hyperphorias and to monitor effects of various interventions.

LENS/PRISM THERAPY

Addition of prism or lens power will change the accommodation vergence interactions. For example, consider an esophoric patient with a greater esophoria at near than distance—convergence excess. Because the patient is overconverged, there is a high amount of convergence-associated accommodation to inhibit. As a result, to maintain clear near vision, accommodative vergence must be used that tends to stimulate more esophoria. Near plus lenses and/or prism are prescribed to make accommodative inhibition easier, reduce the demand to a reasonable amount, and improve binocular responses.

Clinical implications of the model for convergence excess patients are that esophoric patients generally have more blur-driven accommodative demands (AC/A) than exophoric patients whose accommodation comes as a result of convergence (CA/C). Clinical findings have shown that convergence excess patients have more proximal vergence and higher response AC/As than average (48). For esophores, effects of near plus lenses can be determined by considering the estimated lens power, in conjunction with the relationship between the response AC/A and response CA/C ratio. The changing relationship between CA/C and AC/A may also explain why young patients with exodeviations become less symptomatic (49), as their CA/C ratio decreases with age.

CONCLUSION

A model of binocular vision system interactions has been discussed that treats the accommodative and vergence systems as negative feedback systems with "cross talk" between the two systems. This "cross talk" is accommodative vergence and vergence accommodation. The model incorporates proximal vergence, as well as accommodative lag and the depth of focus of the eye, in an attempt to more closely account for common clinical findings.

Clinical implications of this model are best understood by considering the examples in this chapter. Many clinical patients have findings that are accurately explained by the model in Fig. 15.2 (50). The model allows for the common clinical findings of large lags in accommodation and explains why patients can have a large lag and maintain binocularity. Proximal vergence helps explain why presbyopic patients, who lose accommodative vergence, remain asymptomatic. For many patients seen clinically, vergence and accommodative responses are not equal to the stimuli, due to proximal vergence and interactions between accommodative vergence and vergence accommodation. Binocular interactions also help explain why the dissociated and associated phoria frequently differ in magnitude. We based integrative analysis (introduced in Chapter 2) on the model and other current binocular vision research. Integrative analysis thus allows enhanced assessment of binocular findings with improved results over previous systems of analysis.

STUDY QUESTIONS

1. Why is the AC/A derived from calculated measures typically different from that measured using gradient measures?
2. Why is the push-up amplitude of accommodation different when measured monocularly and binocularly?
3. What effect does the CA/C ratio have on measures of fusional vergence?
4. Is the leptokertotic distribution of tonic vergence a significant influence on the distribution of the near phoria?
5. In examining 100 pre-presbyopic patients, what is the single most important factor that determines the distribution of the near phoria?
6. When the patient has a maximum plus refraction and looks from distance to near, how does the accommodation stimulus/response curve predict the amount of accommodative change?
7. How could a patient with a convergence insufficiency (phoria; distance, 1 Δ exo; near, 11 Δ exo) have a normal AC/A when measured with a gradient test?
8. Why might a divergence excess patient report blurred distance vision when he or she fuses? (Hint: present one reason related to CA/C and one to AC/A.)
9. Why are pinholes used when determining the CA/C ratio?
10. How might we explain an increase in esophoria after measures of fusional convergence?

REFERENCES

1. Joubert C. *Proximal vergence and perceived distance* [master's thesis]. Houston, Tex: University of Houston College of Optometry, 1986.
2. Schor CM, Narayen V. Graphical analysis of prism adaptation, convergence accommodation, and accommodative vergence. *Am J Optom Physiol Opt* 1982;59:774–784.
3. Schor CM. The analysis of tonic and accommodative vergence disorders of binocular vision. *Am J Optom Physiol Opt* 1983;59:114.
4. Sheedy JE, Saladin JJ. Association of symptoms with measures of oculomotor deficiencies. *Am J Optom Physiol Opt* 1978;55:670–676.
5. Hoffstetter HW. Graphical analysis. In: Schor CM, Ciuffreda KJ, eds. *Vergence eye movements: basic and clinical aspects.* Boston: Butterworth-Heinemann, 1983:439–462.
6. Hendrickson H. The why of OEP. *J Am Optom Assoc* 1978;49:603–604.
7. Morgan MW. Analysis of clinical data. *Am J Optom Arch Am Acad Optom* 1944;21:477–491.
8. Jones R, Stephens GL. Convergence accommodation and the zone of clear single binocular vision. *Am Acad Optom* Annual Meeting, Dec. 1986.
9. Fry GA. Basic concepts underlying graphical analysis. In: Schor CM, Ciuffreda KJ, eds. *Vergence eye movements: basic and clinical aspects.* Boston: Butterworth-Heinemann, 1983:403–438.
10. Hofstetter HW. The zone of clear single binocular vision. *Am J Optom Arch Am Acad Optom* 1945;22:301–333, 361–384.
11. Hofstetter HW. Orthoptic specification by the graphical method. *Am J Optom Arch Am Acad Optom* 1949;26:439–444.
12. Sheard C. Zones of ocular comfort. *Am J Optom Arch Am Acad Optom* 1930;7:925.
13. Percival AS. *The prescribing of spectacles*, 3rd ed. Bristol, UK: J Wright & Sons, 1928.
14. Manas L. *Visual analysis*, 3rd ed. Chicago: Professional Press, 1965.
15. Haines HF. Normative values of visual functions and their application to case analysis. *Am J Optom Arch Am Acad Optom* 1941;18:18.
16. Goss DA. *Ocular accommodation, convergence, and fixation disparity: a manual of clinical analysis.* New York: Professional Press, 1986.
17. Ogle KN, Martens TG, Dyer JA. *Oculomotor imbalance in binocular vision and fixation disparity.* Philadelphia: Lea & Febiger, 1967.
18. Wick B, Currie D. Dynamic demonstration of proximal vergence and proximal accommodation. *Optom Vis Sci* 1991;68:163–167.
19. Hokoda SC, Ciufreda KJ. Theoretical and clinical importance of proximal vergence and accommodation. In: Schor CM, Ciuffreda KJ, eds. *Vergence eye movements: basic and clinical aspects.* Boston: Butterworth-Heinemann, 1983:75–98.
20. Fisher SK, Ciuffreda KJ, Tannen B, et al. Stability of tonic vergence. *Invest Ophthalmol Vis Sci* 1988;29:1577–1581.
21. Heath GG. Components of accommodation. *Am J Optom Arch Am Acad Optom* 1956;33:569–579.
22. Flom MC. Variations in convergence and accommodation induced by successive spherical lens additions with distance fixation—an investigation. *Am J Optom Arch Am Acad Optom* 1955;32:111–136.
23. Rouse MW, Hutter RF, Shiftlett R. A normative study of the accommodative lag in elementary school children. *Am J Optom Physiol Opt* 1984;61:693–697.
24. Wick B. Clinical factors in proximal vergence. *Am J Optom Physiol Opt* 1985;62:119.
25. Joubert C, Bedell HE. Proximal vergence and perceived distance. *Optom Vis Sci* 1990;67:29–35.
26. Ogle KN. *Researches in binocular vision.* New York: Hafner, 1972:76–81.
27. Wick B, Bedell HE. Magnitude and velocity of proximal vergence. *Invest Ophthalmol Vis Sci* 1989;30:755–759.
28. Zuber BL, Stark L. Dynamical characteristics of the fusional vergence eye movement system. *IEEE Trans Syst Man Cybern* 1968;4:72–79.
29. Semmlow JL, Hung GK, Ciuffreda KJ. Quantitative assessment of disparity vergence components. *Invest Ophthalmol Vis Sci* 1986;27:558–564.
30. Hung GK, Semmlow JL, Sun L, et al. Vergence control of central and peripheral disparities. *Exp Neurol* 1991;113:202–211.
31. Morse S, Wick B. Abnormal adaptation to proximal cues influences tonic accommodation. *Invest Ophthalmol Vis Sci* 1991;30[Suppl]:134.
32. Borish I. *Clinical refraction.* Chicago: Professional Press, 1970.
33. Alpern M, Mason GL, Jardinico RE. Vergence and accommodation. V. Pupil size changes associated with changes in accommodative vergence. *Am J Ophthalmol* 1961;52:762–767.
34. Wesson MD, Koenig R. A new clinical method for direct measurement of fixation disparity. *South J Optom* 1983;1:48–52.
35. Hiles DA, Davies GT, Costenbader FR. Longterm observations on unoperated intermittent exotropia. *Arch Ophthalmol* 1968;80:436–442.
36. Morgan MW. Clinical measurements of accommodation and vergence. *Am J Optom* 1944;21:301–313.
37. Eskridge JB. The AC/A ratio and age—a longitudinal study. *Am J Optom Physiol Opt* 1983;60:911–913.
38. Scheiman M, Gallaway M, Coulter R, et al. Prevalence of vision and ocular disease conditions in a clinical pediatric population. *J Am Optom Assoc* 1996;67:193–202.

39. Porcar E, Nartinez-Palomera A. Prevalence of general dysfunctions in a population of university students. *Optom Vis Sci* 1997;74:111–113.
40. Sheedy JE. Fixation disparity analysis of oculomotor imbalance. *Am J Optom Physiol Opt* 1980;57:632–639.
41. Schor CM. Fixation disparity and vergence adaptation. In: Schor CM, Ciuffreda KJ, eds. *Vergence eye movements: basic and clinical aspects*. Boston: Butterworth-Heinemann, 1983:465–516.
42. Fincham EF, Walton J. The reciprocal actions of accommodation and convergence. *J Physiol* 1957;137:488–508.
43. Jones R. Horizontal disparity vergence. In: Schor CM, Ciuffreda KJ, eds. *Vergence eye movements: basic and clinical aspects*. Boston: Butterworth-Heinemann, 1983:297–316.
44. Schor CM, Homer D. Adaptive disorders of accommodation and vergence in binocular dysfunction. *Ophthalmol Physiol Opt* 1989;9:264–268.
45. Schor CM. The influence of rapid prism adaptation upon fixation disparity. *Vision Res* 1979;19:757–765.
46. Carter DB. Studies in fixation disparity—historical review. *Am J Optom Arch Am Acad Optom* 1957;34:320–329.
47. Semmlow JL, Hung GK. Accommodative and fusional components of fixation disparity. *Invest Ophthalmol Vis Sci* 1979;18:1082–1086.
48. Borish IM. *Clinical refraction*, 3rd ed. Chicago: Professional Press, 1975.
49. von Noorden GK, Morris J, Edelman P. Efficacy of bifocals in the treatment of accommodative esotropia. *Am J Ophthalmol* 1978;85:830–834.
50. Ciuffreda KJ. Components of clinical near-vergence testing. *J Behav Optom* 1992;3:313.

16

Refractive Amblyopia

Included among the amblyopic patients are those whose amblyopia results from uncorrected refractive errors. Such amblyopia is of particular clinical importance because of its prevalence, prognosis, and relative ease of management. Since many patients with refractive amblyopia are not strabismic, their treatment requires only slight modification of the binocular procedures described in previous chapters.

The study of amblyopia is frequently a study of the effects of vision deprivation. From the investigations of Wiesel and Hubel (1) to current studies, it is clear that deprivation occurring in early life has dramatic long-lasting effects on the visual system (2). The essence of animal research is that vision deprivation, such as is produced by lid suture, results in a variety of anatomic and physiologic changes throughout the visual pathway (3). Anatomic changes associated with lid suture are typically more extensive at the lateral geniculate nucleus (LGN) (4), while physiologic changes are more pronounced and varied in the visual cortex (5). Detailed reviews of these findings often provide clinically relevant information (6), including two concepts that directly affect the management of anisometropic and isoametropic amblyopia. These concepts—abnormal binocular competition and the critical period—are discussed below in the section on etiology.

In this chapter, we describe examination techniques and differential diagnosis and present a sequential management of refractive amblyopia that extends the treatment period well into adulthood. Virtually all amblyopic patients should have careful diagnosis and aggressive management. It is important to treat these patients and it is not acceptable to simply monitor them because it is possible to dramatically improve visual acuity and binocular function using sequential considerations of (a) correction of the refractive error, (b) added lenses and/or prisms to improve fusion, (c) part time direct occlusion, and (d) vision therapy to improve monocular and binocular function.

ETIOLOGY AND PREVALENCE OF REFRACTIVE AMBLYOPIA

Definition

Amblyopia is defined as a reduction of corrected visual acuity to 20/30 or less in one eye or a two-line difference between the two eyes, in the absence of pathology (7). Refractive amblyopia may be subdivided into two categories, anisometropic and isoametropic. Anisometropic amblyopia occurs as a result of clinically significant and unequal amounts of uncorrected refractive error in each eye (7). The most ametropic eye develops amblyopia as a result of the unilaterally blurred retinal image. Isoametropic amblyopia results from the presence of very high, but clinically equal, uncorrected refractive errors (7). Both eyes become amblyopic as a result of bilateral visual deprivation from the significantly blurred retinal images of each eye.

Classification

Amblyopia has traditionally been classified in a dichotomy between organic and functional with various subclassifications (8) (Table 16.1). Von Noorden suggested classification of functional

TABLE 16.1. *Classification of amblyopia*

von Noorden	Traditional
Amblyopia exanopsia	Amblyopia exanopsia anisometropic strabismic
Anisometropic Ametropic	
	Isoametropic
Hysterical	Hysterical Isoametropic Light deprivation
Strabismic	

amblyopias based on clinical causes (9). Such a classification is based on the clinical conditions thought to be responsible for creating the amblyopia. In this chapter, we discuss two types of amblyopia, classified according to the refractive errors that result in the decrease in acuity, unilateral difference in refractive error (anisometropic), and significant bilateral refractive error (isoametropic).

Etiology

The factors that result in refractive amblyopia have been investigated in experimental studies on the effects of vision deprivation. In general, the primary factor that results in amblyopia is an uncorrected refractive error that does not permit clear retinal images of equal size and/or shape in each eye. These blurred images do not allow adequate stimulation of the visual system and amblyopia develops. Although refractive amblyopia is regarded as functional, as opposed to organic, the basic amblyogenic factors are much better understood than the term functional implies. Indeed, recent investigations have correlated the clinical conditions that result in amblyopia with resulting deficits in the basic underlying neurophysiology.

Abnormal Binocular Competition

The effects of deprivation are most significant when there is an imbalance in the visual input between the eyes. A competitive interaction exists between the two eyes during early visual development (10), and conditions that allow one eye a competitive advantage result in dramatic changes in the visual pathway of the disadvantaged eye. The accepted explanation for these changes involves a competition for synaptic space on cortical neurons (11). Neurons in the visual pathway of the disadvantaged eye decrease in function and number as a result of this competition, and pathways from the advantaged eye gradually gain more synapses. Thus, this basic science research suggests that genetic coding determines the initial neural pathways and early visual experience subsequently refines and maintains these connections. Abnormal visual experience disturbs the basic pattern and reduces visual capabilities in one or both eyes. Visual pathway changes are more difficult to demonstrate when the eyes are equally disadvantaged.

ANISOMETROPIC AMBLYOPIA

In patients with uncorrected anisometropia, the images falling on the two foveas have the same common visual direction and give rise to a single percept. However, the images may be of substantially different clarity. As a result, in uncorrected anisometropia, the foveal image of the most ametropic eye is likely to be suppressed. This cortical suppression or signal inhibition can eventually result in amblyopia, if it occurs for a sufficient time at the appropriate stage in development. Unfortunately, vision deprivation present in uncorrected anisometropia may escape early detection, since one eye sees clearly and there may be no signs or symptoms.

ISOAMETROPIC AMBLYOPIA

When there is an isoametropic refractive error, interference from dissimilar images does not occur. Thus, any resultant loss of acuity must be from lack of proper stimulation of the visual system (bilateral visual deprivation) during early development, rather than a result of congenital or organic amblyopia. For bilateral visual deprivation to occur, there must generally be a significant decrease in the visual input to both eyes. The most dramatic clinical example of bilateral visual deprivation occurs when an infant has congenital cataracts. Unless removal is initiated very early in life, the resultant acuity is substantially below normal (12). Refractive errors can also "deprive" the visual system of proper stimulation, but they must be very large and, even then, the visual loss is seldom severe (13), at least in comparison to that seen in patients with congenital cataracts.

Critical/Sensitive Period

Imbalances between the visual information reaching the two eyes have the most profound results early in development. Animal studies have established that there is a developmental period for anisometropic amblyopia that probably lasts through most of the first decade of life (14,15). Clinical observations also suggest a similar time course for amblyopia development (16,17). This developmental period can be roughly divided into two portions, a critical period and a sensitive period. The critical period is a relatively short duration of time of maximum sensitivity, perhaps lasting until age 3 in humans. During the longer-lasting sensitive period, the visual system is still susceptible to change, but damage is progressively less severe. The sensitive period probably begins at about age 3 and may last until around age 10. Imbalances that occur later have reduced or nonexistent effects. Certain anatomic changes coincide with these periods, allowing vision researchers to predict that human visual development continues through at least the first decade.

Plastic Period

The "critical" period for amblyopia development does not necessarily follow the same time course as the "plastic period," during which the amblyopic visual system is still amenable to successful treatment. Clinical evidence suggests that plasticity of the visual system remains for periods substantially longer than the first few years. For example, the dramatic response of adult patients with anisometropic amblyopia to treatment (18) suggests that residual plasticity remains in the human visual system for much longer periods than the critical period for development of amblyopia. The ability of older patients to recover from cerebral vascular accidents is further evidence that the human nervous system retains some plasticity throughout life. And, recent basic research studies in cats (19) show that the plastic period, during which the visual system can still change, extends well into adulthood.

PREVALENCE

Anisometropic Amblyopia

Flom and Neumaier (20) investigated the prevalence of amblyopia in 2,762 school children from kindergarten to the sixth grade. They found that 1% of the population had amblyopia, using a criterion of monocular uncorrected acuity of 20/40 or worse, with a difference between the eyes of more than one line of acuity. All children with amblyopia had either strabismus (38%), 1 diopter (D) or more of anisometropia (34%), or both conditions (28%).

The prevalence of amblyopia without strabismus was also summarized by Schapero (21), who determined (from data averaged from six studies) that 62% of amblyopes have binocular alignment of the visual axes. Although one cannot assume that all 62% of the nonstrabismic amblyopia was of refractive etiology, amblyopia appears to occur quite frequently in patients without strabismus. Since anisometropia occurs more frequently than unilateral strabismus, it is not surprising that anisometropic amblyopia occurs more frequently than strabismic amblyopia.

Isoametropic Amblyopia

There is little epidemiologic information concerning the prevalence of isoametropic amblyopia. Theodore et al. (22) surveyed 190,012 inducted soldiers; in a group labeled "unexplained amblyopia," they found 14 of 2,509 men (0.56%) had bilateral amblyopia. In a similar study, Agatson (23) found 7 of 20,000 inducted men to have bilateral amblyopia associated with high refractive errors. More recently, Abraham (24) used an amblyopia criterion of correctable acuity less than 20/25 and reported that 162 of 7,225 patients had bilateral amblyopia. He included patients with 5.00 D or more of hyperopia and/or 1.25 D of astigmatism.

Linksz (25) associated bilateral amblyopia with myopia and astigmatism rather than hyperopia. However, Abraham (24) definitively demonstrated that bilateral amblyopia occurs in a substantial number of patients with significant hyperopia and/or astigmatism. Similarly, Friedman et al. (26) suggested that bilateral hyperopia was the most common cause of amblyopia, in a series of 39 patients with marked ametropia.

The above studies suggest that bilateral amblyopia, secondary to uncorrected isoametropia, accounts for approximately 2% of nonstrabismic amblyopia. Although the true prevalence of bilateral amblyopia in the general population is unknown, Griffin (27) implied that the prevalence of isoametropic amblyopia is decreasing in countries where early vision examinations are emphasized.

AMBLYOPIA CHARACTERISTICS

Signs

Unfortunately, there are no reliable signs to make the patient, parent, or clinician suspect the presence of refractive amblyopia. When there is amblyopia, a very young child may rub his or her eyes and an older child or adult may squint to improve vision. However, these signs occur in a variety of refractive conditions and are not reliable indicators of the anisometropia that is most likely to produce refractive amblyopia.

Symptoms

Much of what was presented above also applies to the presence of symptoms. Complaints of blurred vision, headaches, and ocular discomfort are potential symptoms that patients with amblyopia may report, but it is also very likely that there will be no symptoms. There are only a few refractive situations that create the proper conditions for anisometropic or isoametropic amblyopia. The patient's age and visual requirements, along with the refractive status, all combine to determine whatever symptoms may be present, and there are many refractive conditions that cause symptoms without ever producing amblyopia.

CLINICAL CHARACTERISTICS

There are a variety of visual conditions that are characteristic of refractive amblyopia. Clinically, it is necessary to be familiar with the important characteristics of anisometropic or isoametropic amblyopia listed below.

Refractive Error

Jampolsky et al. (28) examined a sample of approximately 200 patients with nonstrabismic amblyopia and reported that the eye with the greater ametropia, regardless of the type of refractive error, had the greatest loss of acuity. However, this statement does not totally reflect the differential effect that hyperopia has on the development of amblyopia.

Hyperopia

Jampolsky et al. (28) found that hyperopia and/or astigmatism have a greater effect on visual acuity loss than myopia. In their study, the difference in power between the horizontal or the vertical meridians of the eyes was closely related to the unequal acuity—that is, the greater the anisometropia, the greater the amblyopia. Sugar (29) found similar results and concluded that hyperopic anisometropia was the predominating factor associated with nonstrabismic amblyopia. Hyperopic anisometropes had more amblyopia, and the amblyopia increased with the amount of hyperopia and the amount of anisometropia.

The reason for the greater prevalence of amblyopia in hyperopic anisometropia is primarily a result of the different image clarity and the accommodative response. The more hyperopic eye has a blurred image and the amount of blur depends on the amount of anisometropia. Since the eye with the lower refractive error typically accommodates for any near target, the more hyperopic eye always remains with a blurred image. Consequently, hyperopic anisometropia, in amounts greater than 1.25 D, may create sufficient long-term blur to cause a form of vision deprivation in the hyperopic eye. If this occurs, during the critical period during development amblyopia may result.

Myopia

The above studies document that the prevalence of amblyopia is greater in patients with hyperopic anisometropia than with myopic anisometropia. Indeed, in simple myopic anisometropia or anisomyopia, an amount of 5 or 6 D (or perhaps more) is necessary before one image is sufficiently and continuously blurred so that form vision deprivation and amblyopia result (28). Horwich (30) concurs that refractive amblyopia is not expected unless the myopia in the amblyopic eye is more than 6 D. He suggests that the possibility of maculopathy be investigated whenever decreased visual acuity is present in the most myopic eye.

Astigmatism

Astigmatic differences between the eyes can also contribute to development of amblyopia. The reduction of acuity for a given amount of uncorrected astigmatism is usually less than would occur with an equal amount of spherical hyperopic anisometropia (31). However, astigmatism may even be a greater deterrent to fusion than simple anisohyperopia when combined with hyperopic anisometropia. It is possible that uncorrected astigmatism of 1.50 D or more (depending on axis position) might cause enough image blur to result in amblyopia, as accommodation is also unable to compensate for this refractive error (32).

Fixation Characteristics

In almost all cases of anisometropic and isoametropic amblyopia, fixation is unsteady and central (33). Given central fixation as a primary characteristic, an important differential diagnosis for refractive amblyopia is objective assessment of fixation. Assessment is facilitated using direct ophthalmoscopes with fixation targets incorporated in the illumination system (34) (Fig. 16.1A). Since a characteristic of central fixation is stable subjective localization of objects in visual space, when the patient with central fixation fixates on the target projected on the retina, the fovea will be within the circular portion of the target (Fig. 16.1B). If eccentric fixation is present during ophthalmoscopy in an eye that is apparently without ocular deviation, a microtropia is probably present (35). This is an important diagnostic point because the prognosis for successful remediation of anisometropic amblyopia is much higher than that for microstrabismus.

Unilateral High Myopia

Patients with unilateral high myopia may be an exception to the rule that there is central fixation in anisometropic amblyopia. A high percentage of anisomyopic patients with amblyopia demonstrate eccentric fixation in the eye with the greatest myopia (36). Eccentric fixation is a common, although not necessarily constant, feature of this type of amblyopia.

Suppression Characteristics

Anisometropic Amblyopia

The suppression characteristics of 13 patients with anisoametropic amblyopia were investigated by Pratt-Johnson et al. (37). Under binocular testing conditions, 10 of 13 patients had small relative foveal suppression areas in the amblyopic eye. The suppression areas were never absolute and stimuli could always be perceived under binocular conditions, regardless of the acuity. While presenting similar results, Jampolsky (38) reported great variability between the age of onset, depth of suppression, fixation distance, and size of the suppression area.

Isoametropic Amblyopia

Pratt-Johnson et al. (37) also reported the suppression characteristics of five patients with isoametropic amblyopia. Three cases had no suppression scotoma one demonstrated alternating suppression, and one showed suppression in the more amblyopic eye. The scotomas were decreases in sensitivity that may have been a function of the existing amblyopia.

Crowding Phenomenon

Crowding phenomenon, or separation difficulty, describes the clinical finding that resolution ability is related to the separation of acuity targets (39). This phenomenon exists in all eyes, although it is particularly important in amblyopes with strabismus. Linksz (40) suggests that,

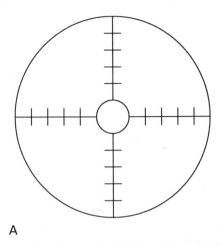

A

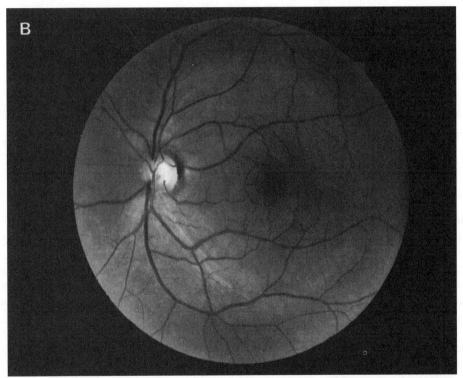

FIG. 16.1. A: Assessment of fixation is facilitated using direct ophthalmoscopes with fixation targets incorporated in the illumination system. The most common clinically available target is a circle with central grid lines. Each line represents 1 Δ of eccentric fixation. **B:** Since a characteristic of anisometropic amblyopia is central fixation, when the patient with central fixation fixates on the target projected on the retina, the fovea will be within the circular portion of the target. The presence of eccentric fixation during ophthalmoscopy generally indicates microtropia if there appears to be binocular alignment.

in cases of hyperopic anisometropic amblyopia, central fixation is present and there is also relatively normal separation difficulty. Maraini et al. (41) found no significant difference in separation difficulty between anisometropic amblyopes and normals. However, strabismic amblyopes had a significant difference in ability to correctly identify single versus crowded E's. The crowding phenomenon is thus a useful method for differential diagnosis of anisometropic or isoametropic amblyopia from strabismic amblyopia.

Electrodiagnostic Tests

Electrodiagnostic tests such as the electroretinogram (ERG) and the visually evoked response (VER) are used in the laboratory to investigate the visual system of subjects with amblyopia (42,43). These tests require a substantial commitment of cash and time and, as such, are not yet useful clinically. There have been differences shown between the responses of patients with strabismic and anisometropic amblyopia on some testing protocols (44) and these tests may prove clinically useful in the future.

COURSE AND PROGNOSIS

The course of refractive amblyopia is that visual acuity remains decreased as long as the underlying refractive condition goes untreated. The severity of the amblyopia depends on age of onset of the refractive error, the amount of anisometropia or isoametropia, changes in refractive error during the critical period, and perhaps to individual differences in sensitivity to vision deprivation.

The prognosis of refractive amblyopia is generally good for the recovery of improved levels of visual acuity. Improvement in visual acuity may also be found well into adulthood (45).

SEQUENTIAL MANAGEMENT PROTOCOL

There are many approaches to treatment of refractive amblyopia [see Amos (32) for a comprehensive review]. The ultimate goal of all therapy protocols for amblyopia is to achieve functional binocular vision with equal visual acuity. According to Flom (46), a functional cure results in equal visual acuity in each eye, along with comfortable single binocular vision at all distances, from the far point to a normal near point of convergence. There should be stereopsis and normal ranges of motor fusion. Corrective lenses and small amounts of prism may be worn if necessary; however, prismatic power is limited to 5 Δ.

In this section, we describe and give the rationale for treatment of refractive amblyopia. Our management recommendation for anisometropic amblyopia is a sequential program that consists of four steps: (a) full refractive correction, (b) added lenses or prism when needed to improve alignment of the visual axes, (c) 2 to 5 hours per day of direct occlusion, and (d) active vision therapy to develop best acuity and improve binocular function (Table 16.2). Isoametropic amblyopia can best be treated by simply prescribing the full refractive correction (13). Occasionally antisuppression therapy is also indicated, but generally the full refractive correction will yield the best possible result; usually there is gradual improvement in vision over the next few years, after the full correction is prescribed.

Determining Compliance

For management to be effective, substantial patient motivation is often required, especially when older children and adults are treated. Indeed, differences in patient compliance may

TABLE 16.2. *Sequential management of anisometropic amblyopia*

1. Full refractive correction
2. Improve alignment of the visual axes when needed
   a. Added lenses if:
      1) High AC/A
      2) Inaccurate or insufficient accommodation
   b. Prism if:
      1) Esophoric at distance (base-out)
      2) Hyperphoric (base-down)
3. Direct occlusion (part-time, 2 to 6 hr/d)
4. Vision therapy
   a. Monocular—maximize monocular acuity
   b. Binocular—improve binocular function

be the most common cause of variation in the results seen when treating amblyopia in older patients. It is important to anticipate patient noncompliance and take precautions to avoid this potentiality. To facilitate patient compliance and motivation, written instructions should accompany home therapy procedures and the therapy should be demonstrated and performed in the office so that the patient fully understands the tasks required. When home therapy is instituted, frequent office follow-up visits (every 2 to 3 weeks) are needed to monitor progress.

Case Study

Case 16.1: Isoametropic Amblyopia

The mother of a 5-year-old girl felt that her daughter sat too close to the television. This was the child's first eye examination. External and internal ocular health was within normal limits. Visual acuity and refraction with cycloplegia was:

RE: $+8.25$ c $- 1.00 \times 25$ 20/200 $- 1$
LE: $+8.75$ c $- 2.00 \times 005$ 20/100 $- 1$ OU 20/100

There was a comitant 5 Δ esophoria at 6 m and 40 cm. Stereopsis was 100 seconds at 40 cm with Randot circles. There was no suppression. Fixation was central with both eyes.

The cycloplegic refractive finding was prescribed and the patient was instructed to return for reevaluation in 1 month. She had worn the correction full time without complaint. Aided visual acuity (VA):

RE: 20/60 $- 2$
LE: 20/60
OU: 20/50

Over the next 3 years, the patient's acuity gradually improved to 20/25$-$, with only small changes in the refractive correction.

Refractive Correction

The first step that we recommend in our treatment sequence for anisometropic amblyopia is to fully correct the refractive error of each eye. A unilaterally blurred retinal image is generally considered to be the primary amblyogenic factor in anisometropic amblyopia, and full refractive corrections are routinely prescribed in treatment of amblyopia in young children. We suggest that a full refractive correction for each eye is required to achieve the maximum result from management for any patient. Thus, our goal is to prescribe, for each eye, the full plus lens power that completely corrects all anisometropia and astigmatism.

Refractive error should be determined with accommodation stabilized in each eye—a potential problem with anisometropic amblyopia, where the amblyopic eye sometimes has very inaccurate accommodation under monocular conditions. We suggest that refraction be performed with either binocular or cycloplegic evaluation. Such examinations are particularly applicable for patients with hyperopic anisometropia, where an eye that appears to be amblyopic under monocular conditions may have normal or nearly normal vision when accommodation is stable and the total hyperopic correction is in place. A viable alternative to binocular refraction that is preferred by many practitioners is cycloplegic refraction.

As discussed in Chapter 3, the full plus prescription might cause significant distance blur for the nonamblyopic eye and be impractical or difficult to wear because the blurred vision makes distance tasks difficult. At times, the refractive findings may need to be reduced so that the nonamblyopic eye can maintain clear distance vision. To achieve this, we recommend slightly reducing only the spherical power of the lenses, thereby retaining the complete anisometropic and astigmatic correction. For example, assume that the patient had reduced distance acuity through the full cycloplegic refraction for the nonamblyopic right eye:

RE: +2.00 c 1.00 × 180   20/30
LE: +6.00 c 2.00 × 5   20/70

If a reduction in the sphere power of the right lens of 0.75 D allowed clear distance vision, then the spherical power of *each* lens can be reduced (retaining the anisometropic and astigmatic correction), resulting in a final prescription of:

RE: +1.25 c 1.00 × 180   20/20
LE: +5.25 c 2.00 × 5   20/70

The refractive error should be reevaluated at each 2- to 3-week follow-up visit. Appropriate lens changes can be made when necessary to maintain the optimum balance and astigmatic correction, while continuing to strive for maximum plus acceptance.

The proportion of patients who can be "cured" with refractive correction alone is unknown. Clinically, we have observed that improvement in resolution of an amblyopic eye occurs with enough frequency, when wearing the best correction, that we always prescribe the full refractive correction as the first step in management. This observation, which is illustrated by the case report below, confirms the reports of Clarke and Noel of spontaneous improvement in acuity for some patients with anisometropic amblyopia who have had only refractive treatment. Our clinical observations suggest that complete improvement occurs in no more than 10% of patients.

Case Study

Case 16.2: Refractive Correction Alone

A 12-year-old girl presented with the chief complaint of blurred vision when looking from reading books to the chalkboard. She also complained of irregular headaches and felt that the left eye bothered her more than the right. Her parents reported that she received a visual examination 2 years previously, but did not wear the prescription. External and internal ocular health was within normal limits. Visual acuity and refraction with cycloplegia was:

OD: plano   20/20 − 1
OS: +3.75 − 2.00 × 005   20/60 − 1   OU 20/20

There was a comitant 5 Δ esophoria at 6 m and 8 Δ esophoria at 40 cm. Stereopsis was 100 seconds at 40 cm with Randot circles. There was no suppression. Fixation was central with both eyes.

The cycloplegic refractive finding was prescribed. The patient was instructed to return for reevaluation in 1 month, but she did not return until 3 months later. She had noticed diplopia for the first 2 days while wearing the new glasses, but now wore them full time without complaint.

Aided VA:

OD: 20/15 − 2
OS: 20/20
OU: 20/15

Eye alignment: 2 Δ esophoria at 6 m and 4 Δ esophoria at 40 cm. Stereopsis was 20 seconds at 40 cm with Random Dot circles.

Refractive correction can be accomplished with either spectacles or contact lenses. In the case of a large difference between the refractive error of the two eyes, contact lenses are often the treatment of choice because thick spectacle lenses may produce intolerable distortions, be cosmetically unappealing, or induce prism when viewing off axis through two lenses of significantly different power. The induced prism (especially vertical prism) may cause diplopia. Induced prism with lateral gaze is minimized with contact lens corrections—a distinct advantage, since reestablishing normal binocularity is a major part of achieving a functional cure. On the other hand, unilateral refractive differences greater than 2.00 D between the spherical equivalents of the two eyes usually result from differences in axial length. Correction of these patients with contact lenses might theoretically cause aniseikonia (Chapter 18). Empirically, however, it has been found that neither form of refractive correction (glasses or contact lenses) prevents binocularity. This suggests that binocular vision is facilitated by clear retinal images, and we suggest that a potential difference in image size with spectacle or contact lens correction should not prevent prescription of the full refractive correction.

Added Lenses and Prisms

After the best refractive correction has been determined, the next step in the sequence of management is to prescribe added lens power or prism if needed to improve eye alignment. Optimum eye alignment should facilitate redevelopment of normal interactions between accommodation and vergence and, therefore, enhance binocularity.

Plus (or Minus) Lens Power in Addition to the Full Refractive Correction

Added lens power can be prescribed to stimulate or relax accommodation and improve eye alignment. Added plus lenses should be prescribed for near work to reduce an esodeviation in the presence of a high AC/A, as described in Chapter 9. Added plus lenses can also be used in the treatment of accommodative insufficiencies or accommodative inaccuracies, which often coexist with amblyopia (47). Added minus lens power may be a consideration during training, if an exodeviation is present and the patient has a high AC/A (Chapter 9).

Prism

If optimum eye alignment is not achieved with the refractive correction and added lenses, small amounts of prism can be included in the prescription. Special attention should be given to correction of any primary vertical phoria or strabismus. Base-out prism can be prescribed for esophoria and vertical prism can be prescribed for hyperphorias. Convergence training is our treatment of choice for exodeviations, and base-in prism is typically not suggested.

Occlusion

Direct occlusion has been used for over 200 years as a treatment for amblyopia. We recommend part-time (rather than constant) occlusion with the rationale, and times are determined on the following basis. Up to 6 hours of direct occlusion can usually be used before there is a sufficient loss of binocularity to result in strabismus. Because patients with anisometropic amblyopia already have some binocularity (and we want to avoid the development of occlusion strabismus), we recommend a maximum of 5 hours of occlusion per day. Schor and Wick (48) demonstrated that even as few as 15 minutes of occlusion will improve visual acuity for some amblyopic subjects. Notwithstanding the results of Schor and Wick, we suggest that the minimum amount of occlusion should not be substantially shorter than a 3-hour period and arbitrarily chose to use a minimum of 2 hours of direct occlusion. Thus, after prescribing the best refractive correction with any added lenses or prism needed to help maintain binocular alignment, we recommend prescription of part-time direct occlusion for 2 to 5 hours per day as the next step in the management sequence. We titrate the initial time that occlusion is prescribed, based on the aided acuity found with the best lens correction at the initial exam.

As shown in Fig. 16.2, when the patient has more severe acuity reduction, we recommend longer occlusion times than when visual acuity is not as compromised. However, when acuity is severely impaired, modification of the schedule is frequently needed because of the problems that patients with substantially reduced acuity have when they try to perform daily tasks while occluded. Thus, we recommend reducing the time of occlusion somewhat when acuity is worse than 20/100. In these instances, however, we also suggest increasing the amount of amblyopia acuity training so that rapid progress will still be made by the patient. Once acuity improves to better than 20/100, the time of occlusion can be increased (Fig. 16.2).

Active Amblyopia and Suppression Therapy

We next prescribe active monocular and binocular amblyopia therapy because active treatment, as opposed to passive management (such as occlusion), has been suggested to significantly reduce the total amount of time that therapy needs to be performed in order to achieve the best visual acuity (49). Figure 16.3 compares the results achieved using occlusion alone with those achieved using occlusion and active therapy (45). Monocular therapy should be designed to provide stimulation of the fovea with resolvable targets. This therapy, which is done while the patient is occluded, should utilize about 20 minutes per day of the monocular stimulation techniques that have previously been shown to enhance amblyopic resolution and foster more normal eye movements and accommodation of the amblyopic eye. Since moderate amounts of central suppression are often present in patients with anisometropic amblyopia, we recommend also prescribing about 15 minutes per day of binocular antisuppression therapy as soon as possible in the management program. This should be designed to force the amblyopic eye

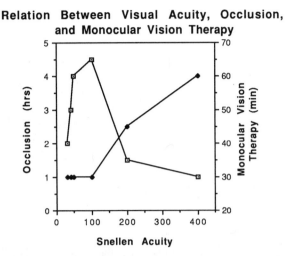

FIG. 16.2. The amount of time spent occluding and/or performing vision therapy is determined by the corrected visual acuity of the patient. When acuity is very poor, relatively more time is spent initially doing active therapy *(black symbols)* and less time occluding *(open squares)*, so that compliance with occlusion can be facilitated and the patient does not have to perform potentially dangerous daily tasks while occluded. As acuity improves, the time spent occluding is increased.

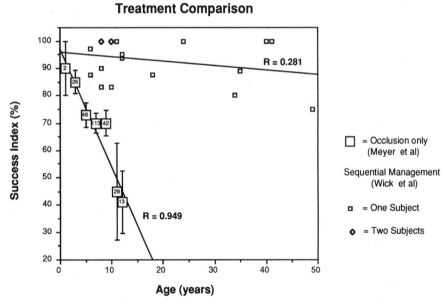

FIG. 16.3. Using only occlusion *(large squares)* results in less acuity improvement than sequential management for older patients *(small squares and diamonds)*. When the patients are young, occlusion alone results in the same ultimate acuity. At all ages, sequential management probably results in the most rapid improvement.

to function in a more natural and competitive binocular situation and to reinforce the normal binocular interactions that are required for a functional cure.

Case Study

Case 16.3: Sequential Management

A 6-year-old boy presented for a routine preschool examination. He had no symptoms. External and internal ocular health was within normal limits. Visual acuity and refraction with cycloplegia was:

$$OD: +3.00 - 1.00 \times 103 \quad 20/60$$
$$OS: +0.25 \qquad\qquad\quad 20/20 \quad OU\ 20/20$$

There was a comitant 3 Δ esophoria at 6 m and 40 cm. Fixation was central with both eyes. There was intermittent suppression of the right eye on Worth dot testing and stereopsis was 140 seconds at 40 cm with Randot circles.

The cycloplegic refractive finding was prescribed. The patient returned for reevaluation in 2 weeks, with acuities unchanged from above. Three hours per day of direct occlusion and binocular antisuppression therapy were prescribed. Binocular therapy consisted of dot-to-dot books with a red pencil, while wearing red/green glasses (red lens over left eye) to enhance the acuity of the right eye and reading using a red/green bar reader to reduce suppression. Accommodative therapy using lens flippers (starting with ±1.25) was included at week 4. Over the next 8 weeks, the print was made progressively smaller, and the accommodative flippers made progressively stronger, as the patient's acuity and binocular status improved as summarized below.

Week	Management	Acuity of Amblyopic Eye	Stereopsis
1	Exam Best prescription (spectacles)	Aided: 20/60	140 seconds
2	Progress visit 2 hr/d direct occlusion. Binocular VT	Aided: 20/60 + 1	140 seconds
4	Binocular and accommodative VT	Aided: 20/40	100 seconds
6	Binocular and accommodative VT	Aided: 20/30	60 seconds
8	Binocular and accommodative VT	Aided: 20/25	40 seconds
10	Binocular and accommodative VT	Aided: 20/20	20 seconds

Sensory Motor Function

For an ideal result, sensory and motor fusion must be maximally enhanced. For patients with anisometropic amblyopia, we recommend prescription of vision therapy to treat the vergence

There was comitant 4 Δ esophoria at 6 m and 40 cm. Stereopsis was 140 seconds at 40 cm with Titmus circles. There was intermittent alternating suppression. Fixation was central with both eyes. The jerk nystagmus had about 6-degree amplitude and a frequency of 1.5 Hz. Foveations were very inaccurate and about 20 ms duration. A +3.00 D near addition gave 0.5 M acuity at 35 cm.

Intermittent photic stimulation was prescribed, as office therapy and vertical line counting was used for home therapy. After 2 months of therapy, visual acuities were 20/30– in each eye using Vectographic testing.

Pleoptics

Pleoptic methods have been advocated by some authors. See Shapiro (35) for a detailed description of pleoptics techniques. Stegall (31) observed that direct occlusion was effective when the amblyopic eye viewed targets through a Kodak No. 92 red filter. Foveal fixation may be stimulated if latent nystagmus is reduced by this method. The red filter and occlusion amblyopia treatment technique of Brinker and Katz (36) may also be a reasonable consideration for treatment of amblyopia complicated by latent nystagmus.

Pharmacological Therapy

The visual sensation of movement (oscillopsia) is an especially distressing symptom that is a common sequellae of acquired nystagmus. When the etiology of nystagmus is an infectious process, a metabolic or toxic disturbance, or a vascular disorder, systemic medication can play a significant role in management. For example, medications are sometimes effective in treatment of the symptoms of oscillopsia and vertigo associated with vestibular nystagmus, downbeat nystagmus, and, on rare occasions, congenital nystagmus. Currie and Matson (37) described ten patients with vertical oscillopsia and downbeat nystagmus that was treated successfully with 1 to 2 mg of clonazepam. The symptoms were reduced for 2 to 6 hours per dose, and one patient experienced 72 hours per dose relief. Side effects of the medication, such as drowsiness and sedation, limit the long-term benefit.

Baclofen, which inhibits the excitatory neurotransmitter system, has been used to decrease oscillopsia in some cases of congenital nystagmus (38), periodic alternating nystagmus (PAN), and seesaw nystagmus. The side effects include dizziness, drowsiness, hypotension, nausea, and weakness. Since most congenital nystagmus patients do not suffer from oscillopsia, this expensive medication is not used often. Baclofen therapy is generally reserved for patients who do not have increases in acuity with the treatments listed above.

Surgery

A frequent cosmetic consequence of nystagmus is a face turn, head tilt, chin elevation, depression, or a combination of these. The patient assumes a head position that moves the eyes into a field of gaze where the nystagmus is lessened and/or visual acuity improves. Kestenbaum (39) designed a surgical technique to move all horizontal rectus muscles, using an identical amount of resection and recession. Successful surgery shifts the null point to the primary position, and any existing face turn is eliminated. Occasionally, there is also increased visual acuity in the primary position, a lessening of the nystagmus intensity, and an increase in the null position over a wider range of gaze (40). Modifications of Kestenbaum's procedure have also been used. For example, when a patient has a vertical head turn, the four vertical rectus muscles are operated on simultaneously (41). The success of these procedures in reducing face turns to within 15 degrees of the primary position is reported to be about 80%.

There are four main points to discuss when counseling patients, regarding the value of surgical intervention for a head turn secondary to congenital nystagmus. First, most authorities only recommend surgery when the face turn is greater than 15 degrees (24). Smaller amounts of anomalous head position are managed with conjugate prisms. Second, consideration is given to both the location of the null point and the amount of head turn. For older patients, these positions may not be the same because social pressure often causes the patient to adopt a helpful, but less than optimum, head position (42). In these cases, surgery is designed to place the null point in the primary position, rather than eliminating the abnormal head position per se. Third, the best surgical results are reported in patients over the age of 4 years. Overcorrections more commonly result when children are younger than 4 years. Fourth, when the head turn patient has strabismus as well as nystagmus, surgery is typically performed on the dominant eye because a change in head position will be mediated by the fixating eye. Surgery is simultaneously or subsequently performed on the other eye to correct the strabismus. The prognosis for a successful result decreases slightly for these more complicated cases.

The esotropia associated with nystagmus blockage syndrome is usually surgically treated after occlusion to eliminate amblyopia and develop normal ocular motility. There is a fair cosmetic prognosis with apparent alignment in the primary position about 50% of the time. There are few functional cures reported, although about 25% have microtropia with some binocular function. Either the Faden operation, with a small recession, or bimedial rectus recessions are used. Surgical results are typically not as good as those in congenital esotropia. Overcorrections and undercorrections are frequent, and the number of reoperations is more than 50%.

SUMMARY

Nystagmus can present a difficult diagnostic challenge. In addition to pathology, the etiologic factors include developmental and genetic anomalies (43). Nystagmus is often caused by (or associated with) afferent and efferent visual defects. Acquired nystagmus, such as opsoclonus, seesaw, vestibular, and many others, requires immediate diagnosis and management of the underlying disease to reduce the long-term consequences. The severity of visual impairment is not always dependant upon the etiology (44).

Although nystagmus cannot generally be cured, we recommend that the clinician aggressively treat nystagmus patients. Using sequential management, the prognosis for functional and cosmetic improvement is often quite high in patients with heterophorias. Treatment consists of (a) correction of the refractive error, using spectacle or contact lenses, (b) prisms to induce convergence or correct a head turn, and (c) vision therapy to enhance fusion. After binocularity is maximally improved, vision therapy to improve fixation stability is used if needed. Medications and surgery play a role in selected cases.

STUDY QUESTIONS

1. Why is a slit lamp helpful in nystagmus diagnosis?
2. What is a foveation and why might it be important to a nystagmus patient?
3. What are the characteristics of PAN?
4. What are important additional case history questions to ask a patient or parent regarding nystagmus?

5. How can you test visual acuity in a patient with latent nystagmus?
6. Describe voluntary nystagmus.
7. Convergence may reduce nystagmus; base-out prism can cause convergence. Support or refute this statement: base-out prism is the treatment for nystagmus.
8. Why might prism base-right in each eye help a patient with nystagmus?
9. Describe how vision therapy for suppression might help a patient with nystagmus.
10. Compare the treatment technique and overall treatment goals of line counting and intermittent photic simulation in treatment of the patient with nystagmus.

REFERENCES

1. Cline D, Hofstetter HW, Griffin JR. *Dictionary of visual science*. Radnor, PA: Chilton, 1989:478.
2. Casteel I, Harris CM, Shawkat F, et al. Nystagmus in infancy. *Br J Ophthalmol* 1992;76:434–437.
3. Gelbart SS, Hoyt CS. Congenital nystagmus: a clinical perspective in infancy. *Graefes Arch Clin Exp Ophthalmol* 1988;226:178–180.
4. Anderson JR. Latent nystagmus and alternating hyperphoria. *Br J Ophthalmol* 1954;38:217–231.
5. Siegel IM. The albino as a low vision patient. In: Faye EE, ed. *Clinical low vision care*. Boston: Little, Brown and Company, 1976:255–261.
6. Schachat WS, Wallace HM, Palmer M, et al. Ophthalmologic findings in children with cerebral palsy. *Pediatrics* 1957;19:623–628.
7. Mehr EB, Freid AN. *Low vision care*. Chicago: Professional Press, 1975:39.
8. Currie DC, Bedell HE, Song S. Visual acuity for optotypes with image motions simulating congenital nystagmus. *Clin Vis Sci* 1993;8:73–84.
9. Dell Osso LF, Daroff RB. Congenital nystagmus waveforms and foveation strategy. *Doc Ophthalmol* 1975;39: 155–182.
10. Eskridge JB, Wick B, Perrigin D. The magnitude of the Hirschberg correction factor. *Am J Optom Physiol Optics* 1988;65:745–750.
11. Gresty MA, Lech J, Sanders M, et al. A study of head and eye movement in *spasmus nutans*. *Br J Ophthalmol* 1976;60:652–654.
12. Pearce WG. Congenital nystagmus—genetic and environmental causes. *Can J Ophthalmol* 1978;13:1.
13. Flom MC, Weymouth FW, Kahneman D. Visual resolution and contour interaction. *J Opt Soc Am* 1963;53:1026–1032.
14. Griffin JR, Cotter SA. The Bruckner test: evaluation of clinical usefulness. *Am J Optom Physiol Optics* 1986;63:957–961.
15. Krimsky E. *The management of binocular imbalance*. Philadelphia: Lea & Febiger, 1948:204.
16. Rouse M, London R, Allen D. An evaluation of the monocular estimate method of dynamic retinoscopy. *Am J Optom Physiol Optics* 1982;60:234–239.
17. Parks MM. The monofixation syndrome. In: Symposium on strabismus. *Trans New Orleans Acad Ophthalmol*. St. Louis: Mosby, 1970:121–153.
18. Leigh RJ, Zee DS. *The neurology of eye movements*. Philadelphia: FA Davis Co, 1983.
19. Scheiman MM. Optometric findings in children with cerebral palsy. *Am J Opt Physiol Optics* 1984;61(5):321–323.
20. Ciufreda KJ. Voluntary nystagmus: new findings and clinical implications. *Am J Opt Physiol Optics* 1980;57: 795–800.
21. Anderson JR. Cases and treatment of congenital eccentric nystagmus. *Br J Ophthalmol* 1953;37:267–281.
22. Mallett RFJ. The treatment of congenital idiopathic nystagmus by intermittent photic stimulation. *Ophthalmol Physiol Opt* 1983;3:341–356.
23. Lo C. Brain computed tomographic evaluation of noncomitant strabismus and congenital nystagmus. In: Henkind P, ed. *ACTA 24th International Congress of Ophthalmology*, vol 2. Philadelphia: JB Lippincott Co, 1982:924–928.
24. Shibasaki H, Yamashita Y, Motomura S. Suppression of congenital nystagmus. *J Neurol Neurosurg Psychiatry* 1978;41:1078.
25. Miller NR. *Walsh & Hoyt's clinical neuro ophthalmology*, 4th ed. Baltimore: Williams & Wilkins, 1985.
26. Lavery MA, O'Neill JF, Chu FC, et al. Acquired nystagmus in early childhood: a presenting sign of intracranial tumor. *Ophthalmology* 1984;91(5):425–434.
27. Lavin PJM. Nystagmus. In: Walsh TJ, ed. *Neuroophthalmology: clinical signs and symptoms*, 2nd ed. Philadelphia: Lea & Febiger, 1985.
28. Calcutt C, Crook W. The treatment of amblyopia in patients with latent nystagmus. *Br Orthopt J* 1972;29:70–72.
29. Windsor CE, Burian HM, Milojevic B. Modification of latent nystagmus: part 1. *Arch Ophthalmol* 1968;80: 657–663.
30. Bedell HE, White JM, Abplanalp PL. Variability of foveations in congenital nystagmus. *Clin Vis Sci* 1989;427–452.
31. Stegall FW. Orthoptic aspects of nystagmus. Symposium on nystagmus. *Am Orthoptics J* 1973;23:30–34.

32. Kirschen DG. Auditory feedback in the control of congenital nystagmus. *Am J Opt Physiol Optics* 1983;60(5): 364–368.
33. Ishikawa S, Tanakadate A, Nabatamte K, et al. Biofeedback treatment of congenital nystagmus. *Neuroophthalmology* 1985;2:58–65.
34. Leung V, Wick B, Bedell HE. Multifaceted treatment of congenital nystagmus: a report of 6 cases. *Optom Vis Sci* 1996;73(2):773.
35. Shapiro M. *Amblyopia*. Philadelphia: Chilton, 1971.
36. Brinker WR, Katz SL. A new and practical treatment of eccentric fixation. *Am J Ophthalmol* 1963;55:1033–1035.
37. Currie JN, Matson V. The use of clonazepam in the treatment of nystagmus induced oscillopsia. *Ophthalmology* 1986;93:924–932.
38. Yee RD, Baloh RW, Honrubia V. Effect of baclofen on congenital nystagmus. In: Lennerstrad G, Zee DS, Keller EL, eds. *Functional basis of ocular motility disorders*. Oxford: Pergamon, 1982:151–157.
39. Kestenbaum A. Nouvelle operation de nystagmus. *Bull Soc Ophthalmol Fr* 1953;6:599.
40. Dell Osso LF, Flynn JT. Congenital nystagmus surgery: a quantitative evaluation of the effects. *Arch Ophthalmol* 1979;97:462–469.
41. Scott WE, Kraft SP. Surgical treatment of compensatory head position in congenital nystagmus. *J Pediatr Ophthalmol Strabismus* 1984;21:85–95.
42. Flynn JT, Dell Osso LF. The effects of congenital nystagmus surgery. *Ophthalmology* 1979;86:1414–1427.
43. Russell GE, Wick B, Tang RA. Arnold Chiari malformation. *Optom Vis Sci* 1992;69(3):242–247.
44. Grisham D. Management of nystagmus in young children. *Problems in Optometry* 1990;11:496–527.

18

Aniseikonia

There are few subjects that have been developed with greater care or are supported by more extensive research than that of aniseikonia. However, even though it is relatively common in clinical practice to encounter patients with symptoms of aniseikonia, iseikonic lens designs are seldom prescribed. As a result, it often becomes difficult to recall the procedures needed for diagnosis and treatment. In this chapter, we briefly describe the condition of aniseikonia and present a simplified method for design of iseikonic corrections.

DEFINITIONS OF ANISEIKONIA

Aniseikonia, which means not-equal-images (1), is defined as a condition of binocular vision where there is a relative difference in the size and/or shape of the ocular image of the two eyes (2). A size difference that causes symptoms (generally 0.75% or more) is defined as clinically significant aniseikonia (3). Smaller amounts of image size difference are usually not clinically significant, although they are relatively common. Even large amounts of image size difference do not cause aniseikonic symptoms for some patients.

The size of each ocular image depends on the retinal image formed by the dioptric systems of the eye, the distribution of retinal receptive elements, and the physiological and cortical processes involved in vision. As a result, the two ocular images are seldom, if ever, equal. There are normal differences in image size when looking at objects in left or right gaze and when objects are located at different distances from the eyes (4). These normal image size disparities form the basis of stereopsis and provide a signal representing where one object is with respect to another.

Static Versus Dynamic Aniseikonia

Aniseikonia can be considered to be comprised of two different, but related, magnification-induced problems—static and dynamic aniseikonia (5). Measures of static aniseikonia assess the actual difference in image size between the eyes and it is these measures, rather than the normal or physiological differences in image size, that we are typically concerned with in clinical determinations of aniseikonia. The amount of dynamic aniseikonia is determined by analyzing differences in induced phoria that occur when a patient looks in various fields of gaze through an anisometropic correction (6). A patient can have either static aniseikonia or dynamic aniseikonia, or both problems at one time. For example, a patient with emmetropia or ametropia (with no difference in the refractive correction of each eye) could have measured aniseikonia. This would be static aniseikonia. Another patient, corrected with spectacle lenses for a large myopic anisometropia, would be expected to have dynamic aniseikonia, due to the difference in spectacle lens powers. Obviously, contact lens correction is the preferred method of minimizing dynamic aniseikonia.

HISTORICAL PERSPECTIVE

Prior to 1945, theoretical and clinical courses in aniseikonia were given at the Dartmouth Eye Institute, and a clinician had to be certified by that institute in order to obtain an eikonometer (7).

519

As instrumentation was simplified and techniques for measuring aniseikonia were improved, the obligatory Dartmouth courses were discontinued. However, initial investigations of the Dartmouth group provided the technical and clinical papers that underlie instruction in professional schools and discussion of aniseikonia in textbooks.

Differences in the retinal image size may result from correction of refractive errors, including antimetropia and anisometropia. Donders (8) described the difference in the relative size of the images of the two eyes due to correction of anisometropia and suggested that these differences may interfere with binocular vision. Lippincott (9), Green (10), Friedenwald (11), and Koller (12) also discussed changes in the retinal images resulting from correction of ametropia. Hess (13) believed that symptoms that occur with lens correction of anisometropia are caused by prismatic effects in the lens periphery. Von Rohr (14) calculated image size differences occurring in unilateral aphakia and high anisometropia. Erggelet (15) pointed out that astigmatic corrections also introduce size differences between the retinal images. He considered these size differences unimportant, since they rarely exceed 4% or 5%. Earlier, Erggelet (16) had considered the possibility that a physiological image size difference might result from unequal distribution of the retinal elements in the two eyes. The correctness of this conjecture is illustrated by the statistical analysis of Carleton and Madigan (17), which showed that aniseikonia occurs in bilateral emmetropia and isoametropia, as well as anisometropia.

Knapp's Law

For some clinicians, confusion results from too liberal an application of Knapp's Law, which states that the corrected eye with axial ametropia has a retinal image equal in size to that of an emmetropic eye of equal power, provided the lens is placed at the anterior focal point of the eye (2). However, there are a substantial number of patients with axial anisometropia who cannot successfully wear spectacle lens corrections, suggesting that Knapp's law is more useful as a guideline than a "law." The ultimate determinant of the retinal image size is based on the separation of retinal photoreceptors and on the registration of these in the visual cortex, not solely on the power or form of the refractive correction. As a result, Knapp's law fails in many cases, since simply correcting the anisometropia and providing clear retinal images has a more beneficial effect on binocular fusion than the detrimental effect of the potentially unequal image sizes.

DIAGNOSIS

It is not generally difficult to decide whether a patient has aniseikonia. A careful review of the case history and a few basic clinical tests should give sufficient information to make a tentative diagnosis on nearly all of the patients suspected of having aniseikonia. After reviewing the patient's symptoms, consider the refractive state and corneal curvature. If these do not allow accurate diagnosis, then a period of diagnostic occlusion and/or an iseikonic clip-over should lend further diagnostic support.

The definitive diagnosis of aniseikonia is done by measuring the image sizes with an instrument (such as the Space Eikonometer), if one is available in the office or on referral. When an eikonometer is not available, the aniseikonic correction may be estimated from the refractive correction required or from comparison of the images seen by the two eyes.

History

The symptoms that the patient experiences are important in the diagnosis of aniseikonia. Symptoms of aniseikonic patients are similar to those of patients with uncorrected ametropia and heterophoria. The incidence of symptoms reported by 500 aniseikonic patients is listed below.

Although local eye discomfort (asthenopia) and headaches are the most frequent symptoms, there are a variety of conditions that may produce symptoms similar to aniseikonia (18). As a result, we recommend that other possible causes for a patient's complaints be investigated and treated, before considering iseikonic correction.

Symptoms of aniseikonia patients include:

Asthenopia	67%
Headaches	67%
Photophobia	27%
Reading difficulty	23%
Nausea	15%
Motility difficulty	11%
Nervousness	11%
Dizziness	7%
General fatigue	7%
Distortion of space	6%

To conduct the examination, it is important to determine the patient's primary symptom, along with its duration and frequency. Begin by having the patient describe the current symptoms using questions such as: "In what way do your eyes bother you most?" Directing the patient to give an accurate description of his or her difficulties requires tact and judgment, because some patients are anxious to report any visual phenomenon or relate their numerous visits to various specialists and it is easy to lose track of the problem that brought them.

The most important symptoms are those present when the refractive correction is worn. Ocular symptoms can conveniently be grouped under the term "asthenopia." Typical ocular symptoms include those directly associated with the eyes, such as aching, burning, eye pain, itching, pulling sensations, and tiring. These symptoms may also include subjective observations, such as blurred or doubled vision and even slanting or tipping of level surfaces. Visual experiences such as these may or may not be accompanied by any ache, pain, or other discomfort, but they often greatly concern the patient. Ocular symptoms are usually related to the use of the eyes and are frequently due to uncorrected ametropia, heterophoria, or aniseikonia. As such, they are often readily relieved by properly prescribed visual correction.

Referred symptoms include dizziness, headaches, nausea, and nervousness. Such symptoms are seldom definitively related to the use of the eyes and, when they exist, a refractive or iseikonic correction is less likely to bring relief. These symptoms, which frequently seem to be of ocular origin, prompt patients to consult with an eye specialist in the hope that the headaches may be due to the eyes and that the eye doctor can "cure" them. However, careful questioning by the clinician may reveal that the headaches are due to other causes, such as allergies or sinus conditions. It is the clinician's task to determine whether referred symptoms have an ocular etiology or if the patient should be advised to consult other specialists.

The length of time that symptoms have been present should also be considered. Long-standing symptoms that have been previously investigated without success tend to strongly suggest aniseikonia. This is because a patient with long-standing symptoms has usually sought a variety of treatments. If all previous treatments have been unsuccessful, it tends to rule out other possible causes for the symptoms and increase the chances for aniseikonia.

Refractive Condition

There are a few patients with equal or no refractive error who have aniseikonia and symptoms (19,20). Many of these are patients are those who have had unilateral cataract extraction and are pseudophakic (21). However, in patients who have not had refractive or cataract surgery, the likelihood of aniseikonia is generally not high, unless the patient is anisometropic. Once the anisometropia is corrected, aniseikonia becomes a definite possibility. Aniseikonic symptoms occur infrequently in the presence of uncorrected anisometropia because one of the ocular images is usually so blurred that the patient uses only one eye and aniseikonic symptoms are not present.

Corneal Curvature

A difference in the corneal power of each eye indicates that at least a portion of the anisometropia is refractive. When correcting such patients with spectacles, a difference in image size will result. Astigmatism is virtually always of corneal or, occasionally, lenticular origin. Either type of astigmatism can be considered a refractive problem, where spectacle correction will result in aniseikonia. In refractive anisometropia, correction of refractive errors with contact lenses rather than spectacle lenses will minimize these differences in image size, especially when the anisometropia is not very high [less than 6.00 diopters (D)] and the difference in corneal power matches the amount of anisometropia. The other advantage of contact lens correction for anisometropic patients is the reduction of the amount of variable prism power induced by versional eye movements.

When prescribing spectacle correction for a patient with anisometropia and equal corneal curvatures, there should be minimal problems with static aniseikonia, provided the lenses do not produce undesired shape magnification. This can be avoided by prescribing equal front curves and center thickness. However, the theory behind equalizing the lens front curves and center thickness assumes that the anisometropia must result from a difference in axial length when the corneal curvatures are equal. Unfortunately, this is not always the case, as the anisometropia may be due to a refractive difference associated with the lens or the back surface of the cornea. Aniseikonia cannot be definitely ruled out simply because the corneal curvatures are equal. Further, the problem of dynamic aniseikonia induced by the spectacle lenses is often a significant deterrent to binocular visual function. In general, these factors suggest that contact lenses should be the initial prescription consideration.

Occlusion

Occlusion may be useful as an aid in diagnosis of aniseikonia. If the patient's symptoms are eliminated by wearing a patch, they are probably due to a binocular problem. Once all other binocular problems have been treated or ruled out, aniseikonia is left as the probable cause of the symptoms.

Clip-on Aniseikonic Correction

A clip-on iseikonic correction is often useful to diagnose aniseikonia. Such lenses have plano power, with magnification based on the combination of front curve and center thickness used in their manufacture. When the clip-on reduces the symptoms, aniseikonia is very likely to be the problem. To further test the assumption, the clip-on can be placed on the other eye. If symptoms are exacerbated, the diagnosis is complete. Unfortunately, when a clip-on lens does not help, aniseikonia may still be the problem, since symptoms may result from the weight and additional reflections caused by the clip-on lens. Table 18.1 shows the lens thickness/curve combinations for various iseikonic clip-on lenses (22).

TABLE 18.1. *Specifications for plastic size lenses[a]*

Percentage magnification	Lens thickness (mm)	Power of first surface	Power of second surface
0.5	3	+2.50	−2.50
1.0	3	+5.00	−5.00
1.5	3	+7.50	−7.62
2.0	4	+7.50	−7.75
2.5	4	+9.37	−9.62
3.0	5	+9.00	−9.25
3.5	5	+10.50	−10.87
4.0	6	+10.00	−10.50
4.5	6	+11.25	−11.75
5.0	6	+12.50	−13.12

[a]Since size lenses are not commercially available, they must be custom fabricated using the parameters listed.

DETERMINATION OF ANISEIKONIA

There are several methods that can be used to determine whether aniseikonia is present. These include estimation of the image size between the two eyes simultaneously, using diplopic images or sequentially using the alternate cover test, Turville testing, the Maddox rod, and double light technique. Assessment can also be made using tests such as the New Aniseikonia test or Space Eikonometry. Although each of these techniques has clinical use, the Space Eikonometer is probably the most accurate and practical.

Size Comparison of Diplopic Images

Comparison of double images is a simple, albeit relatively insensitive, test of the image sizes between the two eyes that can be used to estimate horizontal, vertical, or overall aniseikonia. In this technique:

1. The patient wears the appropriate spectacle correction and views a square target that is doubled, using vertical prism of about 5 Δ. The target will be seen horizontally displaced if any horizontal phoria is present.
2. The patient compares the perceived horizontal extent of the top target with the perceived horizontal extent of the bottom target. A difference suggests horizontal aniseikonia.
3. To estimate the horizontal aniseikonia, a size lens (Table 18.2) is placed in front of the eye with the smallest image. The percentage magnification of the size lens is changed until the two targets appear to be of equal horizontal lengths.
4. The process is repeated for the vertical dimensions.
5. The results are recorded, indicating the magnification needed to equalize the perceived images (e.g., 2.0% on OD-horizontal, 1.0% on OS-vertical OS; 1.5% on OD overall).

Alternate Cover Test

Brecher (23) proposed using the alternating cover test to detect and estimate the magnitude of aniseikonia.

1. Have the patient wear the appropriate spectacle correction and fixate a distance square target that is alone in the visual field.

TABLE 18.2. *Approximate magnification (percent) changes for eyewire distance changes of various lens powers*[a]

Power (V_o)	1 D	2 D	4 D	6 D	8 D	10 D
Eyewire distance (h)						
1 mm	0.1	0.2	0.4	0.6	0.8	1.0
2 mm	0.2	0.4	0.8	1.2	1.6	2.0
3 mm	0.3	0.6	1.2	1.8	2.4	3.0
4 mm	0.4	0.8	1.6	2.4	3.2	4.0
5 mm	0.5	1.0	2.0	3.0	4.0	5.0

[a]Minus lens: moved closer to the eye, increases magnification; moved farther from the eye, decreases magnification.
Plus lens: moved closer to the eye, decreases magnification; moved farther from the eye, increases magnification.

$$\text{Based on: } m\% = \frac{V_o(h)}{10}$$

Where: m% = change in magnification (percent)
    V_o = lens vertex power (diopters)
  Diopter = D
      h = change in eyewire distance (millimeters)
10 results from changing meters to millimeters and expressing magnification in percent.

2. Occlude each eye alternately and ask the patient to compare the horizontal size of the target seen with each eye. The cover paddle should be moved quickly between eyes and held for about 1 second in front of each eye to facilitate comparison of the two images.
3. If there is a difference in perceived size, repeat the test with a size lens in front of the eye with the smaller perceived image. Change the size lens until the image seen with each eye appears to be the same size, as the cover paddle is alternated.
4. The process is repeated for the vertical dimensions.
5. The results are recorded, indicating the magnification needed in each meridian to equalize the perceived images of the two eyes.

Turville Test

The Turville test can be used for detecting and measuring aniseikonia in the vertical meridian using the slide with two horizontal lines that Morgan developed (24) (Fig. 18.1).

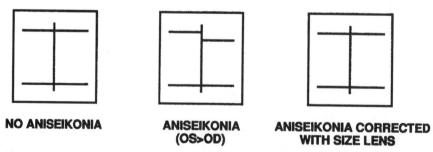

NO ANISEIKONIA   **ANISEIKONIA**   **ANISEIKONIA CORRECTED**
                         (OS>OD)   **WITH SIZE LENS**

FIG. 18.1. The slide, developed by Morgan for Turville testing, appears as two parallel horizontal lines emanating from a central vertical line. The patient's task is to report the relative separation of the horizontal lines on either side of the vertical line. Report of an unequal separation of the lines can be neutralized with a size lens, providing an estimated amount of magnification to prescribe.

1. Position the septum so that the patient sees the right half of the target with the right eye and the left half of the target with the left, while wearing the appropriate spectacle correction.
2. Have the patient compare the vertical separation of the two lines on the right target with the separation of the two lines on the left target. A difference in the perceived vertical separation of the lines on the right side suggests vertical aniseikonia.
3. Aniseikonia can be measured using a size lens in front of the eye with the smallest separation and changing the size lens to equalize the perceived vertical separation of the lines on both sides.
4. This measure of the vertical aniseikonia should be recorded.

Maddox Rod and Two-point Light Sources

1. Two small light sources are placed about 60 cm away, with a horizontal separation of about 20 cm. The patient wears the appropriate spectacle correction and views the lights through a Maddox rod in front of only one eye, with the axis at 180 degrees. One eye sees the two light sources and the other (behind the Maddox rod) sees two vertical luminous lines.
2. Have the patient compare the relative separation of the lights with the relative separation of the luminous streaks. A difference in the separation suggests aniseikonia. Prism can be used to align the light and line on one side, if a lateral heterophoria makes the judgment difficult by causing a displacement of the streaks from the light sources.
3. A size lens in front of the eye that perceives the smallest separation (lights or streaks) can be used to measure aniseikonia. Change the power of the size lens to equalize the separation between the lights and the streaks.
4. The test can be repeated with the light sources separated vertically and the Maddox rod at axis 90 degrees placed in front of only one eye, to determine the presence and measurement of vertical aniseikonia.
5. The size lens that produces the same distance between the lights and the luminous streaks is recorded as a measure of aniseikonia.

The New Aniseikonia Test

1. In the New Aniseikonia test (25), the patient wears red and green filters over the appropriate spectacle correction.
2. Have the patient compare the red and green half-moons in the booklet (Fig. 18.2) to determine the half-moons that seem to have identical vertical diameters.
3. Rotate the booklet to a horizontal position and repeat the test.

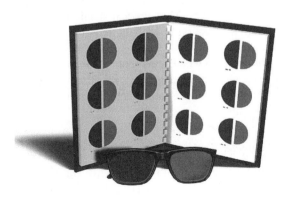

FIG. 18.2. The New Aniseikonia test consists of a book with a number of pairs of red/green half-moons. When viewed with red/green glasses, one of the half-moons is seen by the right eye and the other is seen by the left eye. The patient's task is to determine which pair of targets contains half-moons with the same vertical diameter on each side. This gives an estimate of the amount of magnification to prescribe.

4. The percentage of aniseikonia that is present in each meridian is recorded. This test tends to provide a smaller estimate of the aniseikonia present than the amount measured using a Space Eikonometer.

The Space Eikonometer

The most accurate prescribing for aniseikonia is based on measurement of the image size differences, rather than guessing at the amount of aniseikonia present. From a clinical standpoint, measurement of aniseikonia provides the best means of determining whether a patient's symptoms are related to aniseikonia. These measurements can be made using the Space Eikonometer. Using an eikonometer also facilitates prescription of noniseikonic corrections. For example, practitioners are sometimes reluctant to prescribe an anisometropic correction that might induce aniseikonia. However, the full correction of significant spherical anisometropia does not always result in significant anisekonia. A solution to this dilemma is to use an eikonometer more frequently when aniseikonia is suspected. When the patient's response to the refractive correction is measured with the eikonometer, it is often a pleasant surprise to find little or no aniseikonia. Evaluating the patient's responses to a tentative refractive correction with the eikonometer also allows the clinician to modify the refractive correction to minimize induced aniseikonia, when the visual needs of the patient permit the sacrifice of optimum acuity and binocular function for the sake of comfort or expense.

The Space Eikonometer is extremely accurate—perhaps the most accurate clinical measurement of a binocular function. And, the test is soundly based in physiological optics research on single binocular vision and stereopsis. The Space Eikonometer is no longer currently available for purchase as a new instrument. However, there are a substantial number of used eikonometers available, with an increase in the numbers as practitioners retire. Since this is the only readily available instrument, and many clinicians are not familiar with its use, we have included this short section on use of the eikonometer so that the practitioner who acquires one can more easily become acquainted with the idiosyncrasies of measuring aniseikonia.

Target

The target of the Space Eikonometer appears as two bright white (or yellowish) vertical lines behind a red cross with two dull green vertical lines in front of the cross (Fig. 18.3). The appearance of this target is varied by altering the positions of the controlling levers. The ×90 lever at the top of the instrument (Fig. 18.4) moves the position of the left side of the outside lines closer for right eye magnification or farther for left eye magnification. The ×180 lever moves the relative position of the right sides of the red cross closer for right eye magnification or farther for left eye magnification. The declination wheel rotates the top of the red cross toward the observer for plus settings and away for minus settings. The clinician should familiarize him- or herself with the phenomena described in this section by looking into the instrument, both monocularly and binocularly.

The patient's task during measurement of aniseikonia with the eikonometer is to report the relative positions of the line targets, as changes in the relative magnifications of each are made by moving the controlling levers. The test is complete when the patient reports that all portions of the target are equidistant.

Making Eikonometer Settings

Position the patient comfortably in front of the eikonometer, with the refractive correction in place and the interpupillary distance set on the instrument (Fig. 18.4). Have the patient observe

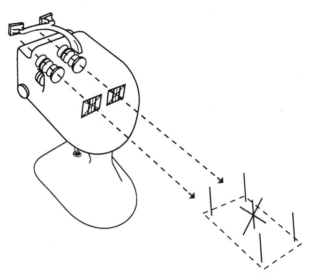

FIG. 18.3. The Space Eikonometer target appears as two bright white (or yellowish) vertical lines behind a red cross with two dull green vertical lines in front of the cross. The patient's task, during measurement of aniseikonia with the eikonometer, is to report the relative positions of the line targets, as changes in the magnifications of each are achieved by moving the controlling levers. The test is complete when the patient reports that all portions of the target are equidistant.

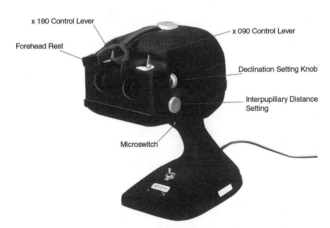

FIG. 18.4. (Top): The appearance of the Space Eikonometer target is determined by altering the positions of the controlling levers. The ×90 lever at the top of the instrument moves the position of the left side of the outside lines closer for right eye magnification or further for left eye magnification. The ×180 lever moves the relative position of the right side of the red cross closer for right eye magnification or further for left eye magnification. The declination wheel rotates the top of the red cross toward the observer for plus settings and away for minus settings. **(Bottom):** Between changes in the controlling levers, visibility of the target is extinguished by using the switch at the bottom of the eikonometer.

the target and report the position of the lines when all settings are on zero. Call attention to the outer lines first. By using a bracketing technique, the ×90 wheel can be moved until the outer lines are seen equidistantly. Extinguishing visibility of the targets with the light switch (Fig. 18.4B), between changes of the lever setting, allows more accurate findings. The measurement procedure is then repeated for the sides of the red cross, using the ×180 lever and, for the tilt of the red cross, using the declination wheel. The method of limits is applied for determining the final location of the levers and declination wheel. The sensitivity of the patient to the three parts of the test is estimated by one half the range within which alignment of the targets are reported. The manual provided with the instrument provides more detail concerning the testing procedure for routine cases.

DETERMINING IMAGE SIZE

After the settings have been determined, the aniseikonic correction is obtained from the three measurements (×90, ×180, and declination) using magnification tables. The decision to prescribe a full, partial, or no aniseikonic correction is based on the measurements and professional judgment regarding the availability of the correction, the cost, and the likelihood that the patient will have successful relief of symptoms. In a following section, these points will be discussed further. Next, however, we discuss some of the difficulties experienced during aniseikonic examination with the eikonometer.

Aniseikonic Examination Difficulties

Monocular Suppression

Patients who lack sufficient stereopsis to respond during eikonometry report that the Space Eikonometer target appears flat. Other indications of monocular suppression is a patient report that the bright white (yellowish) vertical lines appear in front of the red cross or the dull green vertical lines appear behind the red cross. This report indicates that the patient is using the monocular clues of brightness, rather than stereopsis, to evaluate the appearance of the target.

If there is a question as to whether an eye is being suppressed, have the patient observe the target with one eye and then the other. With the right eye, the two right vertical lines are closer together than the two left vertical lines. With the left eye, the left vertical lines appear closer together than the right lines. Thus, with both eyes open, the suppressing eye can be determined by asking the patient whether the right or left vertical lines appear closer together.

Heterophoria

For some patients with good fusion and stereopsis, the Space Eikonometer test indicates the presence of small amounts of heterophoria, most frequently hyperphoria. When there is even as little as 0.5 Δ uncorrected hyperphoria, one of the oblique lines of the cross in the target often appears in front of the other (Fig. 18.5). If this observation is reported, fixation disparity testing should be done to determine the vertical prism required to reduce the fixation disparity to zero (Chapter 14). Then, determine (by the method of bracketing) that the prism ensures exact coincidence of the oblique lines. This is done by placing a 0.5 Δ prism alternately base-down and then base-up before one eye. If there is no remaining hyperphoria, one oblique line will appear in front of the other (and vice versa), as the prism is flipped from base-down to base-up. The proper power prism (it may require more than 0.5 Δ) is then placed in a trial frame and the aniseikonic test is continued.

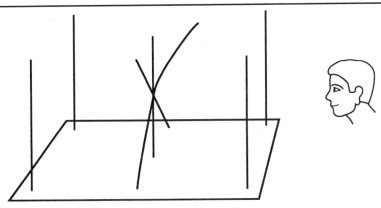

FIG. 18.5. When there is an uncorrected hyperphoria, the Space Eikonometer target may appear to be distorted, and one limb of the cross will tilt toward the observer. Reports of this phenomenon should alert the examiner to place small amounts of vertical prism in front of the hyperphoric eye to restore the perception of a symmetrical cross so that more accurate judgments of the position of the cross can be made.

MANAGEMENT

Prescribing iseikonic corrections requires similar clinical judgment to that used when prescribing refractive and heterophoric corrections. Factors to be considered include the age of the patient, the nature of the previous corrections and the patient's reaction to them, the type of work and hobbies, the patient's temperament and concern about the appearance and expense of the correction, and, above all, the nature of the symptoms and the likelihood of their elimination or reduction by iseikonic correction.

Practical Considerations

In designing iseikonic prescriptions, it is easy to allow the desire to solve the optical problem to overshadow the problems that the patient may have with the correction being prescribed. Remember the primary complaint of the patient and attempt to solve that problem, without creating a new one. A prescription that is optically correct might be considered unwearable by the patient. In certain instances, it is preferable not to prescribe the full refractive findings, but rather to modify them instead of ordering bitoric lenses. A slight change in cylinder axis or power may only reduce the acuity slightly and be preferable to an expensive prescription with unacceptable appearance or weight. In almost all instances, common sense dictates use of the simplest solution and determines the difference between success and failure of management.

Lens Prescription

Although there are no hard and fast rules for prescribing aniseikonic corrections, we recommend considering the following factors when deciding whether or not to recommend an iseikonic correction.

Factors that suggest not prescribing include:

1. Inconsistent or variable measurements of the size difference on repeated trials.
2. Poor depth perception.
3. Aniseikonia in reverse to that expected from the anisometropia.

4. Symptoms that are not related to use of the eyes or have not been improved by refractive or heterophoric corrections.
5. A patient who is comfortable, even with a significant aniseikonia. This can occur if a partial refractive correction for one eye has been worn for several years.

Factors that suggest prescribing include:

1. Aniseikonia that can be measured with a sensitivity smaller than the size difference measured (e.g., 1.0% ±0.50% rather than 0.75% ±1.5%).
2. Definite symptoms related to the use of the eyes.
3. Relief of symptoms with monocular occlusion when there is no significant lateral or vertical heterophoria.
4. Improvement of symptoms while wearing a temporary size lens clip-on for 1 to 2 days.
5. Anisometropia, where the full refractive correction causes (or is likely to cause) discomfort.
6. Failure of other corrections to provide relief of the symptoms.

Prescription Decisions Regarding Patients with Aniseikonia

The issues in designing aniseikonic corrections are comprised of two slightly different points of view—eliminating all estimated magnification difference between the two eyes or eliminating all measured magnification difference between the two eyes. Both of these philosophies have merit and the fact that each "works" clinically indicates that iseikonic lens design is often not an exact science and is frequently more of an art of patient management.

Estimated Magnification Prescriptions

When prescribing to eliminate all estimated magnification (26) difference between the two eyes, the actual aniseikonia is generally not measured, but it is assumed to be related to the difference in the spectacle magnification of the lenses. In practice, this technique is often used when instruments such as the Space Eikonometer are not available. Clinically, practitioners who prescribe, using this philosophy, generally choose to prescribe less magnification than that which would be expected to reduce the magnification difference between the lenses to zero. Typically, around 1.0% per diopter of anisometropia is used to estimate the amount of magnification to prescribe. Unfortunately, this technique tends to be less accurate when prescribing for patients with anisometropic myopia. In general, however, prescriptions designed from this philosophy contain slightly more magnification than those prescribed that are based on actual measures of the aniseikonia.

Measured Aniseikonia Prescriptions

When the aniseikonia present is measured with, for example, a Space Eikonometer, a prescription can be designed that eliminates the measured magnification difference between the two eyes. In this technique, measurements are usually taken through a patient's best spectacle correction. From knowledge of the parameters of the old spectacle correction (eyewire distance, front curve, thickness, and index of refraction), an iseikonic correction is designed by altering these parameters to reduce the measured magnification difference to zero. As long as aniseikonia can be measured, this technique is equally satisfactory for both anisometropic hyperopia and anisometropic myopia. Prescriptions designed that are based on this philosophy usually have slightly less magnification than those that are based on estimates derived from calculation of possible aniseikonia from differences in spectacle lens power.

Regardless of the philosophy of prescribing for patients with aniseikonia, the tables in this chapter can be used to design iseikonic corrections. When prescribing to eliminate an estimated difference in magnification, simply decide how much residual magnification you wish to leave and design a lens that achieves this requirement. If aniseikonia is measured, it is very easy, using the tables, to design an iseikonic correction that reduces the measured difference to zero. The issue of dynamic and static aniseikonia is also not a problem when the aniseikonia is measured, and the measurement includes both static and dynamic components of aniseikonia. The designed iseikonic correction will then be the correction required.

Iseikonic Lens Design

The process of designing lenses to correct aniseikonia, combined with refractive correction (known as "translation"), does not have to be a complex task. When the patient is wearing spectacle lenses, changes in the dimensions of these lenses (front curve, thickness, and position from the eye) can be made to introduce the desired iseikonic correction. This procedure makes it unnecessary to consider the magnification properties of trial lenses and simplifies the design of iseikonic lenses. When patients are already wearing spectacle lenses, the only thing that has to be determined is the amount of magnification needed.

Before considering iseikonic lens design, two steps should be tried. Each of these has merit and together they eliminate the need for many iseikonic corrections. First, prescribe contact lenses whenever possible. Many times a contact lens correction, which eliminates the problem of dynamic aniseikonia, will allow comfortable binocular vision in the presence of a moderate to large amount of static aniseikonia. The success of this premise is illustrated by Case 18.1.

Case Studies

Case 18.1

A 39-year-old woman had radial keratotomy (RK) 2 years previously on her right eye. She did not have the left eye done because of displeasure with the visual results of the first procedure. Her primary complaint was blurred vision at distance and near. She had been about 1 D myopic before RK and had worn spectacles occasionally. She had never worn contact lenses. She had post-RK spectacles, but had broken them. Vision with the spectacles was not satisfactory, due to frequent fluctuations of vision. Refractive error was:

OD: $+7.25$ c $- 2.50 \times 080$ 6/7.5
OS: -1.25 c $- 0.25 \times 090$ 6/6 $+2$
OU: 6/6 $+2$

Keratometric readings were:

OD: 33.25 173, 30.00 at 083   Badly distorted mires
OS: 39.00 173, 38.87 at 083

Because of the large anisometropia, contact lenses were advised. The contact lens for the right eye was fitted to vault the RK-flattened (30.00 D) central cornea, using a front curve of 9.0 mm (38.50 D). This resulted in a high plus refractive tear film which, combined with the contact lens, corrected the refractive error. The power ordered was determined by trial fitting and overrefraction, as is frequently necessary, due to the unreliability of post-RK central keratometry readings.

The patient returned after adapting to the lenses for 3 weeks. She had no trouble during the adaptation period. With the contact lenses, her acuities were:

OD: 6/6 +1   Overrefraction: OD: plano
OS: 6/6 −1   OS: −0.50 6/6

At 6 m, there was no suppression. She was orthophoric, and stereopsis was 2 minutes of arc. At 40 cm, she was orthophoric and stereopsis was 80 seconds of arc (with the AO Vectographic Slide and Near Card series). Space Eikonometry, with her contact lenses in place, revealed little or no aniseikonia, in spite of the anisometropia. She was happy with the vision and had none of the binocular problems that might be expected with anisometropia of this amount. She was advised to continue to increase her wearing time and return in 1 month or as needed.

When a patient does not want to wear contact lenses, judicious changes in the prescription may reduce the potential problem. Thus, our second recommendation is to consider small axis or power alterations for older patients who might be expected to have difficulties with space perception or the moderate changes in astigmatism axis or power that frequently occur. Modification of the correction, when needed, will minimize patient dissatisfaction with a new correction that causes perceptual distortion. Such modifications often alleviate the need to prescribe bitoric iseikonic bifocal lens. Case 18.2 illustrates these tenets.

Case 18.2

H.B., a 61-year-old man, was seen for a routine evaluation. He complained of a slight reduction in distance acuity and some problems reading over the past few months. He was noticing that he could see slightly better at distance when he raised his chin to look through his trifocal. He had glaucoma controlled with Propine (dipivefrin HCL-0.1%), which he started taking after developing severe systemic side effects to Timoptic (Timolol Maleate, MSD—0.25%). His current spectacles were:

R: +0.50 DS   20/40 +2   +2.25 add
L: +0.25 c − 0.25 × 90   20/40   50% trifocal

There was a normal fundus appearance, with very slight early senescent nuclear lens changes in each eye. Interocular pressures were 20 (right eye), 21 (left eye), (American Optical Non-contact Tonometer) (AONCT). Visual fields were full and normal. Refractive error was:

R: +1.25c − 1.00 × 75   20/20 +2
L: +1.00c − 0.75 × 109   20/15 −2

There was a 6 exophoria at 6 m and 14 exophoria at 40 cm through the add. There was no fixation disparity at 6 m and 240 degrees of stereopsis (AO Vectographic Adult slide). A +2.50 add was require for near. Near stereopsis was 200 degrees (Randot) and there was no suppression.

The patient reported clear vision with the new correction in a trial frame, but he noticed that the tabletop slanted and he felt that he had trouble judging where to place his feet when he walked. Modifying the lens correction to change the cylinder axis to 90 degrees and reducing the cylinder power gave satisfactory acuity and eliminated the perceptual distortions. These changes were discussed with him, along with the option for iseikonic lenses to give the clearest acuity and eliminate the distortions. H.B. preferred not to spend the money for an iseikonic correction. The final prescription was:

R: +1.25 c − 0.50 × 90   20/20 −2   +2.25 add
L: +1.00 c − 0.50 × 90   20/20 −1   50% trifocal

The patient returned for a progress evaluation in 2 weeks and reported clear vision with no perceptual distortion with the new correction. Due to the clear acuity without symptoms with a modified conventional correction, no further aniseikonic evaluation was considered.

Fear of potential aniseikonia is NOT appropriate as a rationale for withholding or reducing the power of corrections required by patients with binocular anomalies, such as those who have anisometropic amblyopia that can be successfully treated when they wear the full correction (Chapter 16). For these patients, the benefits of full correction almost invariably outweigh the possible detriments that might occur from induced aniseikonia.

Our third recommendation applies to the commonly seen patient who does not want to wear contact lenses, but who needs the full prescription for clear vision and best binocularity. In these cases, we suggest prescribing spectacles that best correct the refractive error. This is done for two reasons:

1. Some people readily adapt to almost anything (explain a 20 Δ esophoria and a 5 Δ esotropia) and, if the patient adapts comfortably to a conventional correction, the difficulty of designing an iseikonic correction is averted.
2. If the patient cannot adapt to conventional spectacle lenses, then there is a basis for testing, and the parameters of the spectacle lenses can be altered to produce necessary magnification changes. Usually 2 to 4 weeks are sufficient to determine whether the lens correction will be satisfactory. If severe symptoms remain after this time, aniseikonic correction will probably be required.

There are three general rules to follow when altering dimensions of a patient's spectacle lenses, in order to arrive at an approximate correction for aniseikonia (27,28):

1. A change in vertex distance (h) of a lens results in a change in magnification.
2. An increase in the front surface curvature (D_1) of a lens results in an increase in magnification.
3. An increase in the thickness (t) of a lens increases magnification.

There are physical restrictions in the amount of change that can be made in any single variable (e.g., t cannot be reduced to below about 1.5 mm without compromising lens strength). As a result, when designing iseikonic lenses, make small changes in all relevant variables rather than attempting to produce desired magnification changes by modification of only one parameter.

MAGNIFICATION BY CHANGING EYEWIRE DISTANCE AND BEVEL

Eyewire Distance Changes

Table 18.2 shows the approximate percentage changes in magnification that can be achieved with change of eyewire distance (Δh) for various refractive powers. When the spectacle frame

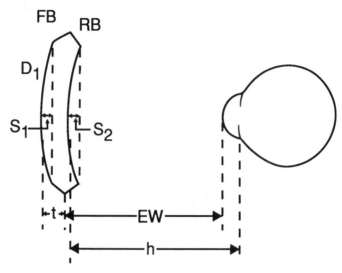

FIG. 18.6. A change in vertex distance (Δh) of a lens results in a change in magnification. Change in eyewire distance (Δh) is positive when the spectacle frame is moved away from the eyes. Eyewire distance is not h, but is considered close enough for calculations determining image size change based on changes in lens position. (D_1, front surface curve; t, lens center thickness; h, vertex distance that is from the posterior pole of the lens to the entrance pupil; FR, front bevel; RB, rear bevel; S_1, front sag; S_2, rear sag.)

is moved away from the eyes, Δh is positive. Eyewire distance is not h (Fig. 18.6), but it can be considered close enough for these calculations.

As an example of the usefulness of Table 18.2, suppose a patient is wearing:

> R: −6.00 D.S. (diopter sphere)   14.5 mm eyewire distance
> L: −2.00 D.S.

Overall magnification of 1.25% (right eye) is decided upon, based on clinical judgment that less than the estimated 4% (4 D anisometropia × 1% per diopter) can be worn comfortably. Repositioning both lenses closer to the eyes will increase the magnification of each lens, but it will be more for the right than the left because of its greater power. This is independent of the fact that no change is made in the front curves and center thicknesses. If the lenses are moved nearer to the eyes by 3 mm (to an eyewire distance of 11.5 mm), the magnification change (Table 18.2) will be +1.8% for the right lens and +0.6 for the left lens. The difference [(+1.8%) − (+0.6%)] is +1.2% more magnification for the right lens, approximately the desired change.

Bevel Changes

The thicker edges of minus lenses make it possible to change magnification by shifting the bevel of the right and left lenses. Table 18.3 shows magnification changes realized by changing from a center bevel to a 1/3 − 2/3 or 2/3 − 1/3 bevel. A 1/3 − 2/3 bevel moves a lens nearer to the eye and increases the magnification of minus lenses, while an anterior bevel (2/3 − 1/3) moves a lens away and decreases the magnification of a minus lens.

The effects of bevel changes are apparent when considering the patient wearing:

R: −8.00 D.S. (center bevel)
L: −8.00 D.S.

TABLE 18.3. *Approximate magnification (percent) changes by changing lens bevel from center to 1/3–2/3 or 2/3–1/3 (2.1 mm center thickness)[a]*

Power (D)	−1.00	−2.00	−4.00	−6.00	−8.00	−10.00
Eye size (mm)						
36	0.03	0.10	0.22	0.37	0.56	0.77
38	0.03	0.10	0.23	0.40	0.61	0.84
40	0.04	0.10	0.24	0.43	0.67	0.92
42	0.04	0.10	0.25	0.46	0.72	1.05
44	0.04	0.10	0.26	0.49	0.78	1.13
46	0.04	0.11	0.28	0.52	0.82	1.19
48	0.04	0.11	0.29	0.54	0.87	1.26
50	0.05	0.11	0.30	0.57	0.92	1.36
52	0.05	0.11	0.31	0.60	0.96	1.44

[a]Minus lens: moved closer to the eye, increases magnification; moved farther from the eye, decreases magnification.
Based on calculating lens edge thickness:

$$\text{edge thickness} = 2.1 - \frac{V_o h_2}{2(tn)}$$

Where: 2.1 = lens center thickness (millimeters)
V_o = lens vertex power (diopters)
Diopter = D
h = lens radius (millimeters)
n = the index of refraction of the lens material (glass = 1.523) minus the index of refraction of air (1.000).

The amount that a bevel change can vary lens position (h) is then calculated and used in the formula m(magnification)% = V_o(h)/10 (Table 18.1), to calculate the change in magnification that can be realized from a bevel change.

The smallest measurement of the frame determines the amount of effect in magnification that bevel alteration will give for minus lenses (the opposite is true for plus lenses). For a frame that measures 44 × 40 mm, the 40 mm measurement determines the amount the bevel can be varied and, thus, the magnification change for a minus lens.

Adjusting the bevels so that the right lens is moved closer (1/3 − 2/3 bevel) and the left farther (2/3 − 1/3 bevel) causes a magnification change of nearly 2.0% (1.92%) for a 52-mm eye size frame.

MAGNIFICATION BY CHANGING BASE CURVE

The change in magnification of a lens when the front surface power (D_1 − front curve) is changed is shown in Table 18.3. This table is based on 2.1-mm minimum lens thickness. The magnification gains of increasing lens front curve are greatest for patients wearing plus (hyperopic) corrections. Myopic corrections with powers greater than −2.50 D have a decrease of magnification, with an increase in front curve (if other parameters remain the same), because the front curve increase moves the lens vertex farther from the eye. The magnification change from an increased vertex distance with increased front curve is additive for hyperopic corrections. For minus lenses, the increase in magnification from a front curve increase is offset by a magnification decrease due to vertex distance changes.

As an example of modifying lens front curve to increase magnification, consider a patient wearing:

R: +3.00 D.S. + 7.50 front curve
L: +5.00 D.S. + 9.50 front curve

Magnification of 1.5% is to be added to the right lens. From Table 18.4, a +4 D increase in the front curve of the right lens (to +11.50) will be enough to give approximately the desired 1.5% increase. A 4 D front curve change for a +2.00 D lens would give a 1.13% increase, while changing a +4.00 D lens would give 1.9%. Thus, about 1.57% is achieved for a +3.00 D lens [(1.13 + 1.9)/2 = 1.57)]. Since the table goes in 2 D power steps, results for intermediate changes must be determined by interpolation.

MAGNIFICATION BY CHANGING LENS THICKNESS

Tables 18.5 and 18.6 show the magnification changes that result from a change in thickness (Δt) of a lens of specific front curve and power when other factors (bevel, vertex distance, etc.) are held constant. These tables also represent the fact that a change in vertex distance (Δh) results from an increase in Δt.

To use Tables 18.5 and 18.6, consider the patient wearing:

R: plano/+6.25 front curve/2.1 mm thickness
L: −2.00 D.S./+4.50 front curve/2.1 mm thickness

A 0.75% increase in magnification is desired on the left lens. To use the tables requires subtraction of the value from Table 18.6 from that in Table 18.5 to determine the percentage change in magnification. Increasing thickness increases magnification and, to achieve our desired magnification, the thickness of the left lens must be increased. From Table 18.5, for a front curve of +4.50 and a thickness increase of +2.0 mm, the value is +0.600%. From Table 18.6, for a lens power of −2.00 and a thickness increase of +2.0 mm, the value is −0.20. The +0.80% [A (+0.600) − B (−0.20)] change in magnification achieved approximates the +0.75% desired.

Increasing lens thickness gives a corresponding increase in edge thickness. This increased edge thickness can be used by changing the bevel to gain a change in magnification. Table 18.7 shows changes in magnification that result from a bevel change after the lens thickness has been increased. This effect is most significant when lens vertex power is greater than −4.00 or +6.00 D or when a significant increase in thickness has been prescribed.

CONSIDERATIONS FOR ISEIKONIC PRESCRIPTIONS

A +2.0 mm thickness increase and a front curve increase of +4 D both represent large changes. As a result, all three variables—eyewire distance (h), front curve (D_1), and thickness (t)—should be altered to achieve desired magnification changes. In this manner, smaller changes can be made to each, and the resulting prescription will be more cosmetically satisfactory. Table 18.8 gives a summary of the effects that can be realized by changing the various parameters. However, in spite of all precautions, very steep front curves and/or very thick lenses are sometimes needed to achieve desired magnification effects. To achieve the most cosmetically appealing result, care should be taken to use lens coatings and a minimum frame size.

Antireflective Coating and Lens Edge Coating

Steep front curves and/or increased lens thickness can cause unwanted internal reflections, as well as resulting in a rather strange looking pair of spectacles. Antireflective coatings are a useful technique that can be used to eliminate a number of excessive reflections. An antireflective coating and a frame-matching edge coat on lenses with an edge thickness over

TABLE 18.4. Approximate magnification (percent) changes associated with various lens powers and changes in front surface curvature[a]

Power (D)	-10 t = 2.1	-8 t = 2.1	-6 t = 2.1	-4 t = 2.1	-2 t = 2.1	-1 t = 2.1	0 t = 2.1	+1 t = 2.6	+2 t = 3.1	+4 t = 4.1	+6 t = 5.1	+8 t = 6.1	+10 t = 7.1
ΔBase curve (D₁)													
-4	+1.46	+1.04	+0.64	+0.24	-0.16	-0.36	-0.56	-0.90	-1.23	-1.90	-2.56	-3.24	-3.88
-2	+0.72	+0.52	+0.32	+0.12	-0.08	-0.18	-0.28	-0.45	-0.61	-0.95	-1.28	-1.62	-1.94
+2	-0.72	-0.52	-0.32	-0.12	+0.08	+0.18	+0.28	+0.45	+0.61	+0.95	+1.28	+1.62	+1.94
+4	-1.46	-1.04	-0.64	-0.24	+0.16	+0.36	+0.56	+0.90	+1.23	+1.90	+2.56	+3.24	+3.88
+6	-2.18	-1.56	-0.96	-0.36	+0.24	+0.54	+0.84	+1.35	+1.84	+2.85	+3.84	+4.86	+5.82
+8	-2.92	-2.08	-1.28	-0.48	+0.32	+0.72	+1.12	+1.80	+2.46	+3.80	+5.12	+6.48	+7.76

[a]Based on: $\Delta m\% = \Delta D_1 [\frac{t}{15} + 0.05 V_o]$

Where: $\Delta m\%$ = change in magnification (percent)

ΔD_1 = the change in lens front surface curve (diopters)

t = lens center thickness (millimeters)

D = diopter

15 = a corrected constant; made up of the index of refraction of glass corrected for the fact that magnification is expressed in percent and lens thickness is expressed in millimeters

0.05 = the change in vertex distance (approximate) for a change in front surface curvature of ΔD_1

V_o = lens vertex power (diopters)

TABLE 18.5. *Magnification changes that result from a change in thickness and front curve*

Base curve	0.50	1.50	2.50	3.50	4.50	5.50	6.50	7.50	8.50	9.50	10.50	11.50	12.50	13.50
ΔThickness (mm)[a]														
-1.5	-0.05	-0.15	-0.25	-0.35	-0.45	-0.55	-0.65	-0.75	-0.85	-0.95	-1.05	-1.15	-1.25	-1.35
-1.0	-0.03	-0.10	-0.17	-0.23	-0.30	-0.37	-0.43	-0.50	-0.57	-0.63	-0.70	-0.77	-0.83	-0.90
-0.5	-0.02	-0.05	-0.08	-0.17	-0.15	-0.18	-0.22	-0.25	-0.28	-0.32	-0.35	-0.38	-0.42	-0.45
+0.5	+0.02	+0.05	+0.08	+0.17	+0.15	+0.18	+0.22	+0.25	+0.28	+0.32	+0.35	+0.38	+0.42	+0.45
+1.0	+0.03	+0.10	+0.17	+0.23	+0.30	+0.37	+0.43	+0.50	+0.57	+0.63	+0.70	+0.77	+0.83	+0.90
+1.5	+0.05	+0.15	+0.25	+0.35	+0.45	+0.55	+0.65	+0.75	+0.85	+0.95	+1.05	+1.15	+1.25	+1.35
+2.0	+0.06	+0.20	+0.33	+0.47	+0.60	+0.72	+0.87	+1.00	+1.13	+1.26	+1.40	+1.52	+1.66	+1.80
+2.5	+0.08	+0.25	+0.42	+0.58	+0.75	+0.92	+1.08	+1.25	+1.41	+1.58	+1.75	+1.92	+2.08	+2.25
+3.0	+0.10	+0.30	+0.50	+0.70	+0.90	+1.10	+1.30	+1.50	+1.70	+1.90	+2.10	+2.30	+2.50	+2.69
+3.5	+0.11	+0.35	+0.58	+0.82	+1.05	+1.28	+1.52	+1.75	+1.98	+2.21	+2.45	+2.68	+2.91	+3.14
+4.0	+0.13	+0.40	+0.67	+0.92	+1.20	+1.46	+1.73	+2.00	+2.26	+2.52	+2.80	+3.06	+3.33	+3.59
+4.5	+0.14	+0.45	+0.84	+1.03	+1.35	+1.65	+1.95	+2.25	+2.54	+2.84	+3.15	+3.48	+3.74	+4.03

[a] + = thickness increase; − = thickness decrease.

TABLE 18.6. *Magnification changes that result from a change in thickness for a given lens power[a]*

Lens power (D)	−10	−8	−6	−4	−2	0	+2	+4	+6	+8	+10
ΔThickness (mm)											
−1.5	+0.75	+0.60	+0.45	+0.30	+0.15	0.0	−0.15	−0.30	−0.45	−0.60	−0.75
−1.0	+0.50	+0.40	+0.30	+0.20	+0.10	0.0	−0.10	−0.20	−0.30	−0.40	−0.50
−0.5	+0.25	+0.20	+0.15	+0.10	+0.05	0.0	−0.05	−0.10	−0.15	−0.20	−0.25
+0.5	−0.25	−0.20	−0.15	−0.10	−0.05	0.0	+0.05	+0.10	+0.15	+0.20	+0.25
+1.0	−0.50	−0.40	−0.30	−0.20	−0.10	0.0	+0.10	+0.20	+0.30	+0.40	+0.50
+1.5	−0.75	−0.60	−0.45	−0.30	−0.15	0.0	+0.15	+0.30	+0.45	+0.60	+0.75
+2.0	−1.00	−0.80	−0.60	−0.40	−0.20	0.0	+0.20	+0.40	+0.60	+0.80	+1.00
+2.5	−1.25	−1.00	−0.75	−0.50	−0.25	0.0	+0.25	+0.50	+0.75	+1.00	+1.25
+3.0	−1.50	−1.20	−0.90	−0.60	−0.30	0.0	+0.30	+0.60	+0.90	+1.20	+1.50
+3.5	−1.75	−1.40	−1.05	−0.70	−0.35	0.0	+0.35	+0.70	+1.05	+1.40	+1.75
+4.0	−2.00	−1.60	−1.20	−0.80	−0.40	0.0	+0.40	+0.80	+1.20	+1.60	+2.00
+4.5	−2.25	−1.80	−1.35	−0.90	−0.45	0.0	+0.45	+0.90	+1.35	+1.80	+2.25

[a]A and B = Δm% for a given base curve, thickness change, and lens power

$$\text{Based on } \Delta m\% = \frac{\Delta t D_1}{15} + \frac{2 V_o}{10}$$

This holds true when the bevel of a lens is centered and lens thickness is increased without changing lens curvature or eyewire distance.

Where: Δm% = change in magnification (percent)
  Δt = change in lens thickness (millimeters)
  D_1 = lens front surface curve (diopters)
  Diopter = D
  15 = a corrected constant; made up of the index of glass corrected for the fact that magnification is expressed in percent and lens thickness in millimeters.
  V_o = lens vertex power (diopters)
  10 results from changing meters to millimeters and expressing magnification in percent

To calculate Δm% the data from Table 18.5 is labeled "A" and is subtracted from the data from Table 18.6 (labeled "B").

TABLE 18.7. *Approximate changes in magnification (percent) by changing lens bevel from center to 1/3–2/3 or 2/3–1/3 when the thickness has been changed in fixed steps from standard (2.1 mm minimum) thickness (based on 46 mm eye size minus lenses)[a]*

Power (D)	−10	−8	−6	−4	−2	−1	0	+1	+2	+4	+6	+8	+10
ΔThickness (mm)													
−1.5	0.94	0.62	0.36	0.18	0.05	0.02	0.00	0.01	0.02	0.04	0.06	0.08	0.10
−1.0	1.02	0.68	0.41	0.21	0.07	0.03	0.00	0.02	0.04	0.07	0.11	0.14	0.18
−0.5	1.11	0.75	0.46	0.24	0.09	0.04	0.00	0.03	0.05	0.11	0.16	0.22	0.27
+0.5	1.28	0.89	0.56	0.31	0.12	0.05	0.00	0.04	0.09	0.18	0.26	0.35	0.44
+1.0	1.36	0.95	0.61	0.34	0.14	0.06	0.00	0.05	0.10	0.21	0.31	0.42	0.52
+1.5	1.45	1.02	0.67	0.38	0.15	0.07	0.00	0.06	0.12	0.24	0.36	0.48	0.60
+2.0	1.52	1.09	0.71	0.41	0.17	0.08	0.00	0.07	0.14	0.28	0.41	0.55	0.69
+2.5	1.61	1.16	0.77	0.44	0.19	0.09	0.00	0.08	0.16	0.31	0.46	0.62	0.77
+3.0	1.68	1.22	0.82	0.48	0.20	0.09	0.00	0.09	0.17	0.34	0.51	0.68	0.85
+3.5	1.78	1.29	0.87	0.51	0.22	0.10	0.00	0.09	0.19	0.38	0.56	0.75	0.94
+4.0	1.85	1.35	0.91	0.54	0.24	0.11	0.00	0.10	0.20	0.41	0.61	0.82	1.02
+4.5	1.94	1.42	0.96	0.57	0.26	0.11	0.00	0.10	0.21	0.44	0.66	0.89	1.10

[a]Minus lens: moved closer to the eye, increases magnification; moved farther from the eye, decreases magnification.
Plus lens: moved closer to the eye, decreases magnification; moved farther from the eye, increases magnification.
Based on calculating lens edge thickness:

$$\text{Minus lens edge thickness} = 2.1 - \frac{V_o h^2}{2(\Delta n)} + \Delta t$$

$$\text{Plus lens edge thickness} = 2.1 + \Delta t$$

Where: 2.1 = minimum lens thickness (millimeters)
V_o = lens vertex power (diopters)
h = lens radius (millimeters)
Δn = the index of refraction of the lens material (glass = 1.523) minus the index of refraction of air (1.000).
Δt is change in lens thickness (millimeters)
The amount that a bevel change can vary lens position (Δh) is then calculated and used in the formula from
Table 18.1 to calculate the change in magnification that can be realized from a bevel change.

TABLE 18.8. *How changes in lens parameters affect lens magnification*

	Strong minus lens	Weak minus lens	Weak plus lens	Strong plus lens
Vertex distance				
Further	Decrease	Little	Little	Increase
Closer	Increase	effect	effect	Decrease
Bevel				
Forward	Increase	Little	Little	Decrease
Backward	Decrease	effect	effect	Increase
Front surface				
Steeper	Small decrease	Increase	Increase	Increase
Flatter	Small increase	Decrease	Decrease	Decrease
Thickness				
Thicker	Increase	Increase	Increase	Increase
Thinner	Decrease	Decrease	Decrease	Decrease

Index	Material
1.4985	CR-39 Plastic
1.523	Crown Glass
1.556	Hi Lite
1.577	True-Lite
1.586	Polycarbonate plastic
1.601	Glass/plastic
1.701	High Index Glass
1.805	Index Eight

2.6 to 3.1 mm will greatly enhance acceptability of iseikonic prescriptions by reducing internal reflections and improving cosmetic appearance.

Frame Size and Material

Careful consideration to selection of frames for iseikonic prescriptions is very important. A fairly heavy frame that fits well will be a good choice because a small change in eyewire distance has a large effect on magnification, especially for patients with anisometropia. To achieve minimum lens thickness and weight, the frame should have as small an eye size as possible. Thick edges of iseikonic lenses can be better concealed by a zyl frame than by a rimless or metal frame.

Examples of Lens Design

The procedures used to achieve desired magnification are complex enough to warrant detailed examples. Two cases, one spherical and one astigmatic, will be discussed. To obtain accurate results, use the following sequence (27):

1. Changes in eyewire distance are preferred because they are most acceptable cosmetically. Thus, we recommend maximally changing eyewire distance (Table 18.2) initially, so that as much magnification change as possible can be realized from this change. When the aniseikonic correction is in the same direction as the anisometropia, reduce eyewire distance as much as possible (keeping in mind that 9 to 10 mm is the practical minimum). Increase the eyewire distance as much as possible when the aniseikonic correction is opposite to that expected from the anisometropia.

2. Change front curve (Table 18.4) as much as possible. Very steep or very flat front curves are not cosmetically appealing, so attempt to stay between +10.50 D and +2.00 D. Selecting front curves that correspond to those available from local laboratories will save both time and money.

3. Change the thickness of the lens (Tables 18.5 and 18.6), using the selected front curve from step 2.

4. Make bevel alterations as necessary, using Tables 18.3 and/or 18.7.

Case Studies

Case 18.3: Design from Estimation

A 23-year-old woman is referred with complaints of long-standing symptoms of headaches and asthenopia when wearing her spectacle correction. She has tried contact lenses, with relief of the asthenopia, but allergies have forced her to discontinue contact lens wear. Her refractive correction is:

R: −1.00 DS
2.1-mm minimum (center) thickness   +5.25 front curve center bevel
15-mm eyewire distance
L: −4.00 DS
2.1-mm minimum (center) thickness   +3.50 front curve center bevel
15-mm eyewire distance
K (keratometer) readings are:
R: 44/50/180 44.75
L: 46.25/180 46.50

Based on the corneal curvatures, the anisometropia of the patient in Case 18.3 is at least partially of dioptric origin. Ogle (29) stated that 1.5% aniseikonia per diopter of anisometropia is the usual amount expected. Since anisometropia is usually due (at least partially) to axial length differences, and underprescribing is the rule rather than the exception, we decided to give 3.0% magnification increase to the left eye rather than 4.5%. To do this, follow the steps set forth earlier:

1. Decrease the eyewire distance (Table 18.2) from 15 mm to 10 mm (either by readjusting the present frame or selecting a new one), to increase magnification +0.5% for the right lens and +2.0% for the left. This is a difference [(+2.0) − (+0.5)] of +1.5%—an increase in magnification relative to the left lens.

2. Change front curve (Table 18.4). Increasing the front curve helps because more magnification can then be gained when thickness changes are made. However, Table 18.4 suggests that little change will occur, and we decided to follow the table and make no front curve change.

3. Change thickness (Tables 18.5 and 18.6). The final desired magnification depends primarily on increasing the thickness of the left lens. For a front curve of +3.50 and a thickness change of +2.5 mm, Table 18.5 equals 0.582 and Table 18.6 equals −0.50, when the thickness of a −4.00 D lens has been changed +2.5 mm. Consequently, the magnification change for changing thickness +2.5 mm [A (+0.582) − B (−0.50)] is + 1.082%.

4. Changing the bevel (Table 18.7) of a −4.00 D.S. lens, which has had a thickness increase of +2.5 mm to move the lens closer (change from center to 1/3 − 2/3 bevel), gives a magnification change of +0.44%.

Alterations of lens parameters have changed the magnification of both lenses to give a net increase of 3.02% magnification overall, left eye. This is determined from:

Change eyewire distance	1.50%
Change front curve	No change made
Change thickness	1.08%
Change bevel	0.44%

Case 18.3: Final Prescription

R: −1.00 D.S.
2.1-mm (center) thickness   +5.25 front curve center bevel
10-mm eyewire distance
L: −4.00 D.S.
4.6-mm (center) thickness   +3.50 front curve 1/3 − 2/3 bevel
10-mm eyewire distance
Antireflective coat; edge coat

Bitoric Lenses

The bitoric lens has different amounts of magnification, in different meridians, within the same lens. In general, iseikonic bitoric lenses are designed so that the same meridians are used for the front cylinder and for the refractive astigmatic correction. Thus, to correct the refractive error and give the desired magnification, both lenses will typically have cylindrical front and back surfaces, since only one center thickness is possible on a lens. The cylinder axes on the front and back of each lens must be aligned exactly to produce the desired lens power. Even a 0.5-degree misalignment can cause significant power deviation from that required. Bitoric lenses are difficult to fabricate and there are few laboratories equipped to do this type of work. When ordering a bitoric lens from a lab, it is best to simplify the order so that it is more easily understood—for example, by using a power diagram (optical cross). Specify the front curves, center thickness, and total power. The lab will determine the proper back curves. To check the lenses when they are received, simply verify the refractive power (using the lensometer), determine that the center thickness matches your order, and check that the front curves have the proper powers and axes.

Case 18.4

A 19-year-old uncorrected symptomatic woman has a 2 Δ exophoria at distance and near. Her refractive correction and acuity are the same as her current correction. Her current correction is:

R: +1.00   20/20−   PD = 62
L: +1.00 c − 2.00 ×180   20/20
Front curve: +6.50 OD and +4.50 OS
Center thickness: 2.6 mm OD and 2.1 mm OS
Eyewire distance: 14.0 mm

Twenty-four hours of diagnostic occlusion eliminated the patient's symptoms. No significant lateral or vertical heterophoria was found. Space Eikonometry reveals the need for:

left 1.25% O.A.c 1.75% × 180

> There are moderate to severe seasonal allergies, and slit lamp examination reveals moderate follicles under both upper lids.

Since contact lens fitting is not appropriate due to allergy and lid appearance, an iseikonic prescription will be designed. When there is a meridional correction required, each principal meridian must be considered separately. For the right lens, the power is the same in all meridians: +1.00 in the 90-degree meridian and the same for the 180-degree meridian. For the left lens, the power in the 90-degree meridian is −3.00; in the 180-degree meridian, it is −1.00.

To design the lenses, follow the steps set forth earlier, but, this time, corresponding principal meridians must be compared.

Horizontal Meridian

1. Change eyewire distance (Table 18.2). Moving a +1.00 lens 4 mm closer decreases magnification in that meridian −0.4%. Moving a −1.00 (left lens, 180-degree meridian) lens 4 mm closer increases magnification +0.4%. This is a difference of 0.8%—a +0.8% increase in the 180-degree meridian, relative to the left lens.

2. Change front curve (Table 18.4). Because the +0.8% increase in magnification in the horizontal meridian (left lens) is most of the desired 1.25% change for that meridian, no front curve change will be made until the effect of the thickness change of step 3 is evaluated.

3. Change the thickness (Tables 18.5 and 18.6). From Tables 18.5 and 18.6, increasing the thickness of a −1.00 lens (with a +4.50 front curve) +1.5 mm gives an increase in magnification [A (+0.450) − B (−0.07)] of +0.52% (left lens, 180-degree meridian).

Vertical Meridian

1. Change eyewire distance (Table 18.2). Eyewire distance was reduced 4 mm in step 1 of the 180-degree meridian and this reduction must also be used in analysis of the 90-degree meridian. Reducing the eyewire distance from 14.0 to 10.0 mm decreases magnification—0.4% for the right (+1.00/90 degree) and increases magnification +1.2% for the left (−3.00/90 degree) lens. This is a difference of 1.6%—an increase of +1.6% in the 90-degree meridian, relative to the left lens.

2. Change front curve (Table 18.4). Decreasing the front curve (90-degree meridian) of the right (+1.00) lens by −2 D decreases magnification −0.45%. Previous discussion of increasing front curve of a lens of −2.50 D or greater showed that a decrease in magnification would result. However, with a steep front curve, an increase in thickness becomes much more significant. Thus, the front curve of the left (−3.00/ 90) lens should be increased. With a +4 D increase in front curve for the −3.00 lens, a decrease in magnification of −0.04% is realized (interpolated from Table 18.3). This gives a relative magnification increase of +0.41% in the 90-degree meridian of the left lens.

3. Change the thickness (Tables 18.5 and 18.6). Lens thickness was increased +1.5 mm when the 180-degree meridian was analyzed and this thickness change must also be used for calculations in the 90-degree meridian. No change in the front curve was made in the 180-degree meridian with a +8.50 front curve (from the +4 D increase in step 2). Increasing the thickness of a −3.00 lens (left lens, 90-degree meridian) by +1.5 mm gives a magnification increase [A (0.847) − B(−0.225)] of +1.072% in the 90-degree meridian.

4. Bevel change. No bevel change is made until the effects of the other changes are evaluated. Bevel changes should be made as a final step, in order to achieve additional needed magnification.

The magnification Changes are:

	180-degree meridian		90-degree meridian
	0.80%	Eyewire distance	1.60%
	No change	Front Curve	0.41%
	0.52%	Thickness	1.072%
	No change	Bevel	No change
	1.32% increase	Total	3.082% increase
	(left lens)		(left lens)

The result is 1.32% OA c 1.76% × 180, which is quite close to the magnification desired (1.25% OA c 1.75% × 180) for the left eye.

Case 18.4: Final Prescription

R: +1.00 DS
2.6-mm center thickness front curve +6.25/180; +4.25/90
10.5-mm eyewire distance center bevel
L: −1.00 − 2.00 × 180
3.6-mm center thickness front curve +4.50/180; +8.50/90
10.5-mm eyewire distance center bevel
Antireflective coat; edge coat

PATIENTS WITHOUT ANISEIKONIA

If the patient will have no (or minimal) aniseikonia with a spectacle correction, it is important that the new prescription be designed so that it will not create or exacerbate a problem. The primary issue to consider is whether the patient is currently wearing a correction or not. If the patient is already wearing a spectacle correction that is similar to the new one, prescribing front curves and center thickness that are equal to the old correction will generally create few problems. If there is a large change in correction or a first correction, then prescribing equal front curve and center thickness lenses in minus cylinder form will typically be sufficient when the prescription is for hyperopic anisometropia. When both lenses have minus power, it is usually superior practice to order stock lenses rather than equal front curve and center thickness, since stock lenses almost always have equal center thickness. Stock front curve lenses also have the proper corrected curves for the minus refractive powers prescribed. Further, the standard front curves used on stock minus power lenses provide a small amount of magnification to the eye, requiring more minus due to the flatter front curve on the more minus lens. If this small amount of magnification is not desired, equal front curves and center thickness should be ordered.

There are other ways that aniseikonia may be inadvertently induced by prescription of a new spectacle correction. This can occur, even when the actual change in refractive error is very small or the only change is that a patient chooses a new frame and the lens power is the same. These inadvertent iseikonic corrections occur because of changes in frame eye size and/or differences in the refractive index of the new and old prescription (e.g., glass lenses in the old correction and polycarbonate lenses in the new one).

Frame Eye Size Changes

When a new frame is chosen that has a substantially different eye size than the previous correction, aniseikonia may be inadvertently induced. In these instances, the patient experiences

TABLE 18.9. *Lens sag (millimeters) for various lens sizes and surface curvature*[a]

Surface curvature	1.50	2.50	3.50	4.50	5.50	6.50	7.50	8.50	9.50	10.50	11.50	12.50
Eye size (mm)												
36	0.4	0.7	1.0	1.4	1.7	2.0	2.3	2.6	2.9	3.3	3.6	3.9
38	0.4	0.8	1.1	1.5	1.9	2.2	2.6	2.9	3.3	3.6	4.0	4.3
40	0.5	0.9	1.3	1.7	2.1	2.5	2.9	3.3	3.7	4.1	4.4	4.8
42	0.5	1.0	1.5	1.9	2.3	2.7	3.2	3.6	4.0	4.5	4.9	5.3
44	0.5	1.1	1.5	2.0	2.5	3.0	3.5	4.0	4.4	4.9	5.4	5.9
46	0.6	1.2	1.8	2.2	2.8	3.3	3.8	4.4	4.9	5.4	6.0	6.5
48	0.7	1.3	1.9	2.4	3.0	3.6	4.2	4.7	5.3	5.9	6.5	7.1
50	0.7	1.4	2.1	2.6	3.2	3.9	4.5	5.2	5.8	6.5	7.1	7.8
52	0.8	1.5	2.2	2.8	3.5	4.2	4.9	5.6	6.3	7.1	7.8	8.6
54	1.0	1.7	2.4	3.1	3.8	4.6	5.3	6.1	6.9	7.7	8.4	9.3

[a]With a change in frame size, the type of correction determines the sag effect. For minus lenses, the smaller frame measurement determines the sag effect; for plus lenses, the larger frame measurement determines the sag effect.

a significant change in the magnification of the lens due to the change in vertex distance induced by the change in lens eye size. A larger lens eye size causes the lens to be located farther away, due to the change in lens sag (Fig. 18.7). Table 18.9 shows the changes in sag that occur when lenses of various size and front surface curvature are used. The change in sag causes the lens to be moved to a different distance from the eye and alters the magnification that the patient experiences.

As an example of the usefulness of Table 18.9, consider the patient wearing:

> R: +1.00 2.6-mm center thickness   +6.50 front curve center bevel
> 14-mm eyewire distance
> L: +4.00 4.1-mm center thickness   +10.50 front curve center bevel
> 14-mm eyewire distance
> Frame size: 42 × 40 mm

There is no change in correction and the patient wants a new and more stylish frame. No change in lens parameters will be made, but if the patient selects a new 52 × 48 mm frame, the lens sag will be increased for both lenses. Because both lenses are plus, the largest measurement of the frames determines the amount of sag. A +1.00 D lens with a +6.50 D front curve has a −5.50 D back curve. A +4.00 D lens with a +10.50 D front curve has a −6.50 D back curve.

From Table 18.9, for the right lens, the back curve is −5.50 and 42-mm "key" eye size sag is 2.3 mm. When frame eye size is increased to 52 mm, the sag is 3.5 mm. The difference is an increase in sag (vertex distance) of 1.2 mm (3.5 − 2.3). This causes a magnification increase of 0.12% (Table 18.2). From Table 18.9, the back curve for the left lens is −6.50 when eye size is 42 mm; the sag is 2.7 mm. Increasing the eye size to 52 mm increases sag to 4.2 mm. The difference (4.2 − 2.7) is an increase in sag (vertex distance) of 1.5 mm. This causes a magnification increase of 0.6% (Table 18.2). Thus, the change in frame eye size alone causes an increase in magnification of 0.48% (0.6 − 0.12) relative to the left lens. This difference may cause perceptual problems for the patient, with a possibility that he or she could never adjust unless other changes were made. The simplest change would be readjustment of the frame. If it were adjusted 1.5 mm closer (to an eyewire distance of 12.5 mm), the increase in magnification caused by the larger frame (+0.48%) would be offset by a decrease in magnification from moving the lenses closer to the eyes (−0.45%) (Table 18.2).

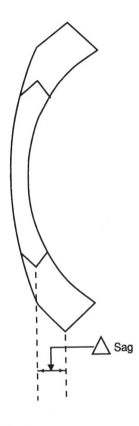

FIG. 18.7. An increase in lens eye size causes a change in lens sag. This change in sag places the lens at a different vertex distance and alters the magnification experienced by the patient. As a result of this factor, aniseikonia may be inadvertently induced when a new frame is chosen that has a substantially different eye size than the previous correction.

The same effect is present in minus corrections. As frame size increases, lens sag (vertex distance) increases and magnification is decreased (Fig. 18.7). For anisometropic corrections, the lens of greatest power has the greatest magnification decrease. This creates a difference in magnification between the two lenses that was not present previously and it may cause perceptual problems. Again, the method of choice for eliminating this effect is to adjust the frame closer to the eyes.

Refractive Index Changes

Changes in the refractive index of the lens also can result in inadvertent iseikonic corrections. Typically, the change in magnification that results from a change of refractive index is small. For example, there is a decrease in magnification of about 0.05% for a change from crown glass to polycarbonate plastic. This decrease in magnification means that, as the index of refraction is increased, the front curve can be made flatter and/or the lens thinner to achieve the same amount of magnification.

A frequent reason for changing to a higher index is to provide improved cosmetic appearance of spectacle lenses. Although the change in magnification is small, many patients complain of altered space perception. This usually results from a combination of the change in material (index of refraction), a decrease in lens center thickness that is often made to minimize edge thickness, and a lack of care in prescribing the front curve of the new prescription. To minimize complaints of altered perception, it is best to make the new minus lens with about 0.50 to 1.00 D more front curve than the old lenses and then to adjust the correction as close to the eyes as possible. Often more face-form (wrap around) and care that the pantoscopic tilt of the frame is the same as the old pair will also help minimize complaints of perceptual distortion due to inadvertent iseikonic correction.

SUMMARY AND CONCLUSION

Although there are a substantial number of patients with symptoms of aniseikonia, iseikonic lenses are not often prescribed. Careful review of the history and clinical tests will provide sufficient information to make a tentative diagnosis of the probability of aniseikonia. When there may be aniseikonia, we recommend first prescribing contact lenses or spectacle correction to determine whether simply correcting the refractive error will solve the patient's problems. Occasionally, for older patients, a small modification of cylinder axis or power may also alleviate symptoms of aniseikonia and eliminate the need for aniseikonic correction.

When iseikonic corrections are required, they can be designed using our general rules to alter dimensions of a patient's spectacle lenses to correct aniseikonia:

1. Changing vertex distance (h) changes magnification.
2. Increasing front surface curvature (D_1) increases magnification.
3. Increasing the thickness (t) increases magnification.
4. Recognition of these factors enables the clinician to determine what lens parameters to change and simplifies design of iseikonic corrections.

STUDY QUESTIONS

1. Why would it be important to differentiate between static and dynamic aniseikonia?
2. What is Knapp's law and why does it not hold true in many suspected cases of aniseikonia?
3. How are symptoms of aniseikonia similar to symptoms of patients with heterophoria?
4. What types of ocular surgery would lead to aniseikonia?
5. What can you do to determine image size difference without an eikonometer or a New Aniseikonia test?
6. Why would 1% be used to estimate the image size difference, when designing a lens correction?
7. In order to increase lens magnification, you need to change which lens factors in what manner?
8. Why does change in base curve not provided a change in magnification for a minus lens?
9. Why is frame eye size important in designing an iseikonic lens?
10. How can you minimize a patient's symptoms of altered space perception, when prescribing new glasses?

REFERENCES

1. Cline D, Hofstetter HW, Griffin JB, eds. *Dictionary of visual science,* 3rd ed. Radnor, PA: Chilton Book, 1989:36.
2. Ogle KN. *Researches in binocular vision.* Philadelphia: WB Saunders, 1950.
3. Bannon RE. *Clinical manual on aniseikonia.* Buffalo, NY: American Optical Co, 1954:100.
4. Reading RW. *Binocular vision foundations and applications.* Boston: Butterworth-Heineman, 1983:219–249.
5. Remole A. Anisophoria and aniseikonia. I. The relation between optical anisophoria and aniseikonia. *Optom Vis Sci* 1989;66:659–670.
6. Remole A. Anisophoria and aniseikonia. II. The management of optical anisophoria. *Optom Vis Sci* 1989;66: 736–746.
7. Burian HM. History of the Dartmouth Eye Institute. *Arch Ophthalmol* 1948;40(2):163–175.
8. Donders FC. *On the anomalies of accommodation and refraction of the eye.* London: New Sydenham Soc, 1864.
9. Lippincott JA. On the binocular metamorphopsia produced by correcting glasses. *Arch Ophthalmol* 1899;18:18.

10. Green J. On certain stereoscopical illusions evoked by prismatic and cylindrical glasses. *Trans Am Ophthalmol Soc* 1888/1890;5:449–456.
11. Friedenwald H. Binocular metomorphopsia produced by correcting glasses. *Arch Ophthalmol* 1892;21:204.
12. Koller C. The form of retinal images in the astigmatic eye. *Trans Am Ophthalmol Soc* 1892;6:425.
13. Hess C. Anisometropia. *Graefes Handb. d. ges. Augenheild.* ch XII, 1903.
14. Von Rohr. In: Henker. *Introduction to the theory of spectacles.* Jena, Switzerland: Jena School of Optics, 1924.
15. Errgelet H. Ein Beitrag zur Frage der Anisometropie. z. f. Sinnesphysiol 1916;49:326–364.
16. Errgelet H. Kurzes Handb. der Ophthal, vol 2. 1932.
17. Carleton EH, Madigan LF. Relationships between aniseikonia and ametropia—from a statistical study of clinical cases. *Arch Ophthalmol* 1937;18(2):237–247.
18. Bannon RE, Triller W. Aniseikonia—a clinical report covering a ten-year period. *Am J Optom Arch Am Acad Optom* 1944;21(5):173–182.
19. Wray AT. Clinical report of the correction of aniseikonia in cases of low refractive error. *Am J Optom Arch Am Acad Optom* 1955;32:535–539.
20. Wick B. Case report—an emmetrope with aniseikonia. *Am J Optom Physiol Optics* 1974;51:51–55.
21. Wick B. Aniseikonia following unilateral intraocular lens implant. *J Am Optom Assoc* 1983;54:423–424.
22. Eskridge JB. Eikonometry. In: Eskridge JB, Amos JF, Bartlett JD, eds. *Clinical procedures in optometry.* Philadelphia: JB Lippincott, 1991.
23. Brecher GA. A new method for measuring aniseikonia. *Am J Ophthalmol* 1951;34:1016–1021.
24. Morgan MW. The Turville infinity balance technique. *J Am Opton Assoc* 1960;31:447–450.
25. Katsumi O, Miyanaga Y, Hirose T, et al. Binocular function in unilateral aphakia. *Ophthalmology* 1988;95:1088–1093.
26. Polaski M. *Aniseikonia cookbook.* Columbus: The Ohio State University.
27. Wick B. Iseikonic considerations for today's eyewear. *Am J Optom Physiol Optics* 1973;50:952–967.
28. Wick B. Iseikonic considerations for today's eyewear—addendum. *Am J Optom Physiol Optics* 1974;51:683–685.
29. Ogle KN. The problem of the horopter. In: Davson H, ed. *The eye,* vol. 4. New York: Academic Press, 1962:325–348.

19

Binocular and Accommodative Problems Associated with Computer Use

Among the most frequent health-related problems reported by users of computer video display terminals (VDTs) are those related to vision. Working on the computer for long periods can lead to eye discomfort, fatigue, blurred vision, and headaches (1). When patients seek care for complaints related to computer use, it is important to accurately diagnose and treat all of their symptoms, not only the visual problems. Symptoms associated with VDT use can largely be categorized into four primary areas—refractive, binocular vision, ocular and systemic health, and ergonomic. Symptoms resulting from each of these can be resolved with proper care and/or attention to environmental design.

ETIOLOGY AND PREVALENCE OF COMPUTER VISION RELATED PROBLEMS

Surveys show that nearly 15% of patients seeking general eye care schedule their visual examination as a result of VDT-related visual complaints (2). This is not surprising, as an estimated 75 million people in the United States currently use computers on a regular basis, and, in the next few years, that number will surely exceed 100 million (3). Surveys indicate that more than 10% of patients present with symptoms primarily associated with VDT use; more than 20% of them could not receive a definitive diagnosis and treatment plan (4). As recently as the late 1980s, about 30% of the workforce used computers and now that percentage is well above 60%.

And, the problem is not limited to adults. Many children use computers for educational and recreational purposes. The way that children use the computer may make them even more susceptible to development of computer-related vision symptoms. Children often continue performing an enjoyable task, such as video games, without breaks, until near exhaustion. Such prolonged activity can increase eye-focusing problems and eye irritation. An additional issue is that computer workstations are typically arranged for adults. Therefore, a child using a computer, on a typical office desk, must often look up higher than an adult. This may cause problems with a child's vision, as well as resulting in symptoms of arm, neck, and back discomfort.

COMPUTER VISION SYNDROME VERSUS COMPUTER USE COMPLEX

The problems associated with computer use are so frequent and there is so often a visually related symptom that the term "computer vision syndrome" has been suggested as descriptive of the group of problems associated with computer use (5). According to *Stedman's Medical Dictionary* (6), a syndrome is a group of symptoms related to a specific disease. This calls to question the term "computer vision syndrome," as it is likely that symptoms stemming from computer use are not a specific disease related solely to vision. This is especially significant when considering the physical symptoms that also accompany computer use [e.g., neck, back, and wrist problems, such as carpal tunnel disease (1), and visual symptoms that are related to lid disease, lack of blinking, or dry eye rather than vision per se (2)]. In medicine, a group of diseases or symptoms associated with similar etiologies is called a complex (e.g., EHHA complex) (7). Thus, the symptoms associated with computer use are more similar in this respect to a complex than a syndrome. For these reasons, we are introducing the term "computer use complex" (CUC) to include all of the visual and physical signs and symptoms associated with computer use. In this chapter, we primarily discuss visually related signs and symptoms related to CUC—what is often referred to as computer vision syndrome (5).

Characteristics

Symptoms

Most symptoms are associated with computer use, although patients also frequently complain of symptoms with reading or other close work. Common complaints include eyestrain, headaches, blurred vision, diplopia, sleepiness, difficulty concentrating, loss of comprehension over time, a pulling sensation, and movement of the text on the screen.

Signs

Visually related symptoms may be associated with any refractive error. Symptoms of presbyopic patients may be related to the binocular state or to the design of the prescription used for computer use. Thus, it is important for the clinician to evaluate the type of correction (bifocal or single vision) and the ways that the prescription is used.

CHARACTERISTICS OF THE CONDITION

Patients with visually related computer symptoms typically have accommodation-based problems. Although a significant heterophoria at near may also be an important finding in many cases, clinicians should use their judgment and generally rely on characteristics, in addition to the magnitude of the angle at distance and near, to reach a diagnosis.

Analysis of Binocular and Accommodative Data

Direct tests of fusional vergence, including step, smooth, and jump vergences, are important in diagnosis. In addition, tests that indirectly assess fusional vergence should be considered. Tests performed binocularly with minus lenses evaluate the ability to stimulate accommodation and control binocular alignment, using negative fusional vergence (NFV) [e.g., positive relative accommodation (PRA) and binocular accommodative facility (BAF) testing with minus lenses]. A characteristic finding in patients with visually related computer use symptoms is a report of blur as the endpoint on PRA and BAF testing, rather than diplopia.

Reduced PRA or BAF results may stem from inability to stimulate accommodation or from reduced NFV. The differential diagnosis is based on assessment of accommodation under monocular conditions. Simply cover one eye after the patient reports blur on the PRA test; if blur persists, the problem is usually accommodative (accommodative insufficiency or ill-sustained accommodation). If the vision clears, the problem is associated with binocular vision (NFV). Normal monocular accommodative ability on accommodative facility testing suggests reduced NFV.

Another important indirect test of NFV is monocular estimation method (MEM) retinoscopy. It is not unusual to find an abnormal result on this test on patients with visually related computer

TABLE 19.1. *Symptoms and signs of visually related computer use problems*

Symptoms
These symptoms are related to computer use, although there may also be symptoms with use of the eyes
after reading or other near tasks:

Eyestrain	Difficulty concentrating on reading material
Headaches	Loss of comprehension over time
Blurred vision	A pulling sensation around the eyes
Double vision	Movement of the print
Sleepiness	

Signs—Exophoria	**Signs—Esophoria**
Receded near point of convergence	Receded near point of convergence
Basic exophoria	Basic esophoria
Greater exophoria at near than at distance	Greater esophoria at near than at distance
Low AC/A ratio	High AC/A ratio

Direct measures of positive fusional vergence (PFV)	
Reduced smooth vergence	Reduced smooth vergence
Reduced step vergence	Reduced step vergence
Reduced fusional facility	Reduced fusional facility

Indirect measures of PFV
Low negative relative accommodation
Low monocular estimation method retinoscopy finding
Difficulty with plus lenses during binocular accommodative facility (BAF) testing

If accommodative excess is also present:
Difficulty with plus lenses during monocular accommodative facility (MAF) testing

If accommodative insufficiency is also present:
Difficulty with minus lenses during MAF and BAF testing
Low positive relative accommodation
Low amplitude of accommodation
Possible improvement in near point of convergence testing with plus lenses

uses symptoms. An MEM finding of greater plus than expected suggests that the patient is using as little accommodation as possible to decrease the use of accommodation or accommodative convergence.

Differential Diagnosis

It is typically not necessary to consider serious underlying etiology in cases of visually related CUC symptoms. As with other conditions, differential diagnosis (Table 19.1) depends on the nature of the patient's symptoms. Visual conditions associated with serious underlying disease almost always have an acute onset, with associated medical problems or neurological symptoms. Typically, patients with visually related CUC symptoms present with long-standing chronic complaints. The health history is negative and, although the patient may be taking medication known to affect accommodation (e.g., allergy-related medications such as Claritin [loratadine]), the symptoms usually are not easily related to use of the medication. The primary functional disorders that typically must be differentiated are basic heterophoria (eso-, exo-, and/or hyperphoria), convergence insufficiency, vergence infacility, and visual discomfort secondary to various accommodative anomalies (e.g., infacility, inaccuracy, or insufficiency).

Most visually related CUC symptoms result from benign conditions, with no serious consequences other than visual symptoms (Table 19.1). It is relatively easy to differentiate the binocular vision disorder present. To do so requires a careful analysis of all accommodative and binocular vision data. Cases 2.1 to 2.4 in Chapter 2 provide examples of the analytical process that the clinician should follow.

Ocular inflammation, such as blepharitis and meibomitis, can cause ocular symptoms of blurred vision after near work. This suggests that slit lamp evaluation is an important test in the differential diagnosis of apparent binocular symptoms related to CUC.

OVERVIEW OF GENERAL TREATMENT STRATEGIES FOR VISUALLY RELATED CUC SYMPTOMS

Sequential Management Considerations

The previous concepts discussed for the sequential management considerations (Table 19.2) of binocular vision disorders also apply to problems related to computer use. In the case of visually related symptoms of CUC, the important issues relate to:

Correction of ametropia
Added lenses
Prism
Vision therapy
Ocular health
Ergonomic issues

Correction of Ametropia

Asthenopia and accommodative fatigue are frequent sequellae of uncorrected refractive errors such as hyperopia and astigmatism. For example, a patient with uncorrected hyperopia must accommodate for the computer working distance, as well as an additional amount to overcome the uncorrected hyperopia. Muscular fatigue resulting from prolonged (and occasionally excessive) accommodation may result in accommodative symptoms. Small amounts of uncorrected astigmatism and anisometropia also often result in visual symptoms. And, some myopic patients experience discomfort when working on the computer while wearing eyeglasses. Each of these patient's symptoms may be due to accommodative fatigue, and accurate refractive correction must be considered in any management plan. The first management consideration, therefore, is correction of refractive error. To properly correct the refractive error of any patient, including computer vision users, we recommend the prescribing criteria discussed in Chapter 3.

Added Lenses

Added plus lenses play a very important role in treatment of visually related symptoms of CUC. Of course, patients with a high AC/A ratio, where there is a significant esophoria at near (e.g., convergence excess), benefit from added plus lenses. In addition to the obvious near

TABLE 19.2. *Sequential considerations in the management of computer use complex*

Optical correction of ametropia	Vision therapy for sensory motor function
Added lens power	Horizontal prism
Vertical prism	Surgery
Occlusion for amblyopia	Ocular health management
Vision therapy for amblyopia	Ergonomic issues
Vision therapy for suppression	

vision problems that result from the onset of presbyopia, various accommodative problems associated with pre-presbyopia, such as accommodative insufficiency and ill-sustained accommodation, cause CUC-related symptoms that can frequently be treated with added plus lenses. Accommodative problems, in which the difficulty is with relaxation of (or frequent changes in) accommodation (accommodative excess and accommodative infacility), respond less well to added plus lenses and generally require vision therapy treatments (Chapter 11).

Prism

Prism, which is important in cases of binocular vision disorders, is used for visually related CUC symptoms when there is an associated binocular problem. Thus, esophoric patients and patients with a vertical heterophoria will have a need for prism to be considered as part of the sequential management for the CUC vision-related problem. See Chapters 10 and 14 for prism recommendations for patients with esophoria and vertical heterophoria, respectively.

Vision Therapy

The final binocular vision-related treatment consideration is the use of vision therapy to restore normal binocular function. Vision therapy is generally an important step in the management of accommodative and vergence problems. In many cases, vision therapy is critical in treatment of the binocular difficulties that accompany CUC vision-related problems.

Surgery

Surgery, which is a consideration for some binocular vision problems when there is a very large heterophoria, typically has no role relative to CUC-related vision problems.

Ocular Health

Eyelid health and tear film integrity are very important causes of symptoms in CUC. Because of the intensity of the viewing task, computer users tend to blink less frequently. In some patients, this decreased blink rate can compromise visual comfort after even a few minutes of computer work, especially in the presence of eyelid disease or dry eye. Thus, it is often important to carefully assess eyelid health with the biomicroscope. Evaluate tear integrity and break-up time (BUT) at the same time.

Ergonomic Issues

While examining patients suspected of having CUC-related visual symptoms, it is important to accurately evaluate how they use the computer. Of course, it is possible to develop a rough estimate of viewing distance, by asking a patient to indicate the computer screen distance with his or her arms. This inexact appraisal of the actual working distance may provide an idea of the monitor's distance and position that is useful to help make decisions as to visual correction and added near lens type, power, and style. However, it is also important to address lighting conditions, glare, other working distances, time allotments to various tasks, and viewing angles. Figure 19.1 depicts some important details of the ergonomic setup.

Computer Use Questionnaire

Optimal assessment of ergonomic issues can best be accomplished with a questionnaire that addresses each of the possible problems (Appendix 19.1, Computer Use Questionnaire). It is

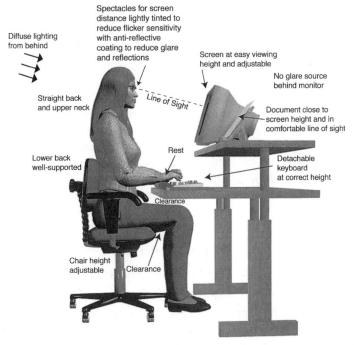

Diffuse lighting from behind

Spectacles for screen distance lightly tinted to reduce flicker sensitivity with anti-reflective coating to reduce glare and reflections

Screen at easy viewing height and adjustable

No glare source behind monitor

Straight back and upper neck

Line of Sight

Document close to screen height and in comfortable line of sight

Lower back well-supported

Rest

Detachable keyboard at correct height

Clearance

Chair height adjustable

Clearance

FIG. 19.1. Evaluation of the use of the computer requires a number of measurements. In addition to those listed in the figure, it is also important to consider the amount of time spent on computer-related tasks.

best to have the patient complete this questionnaire prior to the visual examination; this can be done at the patient's home or office, where he or she has access to all of the measurements and other data required. When the patient tries to fill out the questionnaire during the examination, he or she frequently tries to guess at the distances and often does so inaccurately, making it more difficult to effectively treat symptoms. At times, it may even become necessary for the clinician to visit the workplace to completely resolve the problem (Fig. 19.1).

Course and Prognosis

There have not been studies documenting the overall efficacy of treatment for improving visually related symptoms of CUC. However, as discussed above, treatment of CUC is tied to treatment of refractive errors and binocular vision and accommodative dysfunction, management of eyelid disease and dry eye symptoms, and development of proper ergonomics. Since each of these conditions can typically be successfully treated, it is likely that the symptoms of CUC can be resolved for most patients, provided that each underlying problem that causes symptoms is identified.

Treatment of refractive errors, binocular vision, and accommodative dysfunction is outlined in this chapter and detailed throughout this book. Following a sequential treatment approach for each condition typically leads to successful resolution of the condition, with subsequent lessening of the visually related symptoms of the CUC sufferer. Successful management of eyelid disease and dry eye is almost always possible, with a combination of lid hygiene, medications, and lacrimal occlusion. After faulty ergonomic conditions have been identified (using the questionnaire in Appendix 19.1), management can be initiated.

SUMMARY OF KEY POINTS IN TREATING PATIENTS WITH COMPUTER USE COMPLEX SYMPTOMS

An important feature in the sequential management of the visual symptoms of CUC is the emphasis on proper optical correction and added lenses. Because so much of the problem is associated with prolonged near work, provision of clear vision at distance (best correction) and near (added plus lenses) often has a substantial effect on reducing the symptoms. For the CUC patient, use of prism (horizontal and vertical) and vision therapy are the also important treatment alternatives. Vertical prism is effective when needed to correct a small hyperphoria, and vision therapy is best for treatment of symptoms that result from convergence insufficiency and accommodative dysfunction. Ocular health (specifically eyelid and lash health along, with tear film quality and quantity) needs to be evaluated and any problems treated; such treatment can substantially improve visually related CUC symptoms. The patient's ergonomic computer use should be evaluated and recommendations should be made to improve any problem areas.

Clinical Evaluation

History and Symptoms

In addition to the visual history related to binocular vision and accommodative problems described in Chapter 11, it is important to ask appropriate questions in order to gain the information necessary to make critical judgments regarding the patient's working situation. We recommend questioning every patient regarding these issues. Appendix 19.1 documents the important issues related to computer use. This questionnaire is organized to assess symptoms (visual and physical) and ergonomic issues. When a patient cannot complete the questionnaire prior to an examination, address the appropriate questions during the examination. It is important to ask all patients about computer usage; in addition to the obvious job-related computer use, it is common for children and retired adults to be avid computer users.

Workstation

While examining patients, assess the ergonomics of how they use their computer. For example, Part II of the questionnaire (Work Practices and Environment) provides detailed information about viewing distance, along with the monitor location. The questionnaire also addresses other environmental working issues, including lighting conditions, glare, other working distances, time allotments to various tasks, and viewing angles.

The questionnaire allows the clinician to quickly assess whether workstation issues are a likely source of visually related symptoms of CUC. A workstation that is poorly designed, whether too high or low or with an improperly adjusted chair, can cause substantial symptoms (Fig. 19.1). In addition, a dry office environment and/or poor indoor air quality can aggravate a marginal dry eye problem to the point that symptoms result. The problem of inadequate or poorly directed lighting should not be underestimated. Proper lighting is one of the most overlooked and underemphasized components of our indoor environment. Lighting should be designed to prevent problems, not cause them with reflections and sources of glare.

Evaluation

The customary battery of tests for general binocular vision evaluation, listed in Chapter 3, provides the majority of information required for diagnosing the cause of visually related symptoms of CUC. It is important to consider information gathered via the questionnaire concerning lighting used and the computer workstation setup, when determining whether any modification in testing done might be required. For example, special consideration may need to be given to testing accommodation and vergence under standard 40-cm test conditions, as well as at the computer work distance and under the lighting conditions used by the patient. Modification of the test is frequently needed when making diagnostic decisions based on testing vergence ranges and accommodative accuracy.

Accommodative Ranges (NRA/PRA)

Normal range values have been developed for accommodative assessment of pre-presbyopic patients. However, the norms, which were made for a 40-cm test distance, may not apply to the VDT working distance. A solution is to make measurements at the 40-cm distance and again at the VDT distance; the findings at the VDT distance should be similar to those at 40 cm. An abnormal finding at 40 cm, or an obvious discrepancy between the two findings, indicates a potential problem in this area.

Accommodative Accuracy

Determination of the accuracy of accommodation with MEM retinoscopy (8) is very valuable. This objective test allows measurement of the patient's active accommodative state at 40 cm and under test conditions (room illumination, horizontal gaze, viewing distance, etc.) that closely approximate the VDT environment. When testing at the VDT working distance, use letters that approximate the size of letters on the screen (as determined from questionnaire information). Typically, these are about 20/60 size, although there may be large individual variation.

The PRIO instrument,[a] which is designed to simulate the workstation demand, can be used at the appropriate test distance to determine the accuracy of accommodation with MEM retinoscopy (Fig. 19.2). To use the PRIO, determine the patient's computer work distance (from the answers to Appendix 19.1) and perform MEM retinoscopy at that distance. An abnormal finding can be used as the basis for prescribing a near correction that will yield a more focused

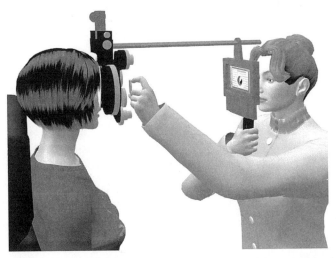

FIG. 19.2. Near retinoscopy by the monocular estimation method can be important when determining a near prescription for computer use. The PRIO instrument provides a target that is similar to the computer screen and allows the clinician to test at the appropriate working distance. Tests (such as the PRIO) may improve patient confidence in the resulting prescription.

computer correction. The PRIO finding and the finding with traditional MEM retinoscopy using the appropriate letter size and test distance are, for the most part, very similar. However, an advantage of the PRIO instrument is that the patient feels that a "special test" is being done that is specifically designed to help visually related CUC symptoms. Such patient impressions are often invaluable (Fig. 19.2).

Other Testing Factors

Pupil Size

While using a computer, a patient needs to view the monitor in normal room illumination (or slightly dimmer). If there is not enough light, a larger pupil will result that can exaggerate distortions of screen letters and decrease depth of focus to the point of distortion. Caution patients of this possibility and make appropriate recommendations concerning VDT brightness and room illumination. Differences in illumination between the monitor and the background should be less than 3:1. Patients will need to monitor this by estimation, as they will seldom be able to measure exact brightness.

Ocular Health

Eye health, specifically tear film integrity, is critical for VDT users. Because of the intensity of the viewing task, computer users tend to blink infrequently. Always evaluate eyelid health and perform a tear BUT if you question tear integrity.

Sequential Management Protocol

Best Refractive Correction

A clear trend has not been identified in the literature in regard to the amount of refractive error that needs to be treated in CUC. Small astigmatism correction, particularly against-the-rule or oblique, seems to be significant for many patients, as do small hyperopic corrections. These factors confirm that the most important first step is to prescribe the best lens correction for the patient. This single step can solve many of the vision-related problems of CUC. The effects of the best correction and the importance of lens design is illustrated by Case 19.1

Case Studies

Case 19.1

History

Samantha, a 30-year-old office worker, presented with complaints of eyestrain and blurred vision after approximately 4 hours of computer use. These problems started when she was required to spend more time working on the computer at work. She never had an eye examination. Her medical history was negative and she was taking Claritin as needed for allergic symptoms (generally in the fall).

Examination Results

History: Computer Use Questionnaire. Samantha reported frequent episodes of blurred near vision and headaches, both of moderate severity. She worked on the VDT for 7 hours per day, with regular breaks. The viewing distance from the eye to keyboard was 17 in. and the distance from the eye to computer monitor was 23 in. Her workroom was medium bright with fluorescent lighting.

VA (distance, uncorrected):	OD: 20/20
	OS: 20/20
VA (near, uncorrected):	OD: 20/20
	OS: 20/20
Near point of convergence:	
Accommodative target:	1 to 2 in.
Penlight:	1 to 2 in.
Cover test (distance):	orthophoria
Cover test (near):	4 esophoria
Subjective:	OD: plano, 20/20
	OS: plano, 20/20
Distance lateral phoria:	orthophoria
Base-in vergence (distance):	X/7/4
Base-out vergence (distance):	14/21/15
Near lateral phoria:	5 esophoria
−1.00 gradient:	12 esophoria
Gradient AC/A ratio:	7:1
Calculated AC/A ratio:	8:1
Base-in vergence (near):	X/8/1
Base-out vergence (near):	11/25/18 Δ
Negative relative accommodation (NRA):	+2.50 D
PRA:	diplopia with −1.75
Accommodative amplitude (push-up):	OD: 15 D, OS: 15 D
Monocular accommodative facility (MAF):	OD: 12 cpm, OS: 12 cpm
BAF:	diplopia with −2.00
MEM retinoscopy:	+1.50 OD and OS

Pupils were normal, all external and internal health tests were negative, the deviation was comitant, and color vision testing revealed normal function. Eyelid and lash health was normal, as was the tear BUT.

Case Analysis

Based on the small esophoria at near, the best way to approach this case is to analyze the NFV group data. This is especially true, as there were no apparent contributory eye health problems. For Samantha, the direct and indirect findings that investigate NFV were abnormal. The direct finding, NFV at near, is moderately reduced. The indirect tests—PRA, BAF, and MEM retinoscopy—also suggest an esophoria/low NFV problem. The distance orthophoria and the high calculated and gradient AC/A ratios all suggest a diagnosis of convergence excess with normal tonic vergence.

Management

Since there was no refractive error, our initial approach, in this case, was to prescribe added lenses for near. To determine the amount of plus to prescribe, consider the AC/A ratio, NRA/PRA relationship, fusional vergence findings, and MEM retinoscopy. In this case, the

NRA/PRA relationship suggests the need for a near addition of about +1.00, as does MEM retinoscopy. The calculated AC/A ratio suggests that an add of +1.00 would reduce the near phoria to slightly more than 2 exophoria. We prescribed plano distance correction with a near addition of +1.00 OD and OS in progressive bifocal form for all near work.

This case illustrates the frequent scenario of ophthalmic correction for CUC. In the absence of significant distance refractive error, most lens corrections are prescribed for near correction because of a problem with accommodation, esophoria, or presbyopia. When prescribing for visually related symptoms of CUC, an important decision the clinician must make when prescribing added plus lenses is whether to recommend single vision lenses or bifocals. We typically suggest a bifocal prescription so that the patient does not have to remove his or her glasses when looking up from the computer. Although there are frequent exceptions, in our experience, CUC patients wearing single vision near lenses often become disillusioned with their glasses because of the continual need to remove them for clear distance vision.

Although a bifocal is our first recommendation for computer use, we sometimes encounter resistance from patients, especially pre-presbyopic young adults, about wearing a bifocal. When this occurs, we review and demonstrate the benefits of a bifocal and, if the patient remains unconvinced, prescribe a single vision near correction. The patient can always change to a bifocal design later, and often will, after he or she personally experiences the problems associated with frequently having to remove the single vision correction.

Issues of Lens Design, Coatings and Materials

In general, for CUC patients, there is a problem with common flattop bifocal designs where the bifocal height is at or below the lower lid margin. The flattop bifocal requires the patient to raise his or her chin to use the bifocal when looking at the computer. With prolonged computer use, this head position causes frequent neck and back pain, ultimately reducing work efficiency. This problem can be somewhat relieved by use of progressive addition lenses (PALs), where the progressive addition is started fairly high in the frame (at the center of the pupil). As long as the near addition is equal to or less than +1.50, most patients can assume a head position that allows them to look at the computer and still use the PAL with minimal head and neck symptoms. For Samantha, we recommended a PAL with the progressive addition starting at the center of the pupil.

As the patient ages (advancing presbyopia), specialized PALs or intermediate/near power bifocals become important considerations. For advanced presbyopia, the standard PAL tends to have intermediate corridor of narrow width (or, if the corridor is wide, the near portion is too low in the frame to be easily used). Of course, these issues are related to the amount of time spent using the computer. For advancing presbyopic patients who spend more than 2 hours per day on the computer, a PAL with the top portion having an intermediate power for computer use and the lower portion with the appropriate near power for reading, is generally the lens of choice. Thus, when an absolute presbyope needs a prescription of plano at distance with a +2.50 near addition, a useful computer prescription might be a computer-designed intermediate/near lens (e.g., +1.25 with a +1.25 near addition) in PAL form (Fig. 19.3). When less than 1 to 2 hours per day is spent on computer use, the advanced presbyopic patient often elects to "get by" with a less than optimal correction, due to the costs involved when more than one pair of lenses is needed. An inexpensive option for the presbyopic patient who cannot afford a specific computer correction is the PC Peeker[b], a +1.12 lens designed to fit behind the spectacle correction and focus the computer monitor (Fig. 19.3).

Lens coatings, such as ultraviolet (UV) protection and antireflective (AR) coatings, are often considered in treatment of visually related symptoms of CUC patients. In general, there

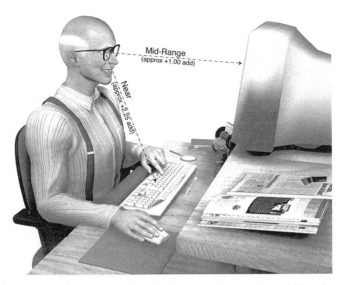

FIG. 19.3. When the presbyopic patient needs a visual correction while using the computer, the lenses are designed so that the bottom portion contains the total near power needed, with the top portion reduced in power so that the focus is on the computer screen. Either a flat top bifocal or progression addition lens design can be used.

is probably no particular need for UV protection for CUC patients who wear their correction only for computer use; if they wear the correction outdoors as well, then the protective issues of UV protection apply. There is little UV radiation from a computer monitor, so UV protection, while it does not hurt, probably does not provide any significant benefit. AR coatings can be helpful for improving vision, especially with large luminance ratios. An AR coating does not reduce screen reflections and we do not feel that AR coating, by itself, will solve problems. However, the AR coating, when combined with the proper lens prescription (such as added lenses) and design (PALs or computer designed intermediate/near lenses) can be of value. Color filters, such as yellow or pink lenses, are mostly cosmetic and of little significant benefit with the advent of color monitors. Samantha's PAL lenses included AR coating.

In Samantha's case, a follow-up visit after 4 weeks revealed that she was doing well with the glasses and had complete relief of symptoms. No additional treatment was recommended.

Prism

Prism is occasionally required for CUC patients, as illustrated in Case 19.2

Case 19.2

History

Diane, a 24-year-old swimming pool designer, presented with a complaint of intermittent double vision when looking up at clients after working on the computer. She had noticed this problem since high school (for at least 7 years), but had not received any treatment. Her health was normal and she was not taking any medication.

Examination Results

History: Computer Use Questionnaire. Diane reported frequent episodes of double vision. She worked on the VDT for 2 to 3 hours per day, with regular breaks. The viewing distance from the eye to keyboard was 17 in. and the distance from the eye to computer monitor was 24 in. Her workroom lighting was variable, as she traveled to client's homes to demonstrate pool designs on her laptop.

IPD:	58 mm
VA (distance, uncorrected):	OD: 20/20
	OS: 20/20
VA (near, uncorrected):	OD: 20/20
	OS: 20/20
Near point of convergence:	1 to 2 in.
Cover test (distance):	7 esophoria
Cover test (near):	6 esophoria
Subjective:	OD: +0.25, 20/20
	OS: +0.25, 20/20
Cycloplegic:	OD: +0.50
	OS: +0.50
Distance lateral phoria:	7 esophoria
Base-in vergence (distance):	diplopia; needs 5 base-out to fuse
Base-out vergence (distance):	diplopia; needs 5 base-out to fuse, breaks at 26 base-out, and recovers at 18 base-out
Near lateral phoria:	6 esophoria
−1.00 gradient:	10 esophoria
Gradient AC/A ratio:	6:1
Calculated AC/A ratio:	5:1
Base-in vergence (near):	X/8/−1
Base-out vergence (near):	X/23/18
NRA:	+2.50
PRA:	−1.25
Accommodative amplitude (push-up):	OD: 12 D, OS: 12 D
MAF:	OD: 10 cpm, OS: 10 cpm
BAF:	intermittent diplopia with −2.00
MEM retinoscopy:	+0.50 OU

Fixation disparity testing with the American Optical (AO) Vectographic slide at distance revealed an associated phoria of 4 base-out.

Pupils were normal, all external and internal health tests were negative, the deviation was comitant, and color vision testing revealed normal function. Eyelid and lash health was normal, as was the tear BUT.

Case Analysis

Because there are no contributory eye health problems, the entry point into analysis of the data, in this case, is the moderate magnitude esophoria at distance and near. NFV at both distance and near are slightly reduced, with diplopia on base-in testing at distance. Diagnosis of basic esophoria is suggested by the equal magnitude esophoria at distance and near, reduced NFV, and normal AC/A ratio.

Management

Even though the management sequence in Table 11.3 suggests first considering best correction, the distance correction would be of little use; correction of this small amount of hyperopia would obviously have little influence on the angle of deviation. Since the best lens correction is of little value, Diane's treatment would have to consist of prism or vision therapy. After considering the options, Diane decided that she did not have sufficient time to devote to vision therapy. Therefore, based on the fixation disparity results, we prescribed a total of 4 Δ base-out prism. The final prescription was OD +0.25 and OS +0.25, with a 2 Δ base-out in each eye. Diane wore these glasses at work for 4 weeks and returned for a reevaluation. She reported complete relief of symptoms, so no further treatment was necessary. After 2 years of wearing the prism correction, she decided to under go a vision therapy program.

Vision Therapy

Vision therapy is often important for treatment of CUC patients. The need for vision therapy is often related to heterophoria problems or accommodative or fusional vergence problems.

Case 19.3

Jack, a 36-year-old stockbroker, presented with complaints of eyestrain and blurred vision after about 2 hours of computer trading. He had experienced these problems for several years, but his previous reading glasses had not been of help to him and he had stopped wearing them after about 4 weeks. His medical history was negative and he was not taking any medication.

Examination Results

Jack reported frequent severe episodes of eyestrain and blurred vision. He worked on the VDT for more that 12 hours per day, with irregular breaks. The viewing distance from the eye to keyboard was 17 in. and the distance from the eye to computer monitor was 24 in. His workroom lighting was fluorescent.

Previous prescription:	+0.50
	+0.50
IPD (interpupillary distance):	62 mm
VA (distance, uncorrected):	OD: 20/20
	OS: 20/20
VA (near, uncorrected):	OD: 20/20
	OS: 20/20
Near point of convergence:	
Accommodative target:	2 to 4 in.
Penlight:	2 to 4 in.
Cover test (distance):	orthophoria
Cover test (near):	3 exophoria
Subjective:	OD: +0.25 − 0.25 × 180, 20/20
	OS: +0.25 − 0.25 × 180, 20/20
Cycloplegic:	OD: +0.75 − 0.25 × 180, 20/20
	OS: +0.75 − 0.25 × 180, 20/20
Distance lateral phoria:	orthophoria

Base-in vergence (distance):	X/4/2
Base-out vergence (distance):	6/10/6
Near lateral phoria:	3 exophoria
−1.00 gradient:	1 esophoria
Gradient AC/A ratio:	4:1
Calculated AC/A ratio:	4.8:1
Base-in vergence (near):	4/8/6
Base-out vergence (near):	6/10/2
NRA:	+1.50
PRA:	−1.25
Accommodative amplitude (push-up):	OD: 9 D, OS: 9 D
MAF:	OD: 11 cpm, OS: 11 cpm
BAF:	2 cpm
MEM retinoscopy:	+0.25

Pupils were normal, all external and internal health tests were negative, the deviation was comitant, and color vision testing revealed normal function. Slit lamp evaluation revealed normal lids and lashes, with no evidence of dry eye or abnormal tear film.

Case Analysis

The normal phoria at both distance and near, normal lids and lashes, and lack of a dry eye condition suggest that an accommodative disorder was the most likely cause for Jack's symptoms. Accordingly, the entry into analysis of this case is data related to accommodative testing, which revealed a normal amplitude, facility, and accommodative response. The NRA and PRA were both low and accommodative function was normal, suggesting a fusional vergence problem. PFV and NFV were reduced on direct and indirect tests. Diagnosis of fusional vergence dysfunction is supported by the low NRA, PRA, and reduced BAF.

Management

We advised Jack that his ametropia was considered insignificant and, since there was no vertical deviation, glasses were not prescribed. His ocular health was normal, indicating no need for treatment in this area either; rather, we suggested a program of vision therapy to normalize fusional vergence findings and eliminate symptoms.

Because he was unwilling to come into the office for therapy, Jack was given vision therapy procedures to practice at home. We followed the sequence outlined in Table 11.8, and six in-office vision therapy progress visits were necessary to evaluate Jack's progress and make changes in his therapy. At the end of therapy, Jack reported that he was able to work on the computer for a full 12 hours without discomfort.

Reevaluation at completion of therapy revealed the following findings:

Base-in vergence (distance):	X/8/6
Base-out vergence (distance):	X/20/16
Near lateral phoria:	2 exophoria
Base-in vergence (near):	14/26/22
Base-out vergence (near):	20/32/28
NRA:	+2.50
PRA:	−2.50
BAF:	10 cpm

The maintenance program suggested in Table 9.9 was recommended. Reevaluation was scheduled in 6 months; Jack returned in 9 months. He revealed that he had stopped maintenance therapy after 3 months. After his symptoms resumed, Jack initiated therapy again on his own. He was again comfortable and his findings remained normal.

Medical Treatment

Many patients who have CUC-related symptoms have ocular health problems that interfere with their vision and cause symptoms. Sometimes the symptoms may seem to come from either a binocular vision or an ocular health problem, and occasionally the symptoms are related to both conditions.

Case 19.4

Jeremiah, a 15-year-old high school sophomore, presented with complaints of eyestrain and blurred vision after about 20 minutes of computer work. He had these problems for 2 years, but his previous visits to eye doctors had not yielded relief. His previous (1-year-old) reading glasses had not helped and Jeremiah had stopped wearing them. His medical history was positive for "eyelid problems," but he was not taking any medication.

Examination Results

Jeremiah reported frequent episodes of moderate eyestrain and intermittent double vision when reading or working on the computer and he felt that these symptoms were worse when he did computer work. Further questioning revealed that the diplopia was a monocular ghosting that remained when he covered either eye. He worked on the VDT for 2 or more hours per day, with irregular breaks. The viewing distance from the eye to keyboard was 18 in. and the distance from the eye to computer monitor was 21 in. His workroom lighting was fluorescent.

Previous prescription:	+0.50 D
	+0.50 D
IPD:	62 mm
VA (distance, uncorrected):	OD: 20/20
	OS: 20/20
VA (near, uncorrected):	OD: 20/20
	OS: 20/20
Near point of convergence:	2 cm
Accommodative target:	2 to 4 in.
Penlight:	2 to 4 in.
Cover test (distance):	Orthophoria
Cover test (near):	2 Δ exophoria
Subjective:	OD: +0.25 − 0.25 × 180, 20/20
	OS: +0.25 − 0.25 × 180, 20/20
Cycloplegic:	OD: +0.75 − 0.25 × 180, 20/20
	OS: +0.75 − 0.25 × 180, 20/20
Distance lateral phoria:	orthophoria
Base-in vergence (distance):	X/6/4
Base-out vergence (distance):	16/21/16
Near lateral phoria:	3 exophoria

−1.00 gradient:	1 esophoria
Gradient AC/A ratio:	4:1
Calculated AC/A ratio:	4.8:1
Base-in vergence (near):	16/21/17
Base-out vergence (near):	16/20/15
NRA:	+2.00 D
PRA:	−1.25 D
Accommodative amplitude (push-up):	OD: 11 D, OS: 11 D
MAF:	OD: 11 cpm, OS: 11 cpm
BAF:	8 cpm
MEM retinoscopy:	+0.25 D

Pupils were normal, all external and internal health tests were negative, the deviation was comitant, and color vision testing revealed normal function. Slit lamp evaluation revealed 2+ blepharitis, with deficient aqueous production in each eye. Tear BUT was 4 seconds in the right eye and 6 seconds in the left.

Case Analysis

Because the phoria was normal at distance and near and accommodative testing was only slightly abnormal, the most likely cause for Jeremiah's symptoms was an ocular health (dry eye) disorder. Analysis of the results of accommodative testing revealed a normal amplitude, facility, and accommodative response. The PRA was low, but, given the normal accommodative function, this probably reflects an aberrant finding rather than a problem with fusional vergence. Another likely hypothesis was fusional vergence dysfunction. PFV and NFV findings were normal on direct measures and indirect tests of fusional vergence. With only a low PRA and normal BAF, the results suggested no problems with fusional vergence; rather, the findings led to a diagnosis of ocular surface health-related CUC problems.

Management

We advised Jeremiah that the previous prescription would not be expected to relieve his problem. The ametropia was considered insignificant and, since there was no vertical deviation, glasses were not recommended. We prescribed a program of eyelid hygiene (lid scrubs twice a day and Blephamide [prednisolone/sulfacetamide] SOP [sterile ophthalmic preparation] HS [bedtime] for 14 days) to normalize his lid and tear health and reduce his symptoms.

Jeremiah was seen in 2 weeks. His blepharitis was substantially improved and he reported that he could read and work on the computer for a longer period of time before experiencing symptoms. Lid scrubs were continued twice a day for 14 days and the Blephamide was discontinued. After 2 more weeks, the blepharitis was under control and Jeremiah was able to read and work on the computer for as long as he wanted, without any discomfort.

Ergonomic Issues

Many patients who have CUC-related symptoms have ergonomic issues related to a computer workstation design that interferes with their work and causes symptoms. Sometimes the symptoms may seem to come from either a binocular vision or an ocular health problem, but the ergonomics of CUC use must be considered in virtually all cases, as illustrated below.

Case 19.5

Jamal is a 23-year-old man who is experiencing head and neck aches after 2 hours of computer work. He is healthy and is not taking any medication. He has been a patient in your practice for several years and his most recent examination was 2 years ago. At that time he had no complaints. He recently started a job that requires him to work on the computer for about 6 hours per day. The findings from the previous and current examinations are listed below.

Examination Results—Computer Questionnaire

In the previous examination, Jamal had no symptoms. At the current examination, he reported headaches, along with neck discomfort, after 3 hours of working on the computer. He worked on the VDT for 6 or more hours per day, with irregular breaks. The viewing distance from the eye to keyboard was 15 in. and the distance from the eye to computer monitor was 15 in. His workroom lighting was fluorescent.

Test	Previous Examination	Current Examination
Near point convergence:	4 to 6 in.	4 to 7 in.
Amplitude of accommodation:	15 D	15 D
Distance phoria:	orthophoria	orthophoria
Near phoria:	5 exophoria	6 exophoria
Calculated AC/A ratio:	4:1	3.6:1
Base-out (near):	10/18/10	14/20/14
NRA:	+2.50	+2.50
PRA:	−2.50	−2.75
BAF:	12 cpm	13 cpm
MEM retinoscopy:	+0.25 OU	+0.50 OU
IPD:	58 mm	58 mm

In both examinations, the pupils were normal, all external and internal health tests were negative, the deviation was comitant, and color vision testing revealed normal function. Slit lamp evaluation revealed normal lid health and good aqueous production in each eye. Tear BUT was normal.

The key findings for the differential diagnosis are the normal binocular vision and ocular health findings. In CUC, these findings may be normal, but the patient may still have symptoms. Given normal binocular vision and ocular health, the CUC-related symptoms that Jamal described are likely to be related to ergonomic issues. The Computer Use Questionnaire revealed that the top of Jamal's 15-in. computer monitor was 9 in. above eye level. He had bright fluorescent room illumination, no glare filter on the screen, and a window behind the monitor. In addition, his work distance was abnormally close (15 in. from the monitor and keyboard). These ergonomic "flaws" are likely to be contributory to Jamal's symptoms.

This case illustrates the importance of proper workstation design to the treatment of CUC-related symptoms. Of course, we want to manage existing binocular vision problems and treat ocular surface disease. However, it is equally important to treat all of the patient's symptoms. This frequently requires considering the effects of the computer workstation. Carefully check the height and arrangement of the computer. The patient's physical stature should determine

TABLE 21.8. *Components of a psychological evaluation*

1. History
2. Cognitive functioning
   IQ level
   Language skills
   Attention and concentration
   Memory
   Visual perceptual skills
   Auditory perceptual skills
   Cognitive style
   Processing speed
3. Academic achievement
   Reading—decoding and comprehension
   Math
   Spelling
   Writing—handwriting, paragraph composition, thematic maturity, grammar, punctuation
4. Emotional functioning
   Self concept
   Frustration tolerance and coping mechanisms
   Relationships with significant others
   Reality testing
   Diagnostic classifications for emotional disturbance

during the testing process. Information must be gathered about three general areas. These include information about the child, school history, and the family. The history obtained by the psychologist is generally summarized in the "background information" section of the written report that he or she provides. The optometrist can utilize this information as the basis for obtaining his or her own history, probing those areas related to the referral question. It is particularly important for the optometrist searching for a connection between vision and reading to understand the age of onset of academic problems and how they became manifest.

Cognitive Testing

Cognitive testing includes assessment of various abilities, including language, memory, auditory and visual perceptual skills, visual–motor abilities, attention and concentration, and cognitive style. This information is gathered by administering an intelligence test as well as supplemental tests. An intelligence test provides an Intelligence Quotient (IQ), as well as information about the various aspects of cognitive functioning mentioned above.

Intellectual functioning is generally classified in the following way: IQ scores have a mean of 100, with a standard deviation (SD) of 15. Thus, about two-thirds of all people obtain an IQ score between 85 and 115 (within 1 SD of the mean) and 95% obtain a score between 70 and 130 (a range of 2 SDs from the mean) (52).

The most commonly used IQ test is the Wechsler Scales (52), which includes 3 tests, the Wechsler Intelligence Scale for Children (WISC-III), the Wechsler Preschool and Primary Scale of Intelligence (WPPSI-R), and the Wechsler Adult Scale of Intelligence (WAIS-R).

The WISC-III, which is administered to children aged 6 through 16, is the test that optometrists are most likely to encounter in a report. It is divided into two scales, the Verbal and Performance scales. Three IQ scores are obtained from this test: verbal IQ, performance IQ, and full scale IQ, which is a combination of the verbal and performance IQs. One is able to compare a child's functioning on verbally related subtests with nonverbal, or more visual–spatial tasks, by comparing the verbal IQ with the performance IQ. The optometrist can determine whether verbal and nonverbal abilities are fairly consistent or whether one area is weaker than the other. This is one important issue to consider when determining whether vision therapy for visual processing skills is indicated. Intervention is indicated when visual processing abilities are significantly weaker than verbal abilities. An example of this would be a verbal IQ of 110 and a performance IQ of 90.

Achievement Testing

Educational testing has an important place in a complete psychoeducational evaluation. Such testing is designed to determine achievement levels in all academic areas. In regard to reading ability, the first stage of the assessment involves evaluation of the child's ability to recognize words and apply word analysis strategies. If the child has significant difficulty in these areas, then there are many implications about how this could affect overall functioning. After analysis of the word recognition and decoding strategies using isolated words and nonsense word patterns, it is beneficial to assess how the child handles word–reading demands while reading in context from representative text material. Finally, reading comprehension is evaluated.

Earlier, we discussed the importance of understanding the nature of the reading problem. The reading assessment provides the information necessary to determine if the visual efficiency problem is related to the reading dysfunction.

Emotional/Personality Testing

Emotional issues can interfere and exacerbate reading problems. For example, reading is a developmental task that cannot be obtained until a youngster is ready. This includes an assumption that the central nervous system is mature enough to handle the complex demands of the act of reading. To some youngsters, taking that next developmental step is intimidating and frightening, and emotional issues surface. Reading may be perceived to be an act that only "the big people do," and this little person may not feel equipped to tackle such an adult activity.

Typical psychoeducational assessments evaluate emotion and personality on a continuum, from objective measures that ask the person directly how he or she feels about a certain issue to much more indirect or projective methods of gaining information. In the more direct method, the person is asked a range of questions in what is called a "clinical interview." Insight from this interview can be gained about the person's feelings about himself, key people in his life, school, and so forth.

Other ways of gaining insight into a person's emotional life include the more projective methods. Sentence completion tests ask that a person complete a sentence stem with the first thing that comes to mind, such as "All my life I. . .". Other methods include projective drawings, where drawings are used to interpret major themes and issues that are relevant to the individual.

When optometrists consider the emotional/personality section of the report, the same basic concepts that were discussed in the achievement section apply. How severe are the emotional problems? What can an optometrist expect from the youngster? Will he or she be very difficult to manage in vision therapy? Is the child overly withdrawn? Is there too much anger and tension in the family system to expect consistent follow-up?

DIAGNOSTIC TESTING/CASE HISTORY

The diagnostic testing for reading-related vision disorders is identical to the testing presented in Chapter 1, with two important exceptions. First, if a child presents with reading problems, it is very useful to perform an infrared eye tracking evaluation while the patient is reading. The clinical instrument available today is the Visagraph II. Objective eye movement recording has several advantages over direct observation and timed/standardized tests. The Visagraph II provides a permanent recording of the evaluation, it is an objective procedure, and it does not depend on the skill of the examiner. The information gained from objective recording is also more sophisticated. It provides information about number of fixations, regressions, duration of fixations, reading rate, relative efficiency, and grade equivalence. All of this information can be compared to established norms for elementary schoolchildren through adulthood. We find it helpful to repeat this testing after intervention, in order to demonstrate changes in reading eye movement patterns.

The other significant modification in the diagnostic routine is the case history, when the concern is whether a vision disorder could be interfering with reading performance. Regarding the case history, Cotter (53) states:

"As a diagnostic tool, its importance cannot be underestimated. An integral part of the evaluation, the case history offers a rich source of data for case formulation that is not available from other forms of assessment."

The case history information shapes the examination strategy, development of the management plan, and the formulation of the prognosis.

Defining the Nature of the Reading/Learning Problem

If the chief complaint is related to reading, it is important for the optometrist to gain as much information as possible about the specific nature of the reading problem. This information can be used to determine if the reading problem may be related to a visual efficiency, visual information processing, or a nonvisual (language) problem. This determination is a critical part of the evaluation and guides the management decisions that must be made. For example, if the history suggests a language problem, part of the treatment plan may include a referral to a psychologist, educator, or speech-language pathologist. If the history suggests that a visual information-processing problem may be related to the child's learning difficulty, further testing would be recommended to evaluate this possibility.

Table 21.9 lists suggested questions that can be asked to help determine whether the reading problem may be related to a visual efficiency, visual information processing, or language disorder. The most basic question is whether the problem started in grades 1 to 3 or in grades 4 and above. Binocular vision, accommodative, and eye movement problems tend to interfere with the reading process when a child reaches the level at which he or she is reading in order to learn, when speed is important, when reading longer passages, and when reading smaller print. As stated earlier, this tends to occur in about the fourth grade and up.

It is also important to ask the series of question suggested in Table 21.9 to try and determine if the reading problem is language-based or visually-based. For example, children who have problems with sounding out words and phonics tend to have auditory-language problems. Reading difficulty that involves comprehension, speed, fatigue with long passages, loss of place, and deterioration with smaller print is more likely to be related to visual efficiency disorders.

Finally, the clinician should inquire about any additional learning issues, such as problems with written language, copying from the board, reversals, and difficulty with letter and number recognition. Positive responses to this series of questions tend to suggest visual information processing problems.

TABLE 21.9. *Educational history to determine nature of reading/learning problem*

Question	Response	Suggests potential problem with:
When did the problem start?	Present since grade 1	Visual processing or language
	Grade 4 and above	Visual efficiency
Does child enjoy when you read to him?	Yes	Visual efficiency
	No	Language
Is child able to verbally discuss reading passage and ask intelligent questions	Yes	Visual efficiency
	No	Language
Trouble sounding out words?	Yes	Language
Trouble with sight vocabulary?	Yes	Visual information processing or language
Trouble with comprehension with long passages?	Yes	Visual efficiency
Trouble with reading speed?	Yes	Visual efficiency
Frequent loss of place, skipping words, lines?	Yes	Visual efficiency
Does your child read better when the print is larger?	Yes	Visual efficiency
Does your child's reading performance deteriorate with time?	Yes	Visual efficiency
Reading level?	More than 2 yr below grade level	Language
	Less than 2 yr below grade level	Visual efficiency
Does your child tend to avoid reading task?	Yes	Visual efficiency
Does your child have difficulty copying from the board?	Yes	Visual information processing
Does your child have difficulty with written work?	Yes	Visual information processing
Does your child tend to reverse or transpose letters, numbers, and words more than expected for his age?	Yes	Visual information processing
Does your child have difficulty with number or letter recognition?	Yes	Visual information processing

Previous Testing

Children with a history of reading problems often have had previous testing from psychologists, special educators, speech-language pathologists, occupational therapists, neurologists, developmental pediatricians, or other physicians. Table 21.10 lists suggested questions to probe for information about previous testing.

The objective is to determine the nature and severity of the reading or learning disorder. Optometric intervention tends to have the most impact when the history indicates that there is an isolated mild to moderate reading problem that appears to be related to speed, comprehension, fatigue, and loss of place when reading. Successful treatment of a visual efficiency problem, in such cases, may lead to better comfort and elimination of fatigue and loss of place. This improved comfort and visual efficiency, along with appropriate reading remediation, will generally have a positive impact on reading performance. Other positive indications would be a normal IQ, minimal difference between the verbal IQ and performance IQ, mild to moderate delays in reading (less than 2 years), and no significant problems in any other areas listed in Table 21.10.

Medical/Developmental Problems and Family History

The final area that should be addressed in the case history is to determine if the child has any medical or developmental problems or a family history that may impact the prognosis for

TABLE 21.10. *Case history—previous testing*

Previous vision care
    History of accommodative, binocular vision, eye movement problems
    History of visual information processing problems
Neurological
    Evidence of neurological problems
    Attention problems
Psychoeducational
    Full scale IQ
    Verbal IQ
    Performance IQ
    Reading, math, spelling grade levels
    Attention and concentration problems
    Emotional, behavior problems
    Diagnosis
    Recommendations
Audiological/speech and language
    Language or speech problems
    Previous speech or auditory processing therapy
Occupational therapy
    Fine motor problems
    Posture
    Muscle tone
    Sensory integration disorder
    History of occupational therapy
Other treatment

treatment or if the child may be "at risk" for reading/learning problems. Cotter (53) defines a child "at risk" as one who has a greater than average chance of developing a sensory–motor deficit or a mental handicap in childhood. "Risk" is not a condition *per se* but a particular circumstance that increases the probability that a certain disorder will occur. These factors are listed in Tables 21.11 and 21.12.

The medical history allows the opportunity to identify particular circumstances that may have contributed to the child's learning difficulties or currently places him or her at risk for future academic problems (53). In addition, the optometrist can use this information to help make decision about treatment and prognosis.

It is important to understand that visual efficiency problems can generally be successfully treated in most patients using lenses, prism, and vision therapy. While the prognosis for successful treatment of the underlying visual efficiency problem is good to excellent in most cases, the impact of this successful treatment on school or reading performance may depend on other factors (e.g., medical or developmental issues and family history). The prognosis for improved reading performance, with appropriate intervention, will certainly be best for a child with normal medical, developmental, and family history, a normal IQ, and only mild to moderate reading problems. Conversely, a child with negative factors in these areas will probably not achieve as much benefit from appropriate intervention.

The use of a parent questionnaire (Figure 21.1) is an efficient way to gather this information. This questionnaire is filled out before the examination, therefore, the optometrist can review the responses, searching for indications of medical or developmental problems that need to be considered when developing a treatment strategy.

We have also included a case history supplement that was suggested by Borsting and Rouse (22) (Figure 21.2). This questionnaire includes 25 questions that require a "yes" or "no" response. The following three areas are covered: school performance (questions 1 and 2), signs and symptoms associated with visual efficiency disorders (questions 3 to 19), and signs and symptoms associated with visual information processing disorders (questions 20 to 25).

TABLE 21.11. *Is the child at risk for reading problems?*

Medical history
    Pre- and perinatal health events
        Problems during pregnancy
        Problems during labor and delivery
        Environmental issues
            Age of mother
            Socioeconomic level
            Use of drugs, smoking during pregnancy
Childhood medical history
    Infections
        Meningitis
        Otitis media
    Metabolic disturbances
    Environmental contaminants
        Lead
        Carbon dioxide poisoning
    Hazardous medical events
        Head injury
        Seizures
        Abuse, neglect
Developmental history
    See Table 21.12
Family history
    Learning/reading problems

From Cotter S. Optometric assessment: case history. In: Scheiman MM, Rouse MW, eds. *Optometric management of learning-related vision problems.* St. Louis: Mosby-Year Book, 1994, with permission.

The use of such a questionnaire allows the optometrist to quickly scan the responses and determine if a visual efficiency problem should be suspected.

TREATMENT

Objectives of Optometric Intervention

If evaluation reveals a reading-related visual efficiency problem, the role of the optometrist is to treat the underlying vision problem. The expectation for intervention should be the reduction or elimination of signs and symptoms associated with the particular visual deficits (4). It is important to reiterate that optometrists do not directly treat the reading or learning problem (5). Rather, remediating these vision problems allows children and adults to benefit more fully from educational intervention (5). The expectation is that, with a reduction in asthenopia and other symptoms, the child will be able to read more comfortably, more quickly, and with better comprehension. The actual effect on reading level and performance, however, depends on the nature of the reading problem and many of the associated issues discussed above.

In the ideal situation, the reading problem is mild to moderate, does not involve decoding, and the child has a normal IQ, good attention span, and no emotional problems. In such cases, the prognosis for improvement in reading, after vision therapy, is good. Very few cases are ideal, however. Most children present with one or more complicating factors that make it very difficult to predict the effect of treatment on the visual efficiency disorder. Therefore, when presenting the treatment alternatives to patients, it is important to clearly define the objectives of treatment. The treatment goal is to eliminate the underlying visual efficiency problem. The rest of the treatment is left to other professionals who are involved with the child's care

TABLE 21.12. *A sampling of developmental milestones*

Skill	Approximate age
Rollover	5–6 mo
Sit up independently	6 mo
Crawling	9–13 mo
Walking independently	12–14 mo
Pedals tricycle	3 yr
Walks up and down stairs (alternate feet)	4 yr
Rides two-wheel bike	7 yr
Fine motor developmental milestones	
Skill	**Approximate age**
Transfers objects from hand to hand	3–5 mo
Holds bottle	6 mo
Pincer grasp	10 mo
Throws objects to floor	12–15 mo
Copies a circle	3 yr
Buttons clothes	3.5 yr
Catches a ball	4–5 yr
Ties shoelaces	5–6 yr
Language: expressive and receptive	
Skill	**Approximate age**
Differential crying for discomfort, pain, and hunger	1 mo
Turns head toward interesting sound	3–6 mo
Pays attention to familiar voices	3–4 mo
Babbling	5–6 mo
"Ma-ma" and "da-da" used appropriately	12 mo
Obeys simple commands	18 mo
Recognizes names of common objects	13–15 mo
Combines words; two-word sentences	2 yr
Simple "kernel sentences" with subjects, verb, and object	3 yr
Names all primary colors accurately	4 yr
Vocabulary of 2,000 to 2,500 words; asks "why?"; defines words, counts to 10	5 yr

From Cotter S. Optometric assessment: case history. In: Scheiman MM, Rouse MW, eds. *Optometric management of learning-related vision problems.* St. Louis: Mosby-Year Book, 1994:249, with permission.

and educational instruction. This may involve reading instruction, psychological counseling, speech-language therapy, occupational therapy, additional optometric intervention for visual information processing disorders, medication for attention hyperactivity deficit disorder, or any combination of these interventions.

Sequential Treatment Approach of Reading-related Visual Efficiency Problems

The sequential treatment approach used will depend on the specific diagnosis. We recommend the specific sequences described earlier in the book for the various binocular vision, accommodative, and eye movement disorders. The one additional issue that must be considered when dealing with reading-related visual efficiency disorders is comanagement with other professionals.

Role with Educators

Hoffman (5) discusses two important responsibilities of the optometrist with educators. The first is to provide general information relative to the effect of vision disorders on learning; the second is to provide specific information about the vision disorders of the educator's student. This might include the suspected relationship with the child's symptoms and signs,

FIG. 21.1. *Questionnaire*

Name: _____   Birthdate: _____
School: _____   Grade: _____
Teacher(s): _____
Parent(s): _____
Occupations: Mother: _____   Father: _____
Medical insurance: _____

A. Entering complaint/major concern:
1) Please state briefly your main concern and the main problem your child is having:
_____
_____
_____
_____

2) Who first noted possible visual difficulties? _____
3) Who referred you to our office? _____

B. Visual history
1) Is this your child's first visual examination? _____
2) If not, when was your child's last examination? _____
Please describe any previous visual treatment your child has received, including glasses, vision therapy, patch, surgery, or medications.
_____
_____
_____

3) Please check any of the following that you or the teacher have noticed or that your child complains about:

__Blurred distance vision
__Double vision
__closes one eye when reading
__Eye turns in, out, up, down
__Fatigue during near visual tasks
__Squints or blinks excessively
__Holds book or paper too close
__Loss of place when reading
__Uses finger or underliner to read
__Poor eye–hand coordination

__Blurred vision during reading
__Words moving or running together
__Tilts head
__Frequent headaches
__Eye strain
__Red or teary eyes
__Avoids close work
__Skips or rereads lines
__Frequent reversals
__trouble learning left from right

__reverses letters and numbers
__mistakes words with similar beginnings
__trouble learning basic math concepts
__poor reading comprehension
__poor recall of visually presented material
__trouble with spelling and sight vocabulary
__sloppy writing skills
__trouble copying from board to book
__erases excessively
__responds better orally than in writing

C. Educational history
1) Has your child repeated any grades? _____
If yes, which one? _____
2) Is your child receiving any extra help in school or in any special classes? Please describe.
_____
_____

3) Have there been any evaluations (psychological, educational, speech/language, occupational therapy, neurological, medical) done at school or by school recommendation?
_____
_____

If yes, please state when and describe the results.
_____
_____

4) Please check if there are difficulties in any of the following areas for your child:
__reading
__spelling
__behavior or motivation

__handwriting
__copying from the board

__math
__attention span

FIG. 21.1. *Continued*

5) Please check if any of the following aspects of reading are difficult or are behaviors you have noted during reading:

__comprehension   __word recognition   __phonics
__slow reading   __loss of place   __fatigue
__uses finger   __avoidance   __comprehension declines the longer he or she reads
__my child has good comprehension when I read to him or her but has difficulty with comprehension
     when reading on his or her own

6) Do you feel your child is performing up to his or her potential in school?

7) Does your child enjoy reading for pleasure?

D. Developmental history
1) Were there any complications with pregnancy or during birth? _____
2) Was the child born prematurely? _____ If yes, how soon? _____
3) Child's birth weight: _____
4) At what age did your child begin walking unassisted? _____
5) At what age did your child begin to say 2- to 3-word phrases? _____
6) Any speech problems now or in the past? _____
7) Any problems with fine motor coordination? _____
8) Is your child clumsy or does your child have difficulty with activities requiring good balance? _____
9) Does your child enjoy and participate in activities such as drawing, coloring, puzzles, block play, etc.?

E. Medical history
1) Have there been any severe childhood illnesses, injuries, or physical impairments?

If yes, please describe _____

2) Has your child had frequent ear infections? _____ If yes, what treatments has your child undergone?

3) Any current health problems?

4) Taking any medications? _____ If yes, list drugs and doctor who prescribed them:

5) Any significant allergies? Please describe:

F. Family history
1) Does anyone in the family have any of the following?

__strabismus (crossed eyes)   __amblyopia (lazy eye)
__high nearsightedness, farsightedness, or astigmatism
__learning or reading problems
__eye disease (please list)

WOULD YOU LIKE A WRITTEN REPORT?

If you would like us to send a report of the examination, please list the names and addresses of the individuals you would like to receive this report:

FIG. 21.2. *Case history supplement*

Patient Name: _____

	Yes	No	
1	—	—	School performance not up to potential.
2	—	—	Attending grade level expected for age.
3	—	—	Skips and rereads words and/or letters.
4	—	—	Complains of blurred vision during reading and writing.
5	—	—	Complains of headaches associated with visual tasks.
6	—	—	Complains of print "running together" or "jumping around."
7	—	—	Reports sensation of eyes "not working together."
8	—	—	One eye turns in or out, up or down at any time.
9	—	—	Experiences unusual fatigue after visual concentration.
10	—	—	Reports pain around or in the eye at any time.
11	—	—	Reddened eyes or lids.
12	—	—	Excessive tearing of eyes or rubs eyes frequently.
13	—	—	Blinks excessively.
14	—	—	Frowns, scowls, or squints.
15	—	—	Tilts or turns head excessively.
16	—	—	Closes or covers one eye in bright light or during visual tasks.
17	—	—	Uses finger as a marker when reading.
18	—	—	Avoids close work.
19	—	—	Holds book too closely.
20	—	—	Reversals when reading (was for saw; on for no) or writing (b for d; p for q).
21	—	—	Poor recall of visually presented materials.
22	—	—	Transposition of letters or numbers (21 for 12).
23	—	—	Poor handwriting.
24	—	—	Clumsiness.
25	—	—	Makes errors in copying from the blackboard to paper.

From Borsting E, Rouse MW, Detecting learning-related visual problems in the primary care setting. *J Am Optom Assoc* 1994; 65: 642–650, with permission.

the recommended treatment, and the estimated length of treatment. Optometrists should also include recommendations for classroom accommodations that the educator can make in the short term, until the vision problem is resolved. Typical classroom accommodations would include: large print materials, line markers, shortened time on tasks, and extended time for written tests.

Role with Other Professionals

In many cases, the patient will have been referred by another professional to rule out a vision problem that could be interfering with learning. In such cases, it is important for the optometrist to provide a written report that summarizes the evaluation results and recommendations and offers suggestions for classroom management. If vision therapy is recommended, it is also important for the optometrist to coordinate the treatment with any other treatment that the patient is receiving.

In some cases, the optometrist may see children who are struggling with reading before any other professional is consulted about the reading problems. In such cases, it is particularly important to determine the nature of the reading dysfunction. If the reading problem appears to be moderate to severe, or language-based, or if the child is difficult to examine because of attention and concentration issues, a referral for psychoeducational testing would be warranted. It is the role of the optometrist to counsel parents and patients about the objectives and importance of such testing and to encourage the family to request the testing from the school or through a private psychologist.

Case Studies

Case 20.1

History

Paul, a 9-year-old fifth grader, was brought in for an examination because his school performance had decreased significantly during the school year. Until the current year, he had been an average student, achieving average grades in all subjects. The specific problem revolved around Paul's inability to read comfortably and difficulty with reading comprehension. He complained that after 10 to 15 minutes of reading, his eyes felt tired and ached. He also reported feelings of burning. If he continued to read, he eventually experienced headaches and finally the words would blur and move on the page. Because of his inability to read comfortably, he was falling behind in his assignments and felt he had to reread passages repeatedly to understand the material. He felt that the amount of required reading had increased significantly during the year.

Because he had been doing well until the current year, there was no recent reading evaluation.

His medical history was negative and he was not taking any medication. He had passed a visual screening with his pediatrician and in school earlier in the school year. He never had a full vision evaluation.

There was no significant family history of learning problems. Both parents were college graduates with high expectations for Paul's education.

Visual Efficiency Testing: Examination Results

VA (distance, uncorrected):	OD: 20/20 −2, OS: 20/20 −2
VA (near, uncorrected):	OD: 20/20, OS: 20/20
Near point of convergence:	penlight: 20 cm break, 30 cm recovery
Cover test (distance):	orthophoria
Cover test (near):	10 exophoria
Subjective	OD: −0.25 DS, 20/20; OS: plano −0.25 × 90, 20/20
Distance lateral phoria:	orthophoria
Base-in vergence (distance):	X/18/10
Base-out vergence (distance):	10/18/10
Near lateral phoria:	9 exophoria
−1.00 gradient:	7 exophoria
Base-in vergence (near):	12/22/10
Base-out vergence (near):	4/6/1
Negative relative accommodation (NRA):	+1.50
Positive relative accommodation (PRA):	−2.50
Accommodative amplitude:	OD: 13D, OS: 13D
Monocular accommodative facility (MAF):	OD: 0 cpm, fails plus, OS: 0 cpm, fails plus
Binocular accommodative facility (BAF):	0 cpm, fails plus
Monocular estimation method (MEM) retinoscopy:	OD: −0.25, OS: −0.25

Assessment and Diagnosis

The history, in this case, was clearly characteristic of a reading problem secondary to a visual efficiency disorder. Analysis of the optometric findings revealed a receded near point of convergence, high exophoria, a low NRA, and difficulty with plus lenses on BAF. Based on these data, we reached a diagnosis of convergence insufficiency. In addition, the patient had a low MEM finding and difficulty with plus lenses on MAF, suggestive of accommodative excess. The patient's symptoms certainly were consistent with the diagnosis, and the recent onset of reading difficulty was not unexpected. It is likely that these visual efficiency problems were present before the current school year. However, with the increased reading demands in the fifth grade—smaller print and the need to read longer passages for comprehension—the child is now symptomatic.

Treatment

We recommended in-office vision therapy based on the approach suggested in Chapter 8. Eighteen 45-minute in-office visits were necessary. After 9 weeks, Paul reported elimination of all of his initial complaints and was able to read more comfortably, faster, and with better comprehension. He did not require any other intervention.

It is important to realize that this case is an exception to the rule. In most cases, the patient presenting with reading disorders has a more significant reading problem with multiple etiological factors. After successful treatment of the visual efficiency problems, the patient may be more comfortable when reading, but the reading dysfunction remains and requires reading remediation.

Case 20.2

History

A psychologist who had just completed a psychoeducational evaluation referred Jimmy, an 8-year-old third grader, for a vision evaluation. Jimmy learned to speak very early and was always a very verbal child. Although his parents' expectations had been very high for him, Jimmy had a history of school-related problems since kindergarten. In kindergarten, he experienced difficulty with letter and number recognition and fine motor coordination. He had great difficulty in first grade with handwriting and copying from the board. He reversed letters and numbers excessively and had difficulty with his sight–word vocabulary. His parents noted that, when they read to him, his comprehension was excellent. Because of these reported difficulties, he was retained in first grade. In spite of retention, he continued to experience problems, and his parents finally brought him to a psychologist for psychoeducational testing. Jimmy claimed to be asymptomatic when reading. However, he rarely read for more than 10 minutes at a time and never read for pleasure.

The parents brought a copy of the psychoeducational evaluation report. This report indicated that there were no significant emotional issues and the WISC-III results included a verbal IQ of 128 and a performance IQ of 104. Jimmy scored almost 2 years behind his chronological age on the Bender Gestalt Test, which is a test of visual motor integration. Auditory processing and language skills were strengths for Jimmy.

Achievement testing was also done as part of the psychoeducational testing. This testing suggested a 1.5-year lag in reading, with weaknesses in sight–word vocabulary, comprehension, and age- or grade-appropriate math skills. In her summary, the psychologist reached a diagnosis of a learning disability with primary weaknesses in visual processing and strengths in language function. She recommended part-time placement in a resource room and tutoring in reading. In addition, she suggested a comprehensive optometric evaluation.

Jimmy's medical history revealed a normal pregnancy, but a very long and difficult labor and delivery by cesarean section. Otherwise, there was no significant medical history. Developmental milestones showed a variable pattern. Language skills developed faster than average. For instance, Jimmy used two-word sentences by 18 months of age and was always a very verbal child. Fine motor skills, however, developed more slowly than expected. He always had difficulty holding a crayon and did not enjoy coloring or playing with puzzles. He could not copy a circle until about 4 years of age.

There did not seem to be any family history of learning problems and there had been no other testing.

Visual Efficiency Testing: Examination Results

VA (distance, uncorrected):	OD: 20/20 −2, OS: 20/20 −2
VA (near, uncorrected):	OD: 20/20, OS: 20/20
Near point of convergence:	penlight: 2.5 cm break, 5 cm recovery
Cover test (distance):	4 esophoria
Cover test (near):	8 esophoria
Subjective:	OD: +1.25, 20/20; OS: +1.25, 20/20
Distance lateral phoria:	orthophoria
Base-in vergence (distance):	X/7/4
Base-out vergence (distance):	10/16/10
Near lateral phoria:	2 esophoria
−1.00 gradient:	14 esophoria
Base-in vergence (near):	8/12/8
Base-out vergence (near):	14/25/14
NRA:	+2.50
PRA:	−2.00
Accommodative amplitude:	OD: 12D, OS: 12D
MAF:	OD: 10 cpm, OS: 10 cpm
BAF:	0 cpm, diplopia with −2.00
MEM retinoscopy:	OD: +0.75, OS: +0.75
Developmental eye movement (DEM) test:	fifteenth percentile (errors)
	fifteenth percentile (ratio)

Assessment and Diagnosis

The optometric evaluation revealed hyperopia and greater esophoria at near, with low direct and indirect negative fusional vergence findings, supporting a diagnosis of hyperopia and convergence excess. Based on the findings from the DEM test, we also reached a diagnosis of ocular motor dysfunction. In contrast to Case 20.1, these findings, although clinically significant, did not adequately explain many of the signs and symptoms experienced by this child. Many of these signs and symptoms were more likely to be related to a visual information processing disorder.

Treatment Plan

We recommended eyeglasses for school and all reading and homework (OD: +1.25 and OS: +1.25). In addition, we recommended a visual information processing evaluation. This testing revealed significant problems in visual–spatial tasks, visual analysis, and visual–motor integration skills. We recommended in-office vision therapy to treat the eye movement disorder and visual information processing problems.

Jimmy required forty-two 45-minute in-office visits. In addition, a considerable amount of therapy was done at home. He was seen twice a week for about 6 months. A reevaluation at that point revealed significant improvements in both the error and ratio scores on the DEM test and visual information processing skills. Jimmy also received help at school and had private tutoring in reading. During the active vision therapy, we asked the teachers to temporarily deemphasize written work, particularly copying from the board.

During 6 months of combined educational and optometric intervention, Jimmy made outstanding progress. At completion of therapy, he found it easier to express his thoughts in writing, copying from the board was considerably better, and he was no longer reversing excessively. His reading level increased by about 18 months, and he was no longer as frustrated in school. We dismissed him from vision therapy and he continued to receive help at school and from his private reading tutor.

This case illustrates a more common presentation in which the learning problems are more complicated and in which both visual efficiency and visual information processing problems are present. In such cases, while it is important to treat the visual efficiency problems, it is also important to make sure that a visual information processing examination is performed and that appropriate educational remediation takes place.

SUMMARY

Management of reading-related visual efficiency problems is one of the more challenging aspects of optometric care. In addition to being able to diagnose and treat visual efficiency problems, the optometrist must be knowledgeable about reading dysfunction, the relationship between vision problems and reading dysfunction, and psychoeducational testing. An understanding of these issues allows the optometrist to ask appropriate questions during the case history, relate test findings to presenting complaints, and make appropriate management decisions.

The other important issue emphasized in this chapter is that optometrists do not treat learning or reading problems. Rather, the primary role is the diagnosis and treatment of vision problems that may interfere with school performance. The expectation is that, with a reduction in asthenopia and other symptoms, the patient will be able to read more comfortably, more quickly, and with better comprehension. Thus, remediating these vision problems allows children and adults to benefit more fully from educational intervention.

STUDY QUESTIONS

1. An optometrist is treating a child with reading-related visual efficiency problems and tells the parents and teacher that he expects the child's reading skills to improve significantly after vision therapy and that no additional intervention should be necessary. State whether you agree or disagree with this statement and explain your reasoning.
2. What aspects of vision should be evaluated when a child presents with a reading-related vision problem?

3. Describe two differences between nonspecific reading dysfunction and dyslexia.
4. Describe three different forms of dyslexia.
5. List five questions that you could ask during the case history that would help determine if the reading problem is related to visual efficiency problems.
6. Explain the concepts "learning to read" versus "reading to learn" and describe how an optometrist would use these concepts in practice.
7. A parent asks you about the effectiveness of colored filters for reading dysfunction. What would your response be?
8. Describe what you would expect to find when reading the results of the IQ test from a psychoeducational report for a child with a significant language problem. What would you expect if there was a problem with visual processing?
9. List the components of the psychoeducational evaluation and describe the significance of each component for an optometrist.
10. List five factors that may place a child "at risk" for reading or learning problems.

REFERENCES

1. Flax N. Vision and learning: optometry and the Academy's early role—an historical overview. *J Optom Vis Dev* 1999;30:105–110.
2. Scheiman MM, Rouse MW. *Optometric management of learning related vision problems*. St. Louis: Mosby-Year Book, 1994:9.
3. American Academy of Optometry, American Optometric Association. Vision, learning and dyslexia: a joint organizational policy statement. *J Am Optom Assoc* 1997;68:284–286.
4. *Optometric clinical practice guideline: care of the patient with learning related vision problems*. St. Louis: American Optometric Association, 2000.
5. Hoffman LG. The role of the optometrist in the diagnosis and management of learning-related vision problems. In: Scheiman MM, Rouse MW, eds. *Optometric management of learning related vision problems*. St. Louis: Mosby-Year Book, 1994:217–225.
6. Garzia RP. *Vision and reading*. St. Louis: Mosby, 1996.
7. Griffin JR, Christenson GN, Wesson MD, et al. *Optometric management of reading dysfunction*. Boston: Butterworth-Heinemann, 1997.
8. Press LJ. *Applied concepts in vision therapy*. St. Louis: Mosby, 1997.
9. Interagency Committee on Learning Disabilities, National Institutes of Health. *Learning disabilities: a report to the U.S. Congress,* 1987. Washington, DC.
10. Solan H. Overview of learning disabilities. In: Scheiman MM, Rouse MW, eds. *Optometric management of learning related vision problems*. St. Louis: Mosby-Year Book, 1994:88–123.
11. Kavale KA, Forness SR. History, definition, and diagnosis. In: Singh NN, Beale IL, eds. *Learning disabilities: nature, theory, and treatment*. New York: Springer-Verlag, 1992.
12. McCormick S. *Remedial and clinical reading instruction*. Columbus, OH: Merrill Publishing, 1987.
13. Solan H. Overview of learning disabilities. In: Scheiman MM, Rouse MW, eds. *Optometric management of learning related vision problems*. St. Louis: Mosby-Year Book, 1994:88–123.
14. Stark LW, Giveen SC, Terdiman JF. Specific dyslexia and eye movements. In: Stein JF, ed. *Vision and visual dyslexia,* vol. 13. Boca Raton, FL: CRC Press, 1991.
15. Griffin JR, Christenson GN, Wesson MD, et al. *Optometric management of reading dysfunction*. Boston: Butterworth-Heinemann, 1997.
16. Griffin JR, Walton HN. *The dyslexia determination test (DDT),* revised ed. Los Angeles: Instructional Materials and Equipment Distributors, 1987.
17. Boder E. Developmental dyslexia: a diagnostic approach based on three atypical reading patterns. *Dev Med Child Neurol* 1973;15:663–687.
18. Boder E, Jarrico S. *The Boder test of reading-spelling patterns*. New York: Grune & Stratton, 1982.
19. Griffin JR, Walton HN, Christenson GN. *The dyslexia screener (TDS)*. Culver City, CA: Reading and Perception Therapy Center, 1988.
20. Christenson GN, Griffin JR, De Land PN. Validity of the dyslexia screener. *Optom Vis Sci* 1991;68:275–281.
21. Flax N. Problems in relating visual function to reading disorder. *Am J Optom Physiol Opt* 1970;47:366–372.
22. Borsting E, Rouse MW. Detecting learning-related visual problems in the primary care setting. *J Am Optom Assoc* 1994;65:642–650.
23. Simons HD, Gassler PA. Vision anomalies and reading skill: a meta-analysis of the literature. *Am J Optom Physiol Opt* 1988;65:893–904.
24. Garzia R. The relationship between visual efficiency problems and learning. In: Scheiman MM, Rouse MW, eds. *Optometric management of learning related vision problems*. St. Louis: Mosby-Year Book, 1994:153–178.

25. Grisham JD, Simons HD. Refractive error and the reading process: a literature analysis. *J Am Optom Assoc* 1986;57:44–55.
26. Simons HD, Grisham JD. Binocular anomalies and reading problems. *J Am Optom Assoc* 1987;58:578–587.
27. Pirozzolo FJ. Eye movements and reading disability. In: Rayner K, ed. *Eye movements in reading.* New York: Academic Press, 1983.
28. Pavlidis G Th. The "dyslexia syndrome" and its objective diagnosis by erratic eye movements. In: Rayner K, ed. *Eye movements in reading.* New York: Academic Press, 1983.
29. Pavlidis G Th. Eye movement differences between dyslexia, normal, and retarded readers while sequentially fixating digits. *Am J Optom Physiol Opt* 1985;62:820–832.
30. Pavlidis G Th. Diagnostic significance and relationship between dyslexia and erratic eye movements. In: Stein JF, ed. *Vision and visual dyslexia.* Boca Raton, FL: CRC Press, 1991.
31. Meares O. Figure/ground, brightness contrast, and reading disabilities. *Visible Lang* 1980;14:13–29.
32. Irlen H. Successful treatment of learning disabilities. Unpublished manuscript presented at the ninety-first annual convention of the American Psychological Association, 1983. Long Beach, CA.
33. Irlen H. Reading by the colors: overcoming dyslexia and other reading disabilities through the Irlen method. Garden City Park, NY: Avery Publishing, 1991.
34. Stanley G. Coloured filters and dyslexia. *Aust J Remed Ed* 1987;19:8–9.
35. Rosner J, Rosner J. The Irlen treatment: a review of the literature. *Optician* 1987;194:26–33.
36. Rosner J, Rosner J. Another cure for dyslexia? *J Am Optom Assoc* 1988;59:832–833.
37. Howell E, Stanley G. Colour and learning disability. *J Clin Exp Optom* 1988;71:66–71.
38. Scheiman M, Blaskey P, et al. Vision characteristics of individuals identified as Irlen Filter candidates. *J Am Optom Assoc* 1990;61:600–604.
39. Irlen H, Lass MJ. Improving reading problems due to symptoms of scotopic sensitivity using Irlen lenses and overlays. *Education* 1989;109:413–417.
40. Hoffman LG, Rouse M. Referral recommendations for binocular and/or developmental perceptual deficiencies. *J Am Optom Assoc* 1980;51:119–125.
41. Lopez R, Yolton RL, Kohl P, et al. Comparison of the Irlen scotopic sensitivity syndrome test results to academic and visual performance data. *J Am Optom Assoc* 1994;65:705–714.
42. Evans BJW, Drasdo N. Tinted lenses and related therapies for learning disabilities—a review. *Ophthalmic Physiol Opt* 1991;11:206–217.
43. Menacker SJ, Breton ME, Breton ML, et al. Do tinted lenses improve the performance of dyslexic children? *Arch Ophthalmol* 1993;111:213–218.
44. Wilkins AJ, Milroy R, Nimmo-Smith I, et al. Preliminary observations concerning treatment of visual discomfort and associated perceptual distortion. *Ophthalmic Physiol Opt* 1992;12:257–263.
45. Wilkins AJ, Evans BJ, Brown J, et al. Double-masked placebo-controlled trial of precision spectral filters in children who use coloured overlays. *Ophthalmic Physiol Opt* 1994;14:365–370.
46. Evans BJW, Wilkins AJ, Brown J, et al. A preliminary investigation into the aetiology of Meares-Irlen syndrome. *Ophthalmic Physiol Opt* 1996;16:286–296.
47. Williams MC, Lecluyse K, Rock-Faucheux A. Effective interventions for reading disability. *J Am Optom Assoc* 1992;63:411–417.
48. Solan HA, Ficarra A, Brannan JR, et al. Eye movement efficiency in normal and reading disabled elementary school children: effects of varying luminance and wavelength. *J Am Optom Assoc* 1998;69:455–464.
49. Wilkins AJ. *Visual stress.* Oxford, UK: Oxford University Press, 1995.
50. Blaskey P, Selznick R. Psychoeducational evaluation. In: Scheiman MM, Rouse MW, eds. *Optometric management of learning-related vision problems.* St. Louis: Mosby-Year Book, 1994:336–371.
51. Silver LB, ed. *The assessment of learning disabilities: preschool through adulthood.* Boston: College Hill Publication, 1989.
52. Wechsler D. *Manual for the WISC-III.* New York: Psychological Corporation, 1990.
53. Cotter S. Optometric assessment: case history. In: Scheiman MM, Rouse MW, eds. *Optometric management of learning-related vision problems.* St. Louis: Mosby-Year Book, 1994:226–266.

at all times. If some letters are missing (suppression), blink your eyes rapidly and look for the missing letters between blinks.

Procedure 3: Repeat procedures 1 and 2, without the aid of the pencil. When you can fuse all four sets of circles (always maintaining the correct response), begin to turn your head slowly from side to side, while you keep the middle circle clear and single and with both colors present. Vary the head movement by rotating it slowly, clockwise and up-and-down.

Note: Keys to improvement:

1. When you can see the central fused circle
2. When you can perform the procedure without using a pencil
3. When the central fused circle is a "mixture" in the color of the red and green circle and appears a shiny or lustrous brown
4. When all of the letters are present in the words "clear these letters"
5. When you can perform the procedure with ease

Procedure 4: Look at a detailed distant object (more than 10 ft away) and make it clear. Then, look at the card and fuse the bottom circle, making it clear and single. Repeat this procedure, until you can look easily from a distant object to the card and easily fuse and clear the most widely separate circles. No pencil is to be used in this therapy. Remember, clear the distance object, then look at the card and fuse the colored circles. When you can do this easily, move the card closer each time you do the therapy. You should fuse the circles at 4 to 6 in. and maintain the correct responses when looking from distance to near. Each time you fuse the circles, the center brownish circle should be clear. When you look at a distance, it should be clear. Do not look from one place to the other until the first place is clear.

First- or Second-degree Targets at 10 to 15 Feet

The purpose of this therapy is to improve your ability to aim and focus your eyes together, which will result in more efficient vision for longer periods of time. The therapy will help you use both eyes together so that you can later obtain all of the benefits of binocular vision. You will know that you are doing the therapy correctly when you can do the procedures quickly and easily, without suppressing.

Perform therapy _____ minutes per day and increase the number of procedures in each session, as you can do them. In the beginning, you may experience discomfort (e.g., headaches, eye strain, etc.) and have to limit the time to a few minutes. As your ability improves, your discomfort will disappear and the time can be increased. Remember that 15 minutes per day is better than 2 hours once a week. Try to establish a routine, so that you always do the therapy at _____ o'clock each day.

Materials required: Set of enlarged first- (nonfusible) or second-degree targets (fusible with suppression checks), yardstick, clock with second hand, and plus/minus flippers.

Setup: Place the second-degree targets on the wall, side by side and touching. Be sure they are not vertically displaced. Hold a yardstick so that its point is between the two targets. Slowly move the yardstick toward your eyes, keeping the tip clear. Notice the targets in the background, behind the yardstick. At a certain point, you should be aware that the targets are beginning to double.

As you continue to bring the yardstick closer, the targets will approach each other and fuse into one so that you will see three sets. To achieve this, you must continue to concentrate on keeping the yardstick clear, while being conscious of the targets in the background. When you have fused the center target, slowly take the yardstick away, concentrating on keeping the center image fused, with the suppression checks present. If you have trouble doing this, bring the yardstick back in, until you can keep the targets fused more easily. This is not an easy task.

Don't get discouraged if you have some trouble; it may take you some time to learn to do it. The targets will appear blurred or you may suppress at first.

If the targets appear blurred, continue concentrating on trying to clear them; the circles will begin to clear and you will be able to read the print. Keep the circles fused and clear at all times.

Procedure 1: Once you can keep the targets in clear focus, walk closer to them, keeping them clear. Move as close to the card as you can, maintaining the fusion. Then walk closer and farther, maintaining the fusion and clarity, and try to increase your range, moving as close as possible. Repeat the therapy _____ times, recording the closest distance you were able to achieve.

Procedure 2: Have an assistant slowly move the cards apart. Continue moving the cards apart, keeping the targets clear and fused as far as you possibly can. Move the cards back together when you have reached your limit, and then bring them apart again, repeating the therapy _____ times. Record the farthest separation you were able to achieve.

Procedure 3: Fuse the targets as before, look at an object in your hand, make sure it is clear and, when it is, look back at the targets and regain the fusion. Continue working in this manner, looking back and forth from the object in your hand to the cards, only switching back when the targets have been fused and cleared. As this therapy becomes easier, move the cards farther and farther apart. Repeat the therapy for _____ jumps, recording the distance from the cards and their separation. Record the time for ten jumps. Rest. Repeat _____ sets.

Procedure 4: Obtain fusion of the targets, while looking through the minus side of the plus/minus lens flipper. Now, quickly remove the flipper so that you are looking through no lenses and regain the fusion response, making sure that the targets are clear and appear in depth. Repeat the alternations, working to re-fuse and clear the targets as quickly and smoothly as possible. Note the time it takes for you to do 20 cycles (40 flips) and record your best time for one set of 20 cycles each day. Do _____ sets each day.

Procedure 5: Repeat procedures 1 to 4, with the first-degree (nonfusible) targets.

Time and recording: Record the amount of time worked and any problems or questions you have, along with your best measured effort for the procedure you did.

Hart Chart—Saccadic Therapy

The purpose of this therapy is to help increase your ability to change the focus of your eyes so that you use each eye to clearly see objects at different distances. The therapy will help you use both eyes together so that you may begin to obtain all of the benefits of binocular vision. You will know that you are doing the therapy correctly when you can do the procedures quickly and easily.

Perform therapy _____ minutes per day and increase the number of procedures in each session, as you can do them. In the beginning, you may experience discomfort (e.g., headaches, eye strain, etc.) and have to limit the time to a few minutes. As your ability improves, your discomfort will disappear and the time can be increased. Remember that 15 minutes per day is better than 2 hours once a week. Try to establish a routine, so that you always do the therapy at _____ o'clock each day.

Materials required: Large Hart chart for distance viewing, small Hart chart for near viewing, and an eye patch.

Procedure 1: Place the Hart chart about 5 to 10 ft away. Occlude the _____ eye with an eye patch. Call out the first letter in column 1 and then the first letter in column 10, the second from the top letter in column 1 and the second letter from the top in column 10, the third letter from the top in column 1 and the third letter from the top in column 10, and so forth. Continue until you have called out all letters from column 1 and 10. As you call out the letters, have an assistant write down your responses and, when the task is completed, check your accuracy. Checking for errors is, in itself, another saccadic therapy technique because you will have to make saccades from far to near to check for errors. Repeat the procedure with the other eye patched.

Procedure 2: Once you can complete procedure 1 in about 15 seconds, without any errors, you can increase the level of difficulty several ways. Continue calling out letters in the other columns. Specifically, after completing columns 1 and 10, call out columns 2 and 9, 3 and 8, 4 and 7, and 5 and 6. The inner columns are more difficult because they are surrounded by other targets.

Procedure 3: An even greater level of difficulty can be achieved by making saccades from the top of one column to the bottom of another. Instead of a left to right and right to left saccade, you will have to make an oblique saccade. For example, call out the top letter in column 1 and then the bottom letter in column 10, the second letter from the top in column 1 and the second letter from the bottom in column 10. Continue this pattern through the entire chart.

Procedure 4: Many other variations to increase the level of difficulty are possible, including incorporating the beat of a metronome and maintaining balance on a balance board, while engaged in the task.

Procedure 5: Repeat the previous procedures, looking from the distance chart to the near one.

Ann Arbor Letter Tracking

The purpose of this therapy is to help increase the accuracy of eye movements from place to place so that you use your eyes as accurately as possible to look at an object. The therapy will help you make accurate movements of your eyes between objects so that you may begin to obtain all of the benefits of accurate vision. You will know that you are doing the therapy correctly when you can do the procedures quickly and easily.

Perform therapy _____ minutes per day and increase the number of procedures in each session, as you can do them. In the beginning, you may experience discomfort (e.g., headaches, eye strain, etc.) and have to limit the time to a few minutes. As your ability improves, your discomfort will disappear and the time can be increased. Remember that 15 minutes per day is better than 2 hours once a week. Try to establish a routine, so that you always do the therapy at _____ o'clock each day.

Materials required: Ann Arbor Letter tracking workbooks, 8.5 × 11 in. plastic sheet, paper clip, pen used for overhead transparencies (washable type), eye patch, and a stop watch.

Procedure 1: To permit the repeated use of the workbooks, cover the page being used with a plastic sheet and secure the plastic with a paper clip. Each page of letter tracking has two or more paragraphs of what appear to be random letters. Occlude the _____ eye. Begin at the upper right and scan from left to right to find the first letter "a;" make a line through the letter "a." Find the very first "b," cross it out, and continue through the entire paragraph, finding the letters in alphabetical order. The goal is to complete this task as quickly as possible; time the therapy procedure and evaluate your accuracy. If you are scanning for the very first letter "d," for instance, and inadvertently miss it and find a "d" later in the paragraph, you will be unable to find the entire alphabet sequence in the paragraph.

After you find and mark a specific letter, lift the pen off the page so that you will have to use eye movements to find the next letter. Repeat the procedure, with the other eye occluded.

Procedure 2: The workbook has letters in five different sizes, creating other levels of difficulty.

ENDPOINT: Discontinue this technique when the performance in each eye is approximately equal and when the patient can successfully complete the paragraphs in about 1 minute.

Visual Tracing

The purpose of this therapy is to help increase the accuracy of eye movements from place to place so that you use your eyes as accurately as possible to look at an object. The therapy will help you make accurate movements of your eyes between objects so that you may begin to obtain all of the benefits of accurate vision. You will know that you are doing the therapy correctly when you can do the procedures quickly and easily.

Perform therapy _____ minutes per day and increase the number of procedures in each session, as you can do them. In the beginning, you may experience discomfort (e.g., headaches, eye strain, etc.) and have to limit the time to a few minutes. As your ability improves, your discomfort will disappear and the time can be increased. Remember that 15 minutes per day is better than 2 hours once a week. Try to establish a routine so that you always do the therapy at _____ o'clock each day.

Materials required: Percon visual tracing workbooks, 8.5 × 11 in. plastic sheet, paper clip, pen used for overhead transparencies (washable type), and an eye patch.

Procedure 1: The workbook contains tracing tasks that gradually increase in level of difficulty from the beginning to the end of the book. Two therapy methods can be used. The easiest procedure is to occlude the _____ eye, place the pen on the letter "A," and trace along the line, until the end of the line. The objective is to determine the number at the end of the line, beginning with the letter "A." Continue until you have found the answer for each line.

Procedure 2: As your accuracy and speed improve, the next level of difficulty can be added. In this technique, perform the same task, using only your eyes. Make an eye movement, without the support of following the line with the pencil.

Loose Lens Rock (Monocular)

The purpose of this therapy is to help increase your ability to change the focus of your eyes so that you use both eyes together to clearly see an object. The therapy will help you use both eyes together so that you may begin to obtain all of the benefits of binocular vision. You will know that you are doing the therapy correctly when you can do the procedures quickly and easily.

Perform therapy _____ minutes per day and increase the number of procedures in each session, as you can do them. In the beginning, you may experience discomfort (e.g., headaches, eye strain, etc.) and have to limit the time to a few minutes. As your ability improves, your discomfort will disappear and the time can be increased. Remember that 15 minutes per day is better than 2 hours once a week. Try to establish a routine so that you always do the therapy at _____ o'clock each day.

Materials required: Age-appropriate reading material of varying sizes (from 20/80 to 20/30), uncut plastic lens blanks (from −6.00 to +2.50, in 0.25 D increments), and an eye patch.

Procedure 1: Occlude the _____ eye and clear and read print that is held at 40 cm, through plus/minus lenses that are alternately held in front of the unoccluded eye. The lenses that will be given to you are based upon the results of the diagnostic testing. In the initial phase of this technique, you have as much time as necessary to clear and read the print. The goal is merely to achieve clear vision, without regard to the time factor. Repeat the procedure, with the other eye patched. Once you can clear the lenses with both eyes, speed becomes the next objective.

Procedure 2: Now, regain clarity as quickly as possible. Begin with low powered lenses and clear the print through +0.50 and −0.50, 20 cycles per minute. When you can accomplish this, increase the power of the lenses until you can perform 20 cycles per minute with +2.00 and −4.00.

Subject Index

References in *italics* indicate figures; those followed by *t* denote tables

A

AC/A ratio
accommodation and vergence
interactions assessed using,
459–461
accommodation control for, 11
added lenses prescription and, 103
assessment of, 10–11
basic exophoria, 326
CA/C ratio and, relationship
between, 461–462, 465,
468
calculated, 10–11
case analysis use of, 71
convergence excess, 11, 271
convergence insufficiency, 230
distribution of, *460,* 461
divergence excess, 11, 285–286
gradient, 10–11
heterophoria and, 62, 452
high
convergence excess (*See*
Convergence excess)
divergence excess (*See*
Divergence excess)
phorias associated with,
268–269
low
binocular vision disorders
associated with, 226
convergence insufficiency (*See*
Convergence insufficiency)
divergence insufficiency (*See*
Divergence insufficiency)
heterophoria with
added lenses for, 224
case studies of, 223–225
description of, 62
phorias associated with, 226
measurement of, 459–461
normal
binocular vision conditions
associated with, 305
phorias associated with, 306
refractive error, 316
response vs. stimulus, 11
von Graefe method for measuring,
37–38

Accommodation
accuracy of, 557–558
lag of, 11
monocular estimation method
retinoscopy evaluations, 25
negative relative, 15–16, 43, 63–64
in nystagmus, 496
positive relative, 15–16, 43
relative, 464–465
spasm of, 272
testing of, 19*t*, 640
vergence and, interactions between
AC/A ratio measurements,
459–461
CA/C ratio measurements,
457–458, *458*
depth of focus, 455
fixation disparity, 466–467
lag of accommodation, 455–456
lens flipper test, 465
lens therapy effects, 467–468
prism therapy effects, 467–468
proximal vergence, 456–457
relative accommodation,
464–465
theoretical findings, 453–455,
454
tonic vergence, 455
vergence adaptation, 466
Accommodation control
for AC/A ratio, 11
for cover test, 6
for von Graefe test, 7–8
Accommodative amplitude, 19*t*–20*t*,
20–21, 46, 67, 293, 360,
464
Accommodative disorders (*See also
specific disorder*)
acquired brain injury and,
576–577
added lens power for, 102–105
assessment methods for
accommodative amplitude,
19*t*–20*t*, 20–21, 46, 67
accommodative facility, 21–24,
47–48
accommodative response,
24–26

general considerations for,
19–20
minus lens amplitude, 21, 46–47
classification of, 334
prevalence of, 334
prognosis for, 335–336
treatment of
plus lenses, 336
prognosis for, 335–336
strategies for, 334–335
vision therapy, 336
vision therapy for, 111–112, 140
Accommodative excess
accommodative data, 351
binocular data, 351
case study of, 356–358
characteristics of, 74*t*
convergence insufficiency and,
241–243, 351, 358
definition of, 349–350
differential diagnosis, 351–352,
352*t*
esophoria and, 351
exophoria and, 351
organic cause of, 352
pseudomyopia vs., 349
signs and symptoms of, 80, 350*t*,
350–351
studies of, 349
treatment of
added lenses, 352
lenses, 352
vision therapy, 353–356
Accommodative facility testing
binocular, 68–69
monocular, 67
technique for, 21–24, 47–48
Accommodative fatigue
astigmatism and, 335
causes of, 335
classification of, 337
Accommodative infacility
accommodative amplitude, 360
accommodative data, 360
binocular data, 360
case study of, 366–367
characteristics of, 74*t*, 358–359
definition of, 358